A PICTORIAL HISTORY OF
MEDICINE

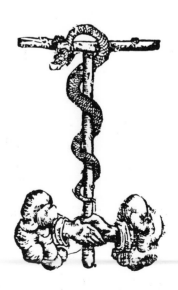

A PICTORIAL

MEDI

(Third Printing)

A brief, nontechnical survey of the healing arts from Aesculapius to Ehrlich — retelling with the aid of select illustrations the lives and deeds of great physicians. . . . . .

CHARLES C THOMAS · PUBLISHER

HISTORY OF
CINE

BY

OTTO L. BETTMANN, Ph. D.

Founder and Director of The Bettmann Archive, New York City

WITH A FOREWORD BY

PHILIP S. HENCH, M. D.

Mayo Clinic, Rochester, Minnesota

. . . a graphic record of the untiring efforts of the medical profession to cure the sick, offer solace, allay pain and secure a better life for all mankind.

SPRINGFIELD · ILLINOIS · U. S. A.

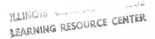

CHARLES C THOMAS · PUBLISHER

BANNERSTONE HOUSE

301-327 East Lawrence Avenue, Springfield, Illinois, U.S.A.

Published simultaneously in the British Commonwealth of Nations by

BLACKWELL SCIENTIFIC PUBLICATIONS, LTD., OXFORD, ENGLAND

Published simultaneously in Canada by

THE RYERSON PRESS, TORONTO

Copyright 1956, by CHARLES C THOMAS — PUBLISHER

Library of Congress Catalog No. 54-10781

First Printing, May, 1956
Second Printing, October, 1956
Third Printing, February, 1962

Printed in the United States of America

"TO ANNE"

FOREWORD

Former President Truman once wrote me: "The best education for a President of the United States comes from an intimate study of the lives, letters, and papers of his predecessors." The study of history can be of as great spiritual and practical value to a physician as to a president.

Dr. Otto Bettmann's *Pictorial History of Medicine* shows the whole extraordinary pageant of healing. If within it are vivid colorings reflecting the scarlet terror of epidemics, the white stillness of death, the gray fog of dark ages, there is also the golden brilliance of discovery. The emotional texture is dramatic, appealing, rich in contrasts: great earnestness and compassion, sometimes cold erudition, and much wishful thinking. If the chronicle of medicine reveals follies, frauds, and foofaraw, one also finds here unsurpassed dedication, integrity, effort incredibly sustained, often heroism and total sacrifice, and thousands of victories wherein no man was loser. In this book Dr. Bettmann has traced the art and science of healing — from the medicine man of ancient times up to the medical man of the twentieth century — in a manner that is both fascinating and scholarly. As a historian he can stand among the peers.

The young doctor of today never meets the greatest of his teachers in person. To be exposed to this incomparable faculty he must go to the pages of medical history: to Hippocrates, Paré, Pasteur, Lister and Osler. These great men are present in everything the doctor does — a fact illustrated by the story of the young physician faced with a difficult case. To bolster the confidence of a patient who was seriously ill, he said, "Why, Mrs. Jones, this morning Pasteur and Roentgen briefed me before I left home; Sydenham and Osler came here with me, and Domagk and Fleming are standing by." To which she replied, "Dear me, won't they cost a lot?"

They will cost nothing. The book of history is open — and free.

Our work rests — more, perhaps, than that of any other profession — on the accomplishments of our predecessors. A knowledge of what they have given to medicine and to humanity should therefore be part of our background, and not for reasons of professional sentiment alone, but for reasons of good common sense.

Pursuing his career, the physician must of course strive to maintain a forward look; for it is ahead that both opportunity and difficulties lie. Yet despite modern complexities, most of our practical problems resemble those of our predecessors. The problems ahead are recurrences, minor variants of those in the past — the past of our elders if not our own. From our point of view they seem to come at us from in front, and to bear a fresh label. But beneath the wrappings there is usually an old problem, already examined and even, sometimes, disposed of. By borrowing experience and wisdom from predecessors we can view certain situations as if in retrospect, and view them with enormous profit.

Physicians will do well, then, to look ahead for problems. Paradoxically, however, they should look "behind" for guidance, and a study of medical history provides an excellent rear-view mirror. Most physicians are unfortunately not conscious of their medical heritage, because few find time to study it. This may not be their fault alone. It must be admitted that many medical histories, however erudite, are not very readable. The author of this book, Dr. Otto Bettmann, has spent a lifetime to remedy this situation. In years of research in art centers all over Europe he has assembled a vast library of medical illustrations, studying, analyzing, and authenticating them so that they could become part of a new medical history: a history of medicine in pictures. This book was designed less for medical historians than for the practicing physician or layman who wishes to inform himself of the background of this profession at a glance.

What is the panorama that opens up before our eyes?

Dr. Bettmann's vista of 50 centuries clearly reveals that the course of medicine has not always been one of advance. If there are volumes of hard-won facts, life-saving ingredients and conclusions, and galaxies of truths and half-truths, there are also despairs, superstitions, and sophistries. Although the over-all direction of medicine has been, at least since the Renaissance, one of improvement, its progress toward betterment has been on countless occasions retarded, or even reversed. Thus it is more accurate to speak of the "history" or the "development" of medicine, rather than of its "progress" or "advance." And for the reader, a chronicle which recounts the ebb as well as the flow of medical art and science is both more accurate and more entertaining than a mere description of clinical and technical advances.

To what extent have physicians, individually or collectively, been responsible for the course of medicine, for its forward spurts or its backward shifts? One view has it that medical progress depends chiefly on discoveries; hence the rate at which medicine advances is determined largely by the appearance of medical leaders and the results of their researches. Another view is that man is more servant of Fate than master, the product rather than the maker of environment. Thus great physicians are not "born medical leaders," but become leaders through the circumstances of their lives. Each period of travail generates its own saviors; each crisis produces discoveries.

Of these two views Dr. Bettmann supports neither extreme wholly. Because the physician is only one of many factors that have influenced the direction of medicine, the story cannot be told in terms of the medical man alone. Our medical benefactors must not be nameless, of course; but they must be seen in perspective, in the company of nonmedical contemporaries — friendly, indifferent, or hostile — whose ambitions and attitudes also require elaboration. Thus the author presents the course of medicine as part of general history. He views it not as a chronology of discoveries, but as only one of the great social forces — a continuing force, but one of fluctuating potency, now dominant, now recessive. This absorbing book shows what impact the physician has had upon each of the great cultural and political areas, and vice versa.

There seems to be no special "climate" for medical discovery; great discoveries have been made almost anywhere and everywhere. No desolate military outpost is too small and disorganized, no research center too large and too organized, to prevent them. Wherever there is a physician, in that place are the potentials for discovery of new medical truths.

To be useful, however, medical truth must be put to work; it must serve. In the last analysis, that can happen only when the informed, dedicated physician and a single patient who needs him actually meet. It is in this place, a sick room, where the truthful dreaming of the theorist, the demonstrations of the experimentalist, the magic of the chemist, the guidance of the laboratory, and the wisdom of the practitioner finally come together for the critical testing.

Such is the story that Dr. Bettmann's book reveals. The product of the author's 30-year pictorial treasure hunt — plus his lifelong study of medical texts — the material displays a richness and variety which stamp it as part of a "collector's collection." Included are previously unpublished original photographs, and many ancient illustrations not heretofore published outside their land of origin.

In view of his vast array of graphic material, the author must have been sorely tempted to appeal chiefly to the eye; to construct his own medical art gallery within cardboards; to let most of the pictures speak for themselves, with mere captions and program-notes for the less articulate of his selections. But Bettmann the specialist in medical art is not subordinate to Bettmann the textual historian. The two combine harmoniously to create a superior form; and the lucid text is brightened by the instructive anecdote, the humorous twist.

Many readers will, I believe, be fascinated by this book without pausing to analyze its special appeal. But those who disregard the identity of that appeal are depriving themselves of what is, in my opinion, an important bonus. Almost daily the physician has to do some teaching of patients, medical school and hospital personnel, fellow-physicians, or public groups. The public's avid interest in health is greatly increasing the physician's responsibilities and opportunities as a teacher and lecturer. He is not often as effective as he could be because he seldom appreciates, or employs fully, the power of visual instruction. "A picture may instantly present what a book could set forth only on a hundred pages." Today's doctor will do well to heed this century-old dictum of Turgeniev — a dictum convincingly exemplified in Dr. Bettmann's *Pictorial History of Medicine*.

Its chapters are subdivided into compact thematic units of text and illustration. Each unit covers a particular subject — perhaps one great leader, an important controversy, or the development of some specialty. But the units keep their logical places in the general text, never losing their connection with related events. Thus there is no break in the continuity of interest and the sense of progression.

A *Pictorial History of Medicine*, then, is no "pictorial souvenir" for the physician to inspect casually and then consign to the patients' waiting room. Instead it should become a permanent member of his small, desk-side privy council: as dependable as the latest medical book or journal. In order to keep the size and cost of the book practicable, Dr. Bettmann concludes his chronicle as the twentieth century begins. Others will share my hope that this is not an end, but a pause, and that a companion volume will tell the fabulous story of medicine's last 50 years.

PHILIP S. HENCH, M.D.

Mayo Clinic
Rochester, Minnesota

CONTENTS

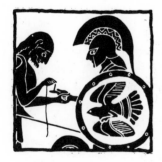

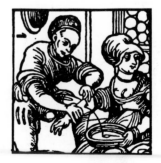

xi

CONTENTS

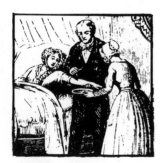

THE NINETEENTH CENTURY II   260

Triumph of Medical Science. Reveille in Germany.   Bernard and Virchow.   Backwoods Doctors.   New Tools for Diagnosis.   Florence Nightingale. Civil War Medicine. Psychiatry Takes Root. Lister Curbs Sepsis.   "Therapy in Bloomers."   In Praise of the Country Doctor.   "For All These Ills. . . ."   Sanitation for Cities—at Last!   Yellow Fever Rips the South.   Pasteur, Peer of Preventive Medicine.   Koch Tracks Down Tuberculosis. The Aseptic Method. Nurses are Needed. Childcare Made a Science. Johns Hopkins: Great Doctors—Great Teachers. Osler: Giant of the Wards.   Rays of Hope.   Towards Chemo-Therapy.

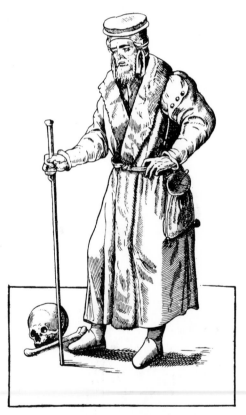

Surfeyte, age, and ficknes, are enemyes all to health,
Medicines to mende the body excell all worldly wealth:
Phyficke ftill flourfie, and in daunger will giue cure,
Till death vnknit the liuely knot no longer wee endure.

A PICTORIAL HISTORY OF
MEDICINE

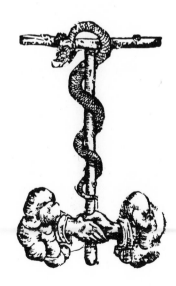

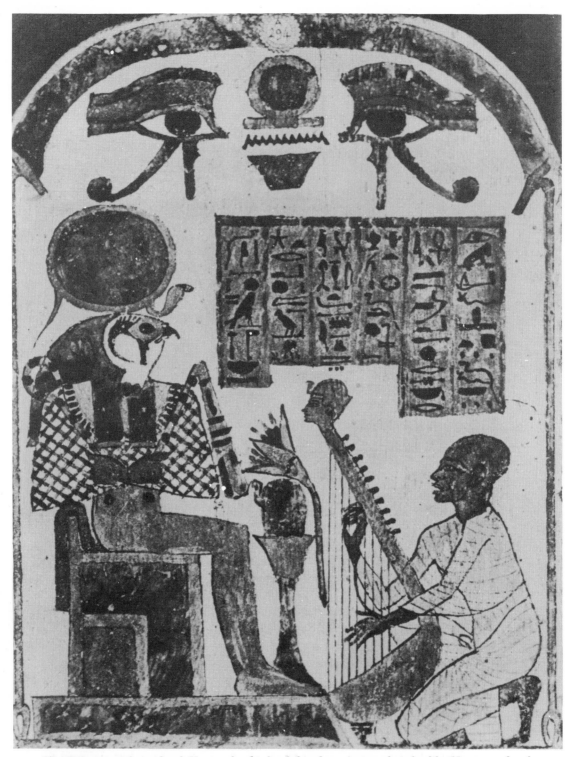

The Egyptian sick implored Horus, the ibis-headed god, to restore their health. Harps made of medicinal wood accompanied their incantations. The Eye of Horus became a symbol of recovery.

From the medicine man of ancient times to the medical man of today · the evolution presents a fascinating study. The line of advance is not always straight and obvious. Yet, no professional owes more to the longago past than does the doctor.

To this day the mystic sign ℞ adorns the top of his prescription. Its origin appears to go back some 5000 years and to be based on the legend of the Eye of Horus. The Egyptians used this magic eye as an amulet to guard them against disease, suffering, and all manners of evil . . . Suffering had made Horus a healing god. As a child, he lost his vision after a vicious attack by Seth, demon of evil. The mother of Horus, <u>Isis,</u> hurriedly called Thoth, scribe and sage to the rescue. Thoth, with his wisdom, promptly restored the eye and its powers. This led the Egyptians to revere the Eye of Horus as a symbol of godly protection and recovery.

During the Middle Ages, the Horus Eye reappeared in a new form resembling our numeral 4. Doctors and alchemists scribbled it on their prescriptions to invoke the benevolent assistance of Jupiter. Gradually, by slow transformation, the Jupiter sign changed into ℞ . . . It is this late descendant of the Eye of Horus which serves to the present day as a link between ancient and modern medicine . . . a true symbol of the durability, strength and beneficence of the healing profession through the ages.

MEDICAL LIFE ALONG THE NILE

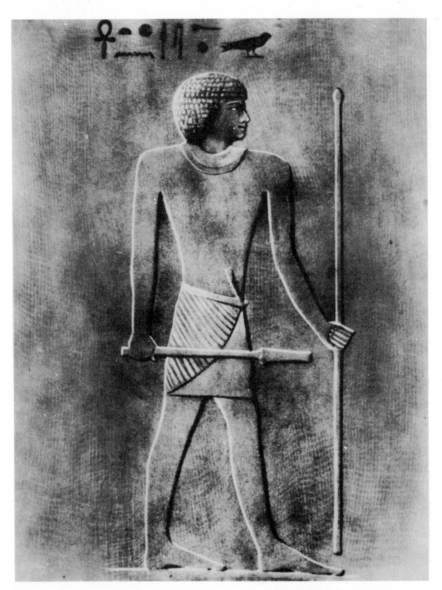

The world's first portrait of a doctor known by name: Sekhet'enanach, chief physician to Pharaoh Sahura (2550 B.C.). The inscription tells us that he gained renown "for curing the king's nostrils." The doctor carries two sceptres, the symbols of power and wisdom. It has been suggested that the king erected this monument to make amends for that age-old failing: tardy payment of the doctor's bill.

In ancient Egypt medicine basked in the sunlight of royal patronage.

The Pharaohs surrounded themselves with a prodigious staff of physicians whose task it was to prolong and protect the ruler's life. Some of the doctors took on definite functions. One served, for instance, as "keeper of the drugs"; another, as "head of the fumigation department." On his tomb near the pyramid of Gizeh, the chief physician Irj (c. 2500 B.C.) is described as "shepherd of the anus." In his reliance on "specialists" an ancestor of Tutankhamen went so far as to appoint a medical guardian for his left eye and another one for his right eye.

Centuries later, Herodotus, the Greek historian, still found Egyptian doctors grouped into specialties: "The practice of medicine is so divided up amongst them," he wrote, "that each physician is a healer of one disease and no more, some of the eye, some of the teeth, some of what pertains to the belly."

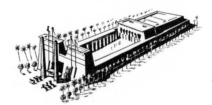

Since Egypt's official doctors belonged to the class of priests, their training centered around the temples, which served as places of worship, medical schools, and hospitals. One hall was reserved for religious services; others were set aside for the instruction of students, and as storerooms for medicines. The rear of the building housed a library.

The novice was initiated into magic and medicine by learning the code of medical precepts by heart. On certain days he attended consultations held by the high priest in the "court of miracles."

According to Egyptian belief, all true medical knowledge was revealed by the gods. Thoth, the healer of Horus, had recorded this knowledge in secret books which contained the list of all human ills and their cures. Thoth, the Hermes of the Romans, had sealed these books "hermetically." Only the priest-physician knew how to read them and apply their wisdom to the care of the sick.

Aside from the priest-physicians, Egypt had magicians who were adept healers. When they visited the sick, they brought along a papyrus roll filled with incantations, and an ample supply of baked earth to make amulets. The belief was prevalent that demons

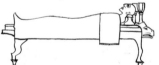

caused disease. Demons, it was thought, entered the patient's body, broke open his bones, sucked out the marrow and slowly devoured his flesh. The trick was to drive out these demons, usually by threats and incantations. "Get back, thou enemy," the doctor might shout, "Horus conjures thee — he cuts thee off, he spits thee out."

These rites were often accompanied by massages, by tramping on the patient's body, or by administering potions noxious enough to nauseate the patient, thus subjecting him to a form of "shock therapy."

Methods that in retrospect appear quite rational were not unknown to these doctors. In the case of an inflamed uterus, for instance, an early form of intravaginal diathermy was applied: The patient had to stand over hot coals sprinkled with scented wax, and the ascending smoke was to reduce the inflammation.

The enema was a common remedy when the patient needed purging. The doctor had no qualms to use it. Thoth himself had revealed the enema one day to a few priest-physicians who were standing on the banks of the Nile. The god of medicine and science had landed on the water in the form of a sacred ibis. Filling his beak with water, he had injected it into his anus. The doctors took the hint, and the result was a great boon to humanity, the Divine Clyster.

The doctor's fee for bedridden patients was at times compounded in a strange if simple way. It was a rule of hygiene among the Egyptians to shave their hair. As they were almost excessively fastidious about it, the barbershops were kept humming. But if a man became sick and was confined to his bed, he let his hair grow. Upon recovery, a barber was called in to cut it. Then the hair was carefully weighed and assessed to determine the doctor's bill. A bald Egyptian, with no basis for assessment, could hardly afford to get sick.

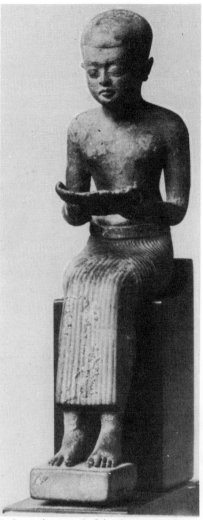

Imhotep (c. 3000 B.C.), physician, states-man, builder, was deified after his death.

In the eyes of the Egyptians Imhotep was the epitome of a great physician. His stature grew with the years until he was raised to full godhood. He visited the sick to give them "peaceful sleep" and in his sanctuaries votive tablets recorded his healing miracles. During his life this physician was also a statesman and builder. As a tomb for his master, King Zoser, he designed the world's oldest free standing structure, the step-pyramid of Sakkara.

3

EMBALMING GIVES CLUES TO SURGEONS

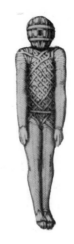

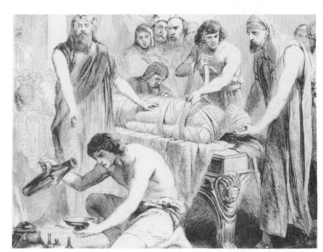

Mummification was a religious custom in Egypt, performed by a special caste of priests. Since it was wholly concerned with death, the doctor kept wisely away from it. Yet surgeons inevitably profited from the techniques of the embalmers.

These men must have been thoroughly familiar with the relation and interdependence of the various organs. The embalmers left the heart and kidneys inside the body, but removed the viscera and usually stored them in precious vases. Special instruments were devised to remove the brain through the nostrils. Such experience advanced the knowledge of anatomy

Mummification ceremony: After immersion in preservatives, corpse was artfully bandaged.

and surgery. At the same time it conditioned the public to the idea of dissection.

Embalming also acquainted the doctor with methods of avoiding bodily decay. Substances with strong antiseptic properties — resins, naptha, natron, liquid pitch — were used in preparing the corpse for the hereafter. This gave the physicians a faint knowledge of antiseptics. Also, the

embalmers swathed the body in the finest of linen impregnated with bituminous substances. Some strips extended over 1000 yards, and compared favorably with modern gauzes. These were arranged with amazing symmetry. As Dr. Augustus Grenville stated in his *Essay on Mummies:* "There is not a single form of bandage known to modern surgery of which swathings are not seen in Egyptian mummies."

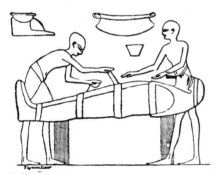

Bald assistants encase mummy in coffin. They also add final touches.

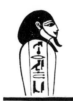 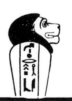 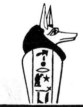

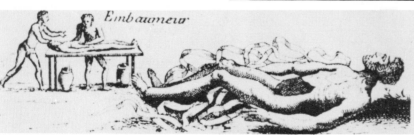

Precious alabaster vases (above) were used to preserve viscera. Animal heads symbolize the sons of Horus.

Mummy powder was used during the Middle Ages to ward off disease. Fakers made powder synthetically to fill demand.

4

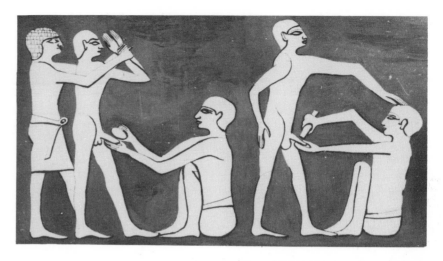

Circumcision of two youths is shown on front of Ankhmahor tomb at Sakkara. According to the inscription, the surgeon reassures the young patient: "I shall do you good." Youth at right replies, "Oh, physician, this is excellent." But his companion balks. "Hold him," the surgeon tells his assistant "do not allow him to stir." The ceremony probably preceded marriage.

Surgery received a further impetus when the introduction of copper raised Egyptian civilization "out of the slough of the Stone Age" and put sharper instruments into the surgeon's hand. The knife and the cautery were freely, if crudely, employed. There were specialists in ophthalmic surgery, and as far back as 4000 B.C. circumcision was practiced, chiefly as a hygienic measure. In the sixth century B.C. Pythagoras was said to have been rejected by a temple school in Egypt unless he agreed to be circumcised.

The papyri indicate that the basic methods for staunching blood, closing wounds and setting fractures were surprisingly sound. Fresh meat was used to stop hemorrhage, and adhesive plaster was known. As a rule operations were preceded by incantations. This magic ceremony had its rational function. Even the bedside manner of the modern physician is a mild form of exorcism designed to give the patient a little moral support.

Political factors proved equally important to surgical progress. The Egyptian empire was thoroughly militaristic, and wars as Hippocrates later pointed out, are the "true school of the surgeon." So the doctors gained added experience on macabre battlefields.

EGYPTIANS SUFFERED LIKE MODERN MAN

Pott's Disease

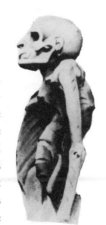

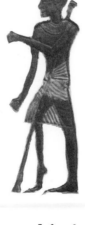

Infantile Paralysis

Thanks to the embalmers' skill and a dry climate, the modern paleo-pathologist can confidently report on the state of health in ancient Egypt. Once unwrapped, many of the well-preserved mummies showed unmistakable signs of rheumatoid arthritis. Professor Elliot Smith found a typical case of Pott's disease, with severe spinal curvature and a large abscess in the region of the loins. Bladder and kidney stones also were identified, and a study by Armand M. Ruffer indicates that arteriosclerosis was a common disease 3500 years ago.

All of this contradicts Herodotus' report that the people of Egypt enjoyed excellent health. They suffered just like modern man. Communal care of the sick also seems to have been known. Many mummies bear out the fact that diseases reached advanced stages, and as Ruffer concludes, "Patients would have died of inanition without some form of nursing care."

5

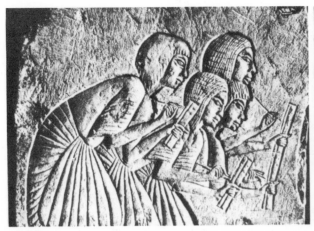

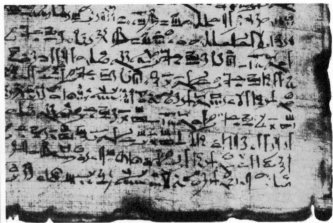

PRESCRIPTIONS COME ON PAPYRUS

Egyptian medicine was further bolstered by the art of writing and the availability of papyrus, a light and durable writing material. These enabled the physician to record his experiences and establish a tradition. The lore of other ancient cultures had proven ephemeral, but the papyri became a natural reservoir for medical wisdom. One scroll acquired by Georg Ebers in 1873, contained 700 remedies for afflictions ranging from crocodile bite to pain in the toenail. Dated c. 1500 B.C., this document indicates that the art of diagnosis had been highly developed for some time. Twenty different ailments were listed for the stomach alone, including constipation. The remedy for this latter scourge — castor oil mixed with beer — seems quite applicable even today.

A second famous papyrus, discovered by Edwin Smith in 1862, has been called "the world's first surgical textbook (c. 1700 B. C.)." It was organized to deal with case problems, and ritual and incantation were kept at a minimum. Forty-eight traumatic lesions were described and thoroughly analyzed, each in the same orderly fashion: examination, diagnosis, advice to the doctor as to whether he should accept the case, and if so, detailed instructions for therapy. For example, a woman suffers "in her abdomen," is unable to menstruate and has "trouble in the upper part of her vulva." The doctor is instructed to tell her she has "obstruction of the blood," and to prescribe as follows: Wam, $\frac{1}{16}$; Grease, $\frac{1}{8}$; Sweet beer, $\frac{1}{8}$; to be cooked and drunk for four days. He is also told to mix an ointment of "oil, tepnenet, eyepaint and sweet frankincense," and finally, to "anoint the organ therewith very frequently."

Other papyri too, indicate that the Egyptians had an amazingly complex materia medica: herbs, minerals, secretions and animal substances, the latter derived from such beasts as the ox, bat, ass, mouse, elephant, crocodile, lion, camel, hyena and vulture. Saliva, urine, bile, faeces and parts of the body also were used, along with worms, snakes and insects. All these were

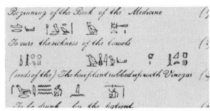

EBERS PAPYRUS
compounded into gargles, salves, snuffs, emollients, pills, inhalations, fumigations, purgatives. In addition, the Egyptians knew the ameliorating effect of yeasts and molds on wounds and recommended the use of opium, hemlocks, squills, castor oil and copper salts.

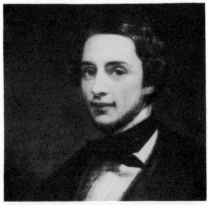

Edwin Smith American Egyptologist acquired surgical papyrus at Luxor (1862).

6

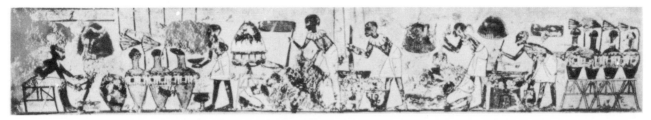

An Egyptian drug establishment in operation; plants, animals and secretions were used in medicaments.

One strange remedy deserves particular mention. Some doctors prescribed dead mice — as a last resort — for infantile ailments, and evidence from the mummies indicates that their advice was followed. Skinned mice were found in the alimentary canals of children's mummies dating as far back as the year 4000 B.C.

Such medicines and therapies were passed along from generation to generation, with folly preserved as well as fact. This proved to be unfortunate, when the tradition hardened into a series of rigid laws which the doctor was compelled to obey. (If he deviated, and his patient died, then the doctor was in grave jeopardy.) Layer upon layer, wisdom and stupidity piled up, and ultimately the latter prevailed. Formalism developed like an encrustation over the field of medicine, as it did over all other fields, and Egyptian civilization finally sank down and died of its own weight.

But the Egyptian doctor, while he lasted, was "cock of the walk" in the Ancient East. Herodotus admired his specialized knowledge. The kings of every nation tried to lure him to their courts. Cyrus sent to Egypt for an oculist, and Darius secured an Egyptian specialist to treat his mother's eye. Moreover, the immense materia medica of Egypt passed into the pharmacopoeia of neighboring countries and spread through the Middle East. Later, the Greeks were to draw heavily upon Egyptian findings to develop their own great medical system. In Roman times, Galen suggested that a sprinkling of Egyptian terms in a prescription would help to fortify the patient's belief in the remedy. And in the 18th century, quacks in the streets of London could still lure crowds to their stumps, simply by displaying "Doctor of Egypt" upon their shingles.

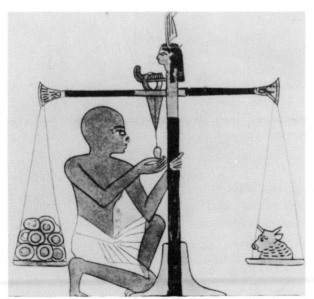

Balance was well known in Egypt. Some experts assert weights were based on the decimal system (1380 B.C.).

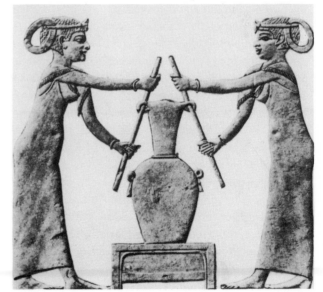

Female druggists squeeze animal skin filled with herbs. Egyptians used this method in making medicinal lotions.

7

BABYLON

ASSYRIA

PRIESTS
CHASE
DISEASE
DEMONS

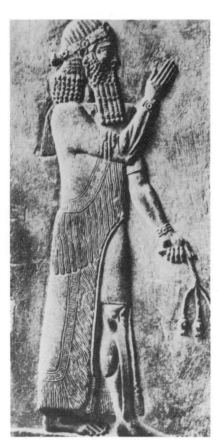

Knotted whip was used by priest to scare off hordes of disease-demons.

Baal-Zebub — God of flies. Babylonians believed insects spread disease.

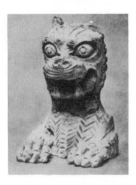

Evil demons, frightened by seeing tiny replicas of themselves, fled.

While the Egyptians concerned themselves a great deal with life after death, the practical Babylonians were more preoccupied with immediate physical needs. Their priest-physicians set out to conquer disease in this world — and to this end they declared war on the demons that caused human suffering.

Grotesque masks and daggers were fashioned to terrorize the imps of sickness. Chains were on hand so that Marduk, lord of magic, might "bind the witch with ropes." A special watch was kept for the vicious "southwest wind," a dog-bodied eagle with lion's paws whose hot breath brought consuming fever to man and beast alike. To ward him off, clay and metal likenesses of this evil doer appeared on every door and window. (He was supposed to be scared at his own sight.)

Such superstitious maneuvers reflect a dim anticipation of preventive medicine and the germ theory. The Baby-

lonians held that disease was an abnormality caused by invisible external agents. If members of a family became ill with similar symptoms, a specific demon was blamed for the contagion. Moreover, Baal-Zebub, the god of flies, gnats and all other insects was directly blamed for ill health by the neighboring Philistines and Phoenicians. A temple was erected at Ekron to appease him. Arad-Nana, the Babylonian court physician warned his master, Assurbanipal, in a letter: "Beware of flies and shun lice in the interest of good health" (c. 660 B.C.). The advice was sound, whatever the superstition behind it.

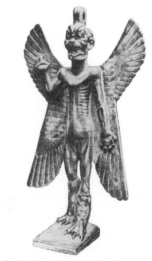

Dog-bodied eagle with lion's paws, "the southwest wind," could consume man and beast with agonizing fever.

TELL-TALE LIVER

The Babylonians also originated a primitive form of medical prognosis. They asked the patient to breathe into a sheep's nose. Then they slaughtered the sheep, took a "reading" of its liver and predicted the outcome of the case.

A "breathed-on" sheep's liver, it was believed, would register the nature of a disease and the prospects for recovery. The priests examined it with great care and recorded their findings by sticking wooden pegs into a clay model of the organ, zoned off into essential regions (right).

The liver also played a part in the fate of men and nations. As the seat of all vital functions, it was the obvious choice of the gods for revealing their intentions. Thus, a tight sheep's liver meant victory in war; a shriveled one forecast defeat. In addition the stars and moon were read for fateful omens. The Babylonians were the first to employ astro-diagnosis.

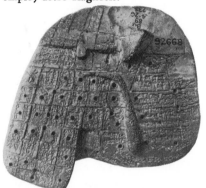

Readings from sheep's liver were pegged into clay model to help foretell patient's future (British Museum).

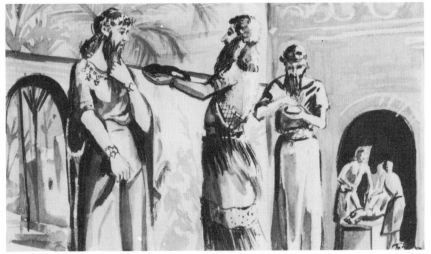

Patient breathed into sheep's nose; then the animal was killed, its liver examined.

SURGEON IN TROUBLE

A priestly class, called ashipu, specialized in the mysterious realm of inner medicine. But surgery, visible sores, fractures and snakebites were handled by practical doctors, called asu. These wise healers were skilled in herbal and mineral cures. According to Hammurabi's code (c. 1950 B.C.), they formed a special non-priestly group which practiced under strict government regulation. A scale of fees was fixed by law, based on the patient's ability to pay and the seriousness of the case. Thus, a nobleman had to pay 10 shekels to have an abscess opened, while a freeman paid five.

Although this income-bracket billing has a modern ring, the code contained some uncomfortable clauses. Payment was made, for instance, only upon recovery. Worse yet, the doctor was punished for failure — again according to scale: Loss of a nobleman's sight meant loss of the doctor's hand; loss of a slave's life, meant a payment, to the owner, of a new slave. There was no margin for error, so the doctor either had to be flawless or lucky.

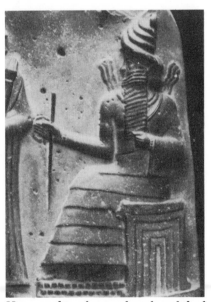

Hammurabi, whose code acknowledged surgeons as a special class, imposed harsh reprisals for operative mishaps.

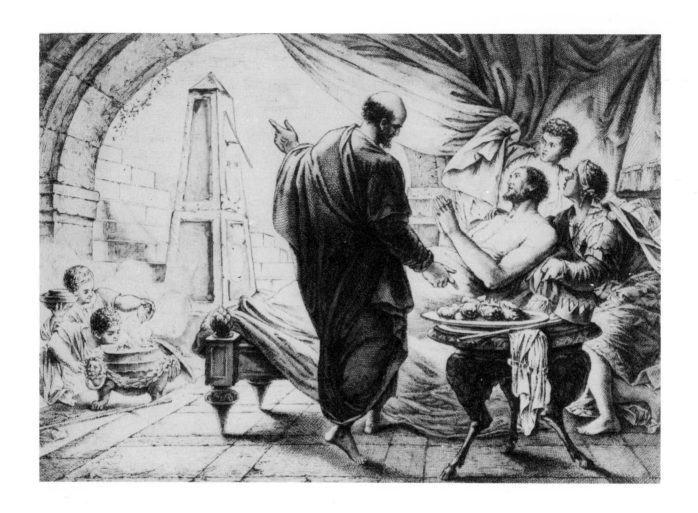

"I, GOD, AM THY PHYSICIAN"

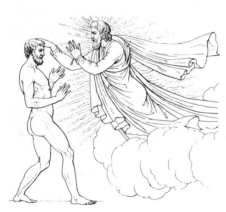

Through monotheism, Jewish medicine kept aloof from the incantations, exorcism and astrology of Babylonia and Egypt. According to the tenets of the Old Testament, God was the only physician, and at the same time, the only source of disease. In the main, the Old Testament reflected a new and purer concept of sickness and health.

For the early Jewish tribes this concept was closely linked to moral-ity. Obedience to God's laws was a passport to good health, while a step off the path of righteousness meant punishment through disease. Illness was the wage of sin: "If thou wilt diligently harken (to) the voice of the Lord . . . I will put none of these diseases upon thee." God was called Rophe Cholim, the supreme healer. Rophe later was to signify the lay physician, or as Luther translated it, "God's own body patcher."

Isaiah (left) shows ailing king Hezekiah that God has set the sun back ten hours as sign of His mercy.

At first with the Department of Health under one Great Physician, there was little room for such "body patchers." Doctors were considered usurpers of the Lord's healing prerogatives. Thus, the Bible speaks censoriously of King Asa (915-875 B.C.) who "sought not the Lord, but the physician" to cure his foot disease. But Asa won out in the long run: he is now hailed as the Bible's first patient to consult a doctor. Only gradually did God "delegate" his healing powers to the prophets, the priests, and finally, to the physicians.

The prophets restored the sick to health through a combination of prayer and a therapy which was at times surprisingly rational. Their prayers helped to strengthen the patient's belief that God's wrath had caused the disease, and that God's mercy

would effect a cure for the disease.

The Bible bears out the efficacy of the faith and common sense methods employed by the prophets. The case of King Hezekiah is a striking example of such therapy. He suffered from some form of furunculosis and was afraid he would die. The prophet Isaiah was called to his bedside. At first, Isaiah held no hope for the king and told him to put his house in order. But Hezekiah pleaded with the Lord for a few more years of life. Mercifully God informed Isaiah that he had granted the king an additional 15 years and to give evidence of his decision, He moved the shade on the king's sun dial back 10 hours. Hezekiah lost his fear of death, and Isaiah was able to apply a "cake of heated figs" to the boils, thereby diminishing the pain and reducing the dangers of septicemia. The king recovered in short order.

The prophet Elisha was equally blessed with faith and wisdom. When he was asked to restore to life the smothered boy of the Shunammite, he

took the child to the roof, and revived him quickly with a form of artificial respiration: Bending over the child, Elisha blew air into his mouth (a method used to this day on newborns) and thereby set off seven sneezes. The sneezes removed an obstruction in the child's trachea, and recovery was almost instantaneous.

The *Book of Kings* (II:5) contains a second example of Elisha's good work as God's medical legate. Naaman, a Syrian general, was afflicted with a skin eruption. He went to Israel on the advice of a Jewish slave girl, who had told him to appeal for recovery to Jehovah, through Elisha. But Elisha refused to see Naaman. He sent word instead that the general should first take seven dips in the Jordan. Grudgingly, the bewildered general complied, and "his flesh came again like unto the flesh of a little child, and he was clean." The grateful patient asked the prophet-physician for two mule loads of Israeli earth to take back to Syria, so he might worship Jehovah "upon His own soil."

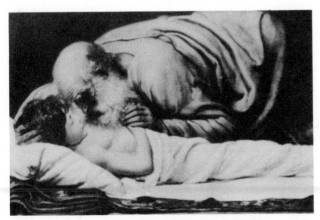

Elisha breathed into mouth of suffocating child. This set off a series of seven sneezes removing obstruction in the boy's trachea.

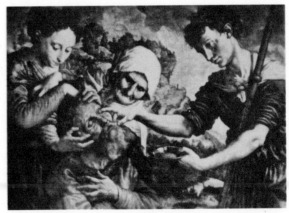

Tobit's son rubbed the eyes of his blinded father with fish-gall. This cleared the cornea and Tobit's sight returned.

11

MOSES - PUBLIC HEALTH LEADER

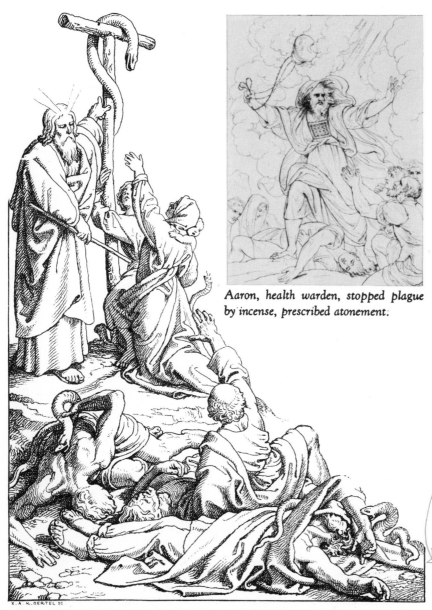

Aaron, health warden, stopped plague by incense, prescribed atonement.

Brazen Serpent erected by Moses at God's command. Those bitten by serpents were to look at this image, reiterate their faith and be healed. All those doubting God's mercy were to be devoured. The idea of counteracting evil by facing it was widespread in antiquity. Patients formed images of hurtful animals and demons, in order to drive them away. Moses linked this belief with the tenet that all healing power rested in God. Faith in him meant recovery.

Mosaic Law contained both the essence of the Jewish religion and at the same time an impressive system of pre-Hippocratic medical thought. Even if Moses did not originate this code all by himself, he remains to this day one of the most farsighted proponents of preventive medicine.

Adopted by the Pharaoh's daughter and raised in the royal household of Egypt, Moses studied hygiene and medicine at the temple school of Os. In the palace he saw the effects of licentious living and acquired his distaste for quacks and magicians. Later he banned quackery in his famous code. The idea of God as the sole physician — left little room for miracle-mongers or magic remedies.

It also left no room for the Pharaoh's refusal to free the Jews from slavery. According to one Biblical theorist, Moses used his knowledge of public hygiene to wage bacterial warfare on the Egyptians. He set off the ten plagues by contaminating the Nile and all other waters. (Others hold that the poisoning was caused by the tail of a descending comet.) The frogs fled the rivers and died in droves on the shores. This attracted swarms of insects: the insects killed many Egyptians, whose cadavers rotted and "the land stunk." In the general confusion, Moses and the Jews left Egypt.

12

Whatever theory of the exodus is accepted, the Jews could not have wandered for the next 40 years without a public health leader of genius. Moses provided them with an excellent code. "For the Lord, thy God, walketh in the midst of thy camp," he told them; "therefore shall it be kept immaculate." To this end, garbage and excreta were disposed of outside the camp; contagious cases were quarantined; spitting was outlawed as unhygienic, and bodily cleanliness became a prerequisite for moral purity. Most important of all, from a modern standpoint, the Jews set aside the Sabbath as a day of rest. Though some of these laws were Egyptian in origin, Moses was the first to codify them and present them as the tenets of one God.

The enforcement of this code was in later years entrusted to the priests of Israel. Unlike their Egyptian predecessors, they avoided actual medical practice and concentrated upon the observance of health rules with regard to food, cleanliness and quarantine. They removed contagious cases from the community and had the victim's clothes burned, their homes scoured. Earthen vessels were broken and wooden ones washed. Then, when the patients began to recover, the priests were expected to look at them to "behold if the plague be dim." If it was, the patients could soon go back to the settlement.

Though God saw to the healing of internal disease, epilepsy and blindness, the lay physician gradually received jurisdiction over self-evident cases. This rise in status was due to the Jews' changeover from nomadic to city life. Afflictions multiplied, and

greater reliance on the lay doctor became imperative. Thus, in *Ecclesiastes*, XXXVIII, written about 200 B.C., the patient is advised to "pray unto the Lord . . . then give place to the physician, for the Lord hath created him (and) thou hast need of him." Jewish temples hired doctors by this time to look after the priests, who had developed an arthritic condition from daily cold baths.

This reliance upon worldly healing power resulted in a strict licensing system. Before he could practice, the Jewish doctor had to obtain his permit from the law courts. Fortunately he was spared from the cruel Babylonian practice of retribution for failure to cure. He even was urged to charge a proper fee, since as the Talmud puts it, "free cures seldom work," and "a physician who charges nothing is worth nothing."

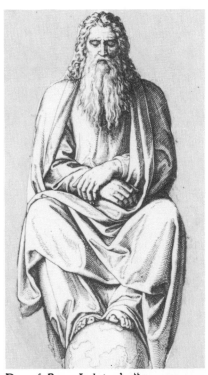

Day of Rest, Judaism's "greatest contribution to human welfare" (Sudhoff).

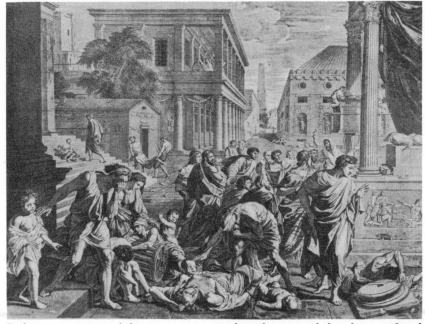

Rodents as carriers of disease are recognized in the story of the plague inflicted by God upon the Philistines after they had robbed the Jews of Ark of the Covenant. The Bible says bubonic plague spread in foe's land after rodents invaded it.

13

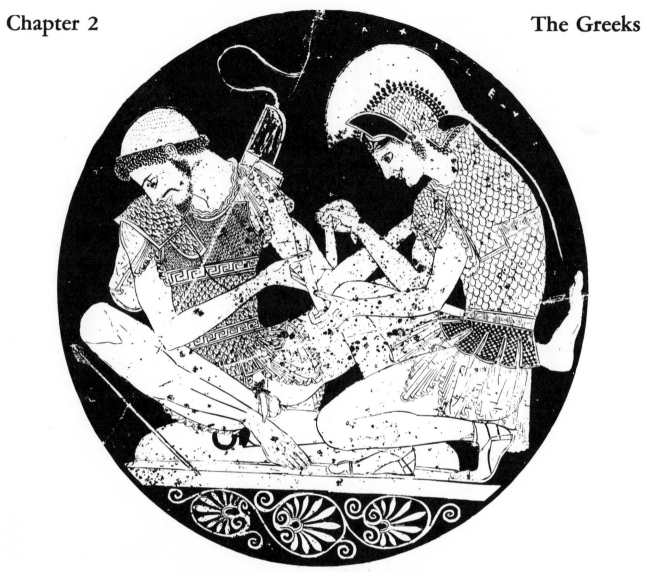

Achilles (right) learned first aid from Chiron, the medical centaur. Here he binds wound of Patroclus.
Fifth Century B.C. vase painting.

The Greeks inherited the medical knowledge of Egypt, Babylonia, Phoenicia and other Eastern countries. They sorted it out, tried to discard magic, and merge the remainder into a rational structure. The new edifice took time to build, and it required new methods: careful observation (in place of blind belief), plus the certainty that disease was a natural phenomenon, and not a divine infliction. But once the structure was up, it stayed up, and remains, even today, one of the most significant landmarks of western civilization.

The Homeric poems, assembled around 1000 B.C., show medicine largely in the hands of practical army surgeons. Then in the succeeding centuries, the priests of Aesculapius made their influence felt. This religious cult propounded magic more than medicine, but even the magic had its common sense elements. Gradually the sounder concepts prevailed and a group of shrewd, analytical practitioners emerged from the temples of Aesculapius. Their teachings molded the mind of Hippocrates, the founding father of rational medicine.

According to the Homeric legends the early Greek physicians were heroes among heroes, skilled in their profession and easily "worth more than armies to the public weal." The expeditionary force at Troy numbered about 100,000 men. There were a good many brave doctors among them, but their battlefield performance was actually quite poor (Froehlich places the mortality rate at 77.6 per cent). Nevertheless Homer praised their work highly. He by-passed the fevers, epidemics and complications which attend all large-scale military ventures, and concentrated instead upon the gallant staunching of bloody wounds, upon surgery under emergency conditions.

Since the besieging army was somewhat short on doctors, the heroes were forced to fall back upon first aid measures like bandaging, the application of balms and of hemostatics. Many such medical skills were rooted in mythology. Chiron, the friendly centaur, had instructed Achilles in medicine, and Achilles had passed this knowledge along to his comrades. This makes Chiron the Greek army's first medical mentor. But let Homer tell it, in Book XI of the *Iliad*, at the point where the wounded Euripylus speaks to Patroclus:

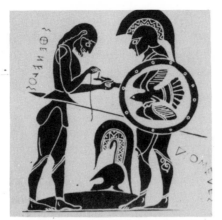

Sthenelos bandages Diomedes' hand as Greeks cope with doctor shortage.

HOMER'S BATTLE SURGEONS

Two regimental surgeons were singled out in Homer's poems as heroic fighters and physicians. Machaon and Podalirius were sons of Aesculapius, but they appeared in the Iliad as solid and worldly, rather than godlike. Machaon served as private physician to Menelaus. When an arrow pierced the latter's armor, Machaon rushed to his side, drew the shaft, "but left the head behind." Then he sucked the blood and applied a "sovereign balm."

Later, Machaon was wounded by Paris, whose elopement with Helen had touched off the war. The Greek camp was deeply concerned as Machaon lay wounded in his tent, in need of "the succor which so oft he lent." It was here that one by-stander, Idomeneus, made the classic remark that one surgeon was worth an army of men:
*A surgeon's skill our wound to heal
Is worth more than armies to the public weal.*

Podalirius, another son of Aesculapius, seems to have specialized in internal medicine. He diagnosed Ajax' madness, for instance, by one look at his flashing eyes.

On his return trip from Troy, Podalirius had a lucky accident. His ship was wrecked on the coast of Caria, but a herdsman rescued him and took him to the royal palace. The king's daughter, Syrna, had just fallen from the roof. All attempts to revive her had failed, but Podalirius bled both her arms and saved her.

The case ended happily for doctor and patient. Podalirius married the king's daughter. Later he built two castles. One was named after his wife the other after the goatherd who had rescued him.

*But thou, Patroclus, act a friendly part
Lead to my ship and draw this deadly
   dart
With lukewarm water wash the gore
   away
With healing balms the raging smart
   alay
Such as sage Chiron fire of Pharmacy
Once taught Achilles and Achilles thee.*

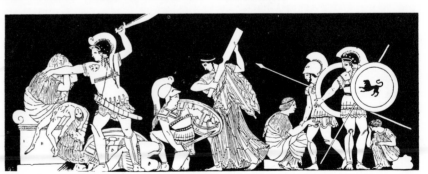

Scene during Trojan War shows variety of weapons used by Greeks. Battle surgeons studied their effects and learned how to cure wounds efficiently.

AESCULAPIUS

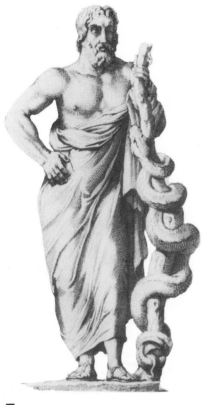

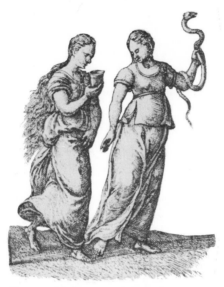

Hygeia and Panacea, daughters of Aesculapius, tend serpents, givers of health.

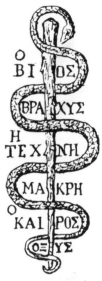

"Life is short; art is long; experience difficult." Original Aesculapian wand.

In Homeric days medicine's supreme diety, Aesculapius was a mere mortal, though an excellent physician. His rise to godhood occurred somewhere between the Trojan war and the ninth century B. C. According to mythology, Apollo had snatched Aesculapius from the womb of his unfaithful earthly mistress, Koronis. Later on, Apollo turned the young god over to Chiron, the centaur who had a gift for healing. Chiron taught the boy all he knew about medicine, but his pupil soon surpassed him as a practitioner. Aesculapius became so successful that Zeus had to smite him with a thunderbolt, so the gods could retain their power over life and death.

The children of Aesculapius carried on his good work. Telesphoros represented as a little hopeful boy was believed responsible for "recovery," while Aesculapius' daughter Panacea possessed deep knowledge of all the earth's remedies. Hygeia performed an equally important task: she fed the serpents who effected the healing miracles. Public welfare was her domain.

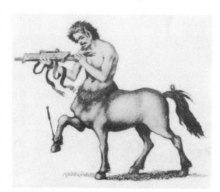

Chiron, chirurgeon — "handman" taught first aid to Aesculapius, Achilles.

The question of who came first, Aesculapius or the serpent, has been settled in favor of the serpent. Reptiles have been considered synonymous with wisdom since time immemorial. The snake, in particular, coming out of the ground, which holds many curative substances, was believed to possess secret healing powers. Consequently, the ancient Greeks ate snake meat to acquire proficiency in the healing arts and even immortality.

The Aesculapian staff has often been confused with the caduceus, the "Herald's Wand" used by Hermes, or Mercury, to open doors between gods and men — but the Aesculapian staff entwined by one snake is regarded by classicists as the true symbol of the profession (above).

16

HIS TEMPLES
WERE CENTERS
OF FAITH HEALING

To worship Aesculapius, the benign healing god, temples sprang up all over Greece. At first, they functioned as places of worship, but as time went on they took on in addition the function of clinics and hospitals. The fame of such medical centers at Epidaurus, Pergamos and Cos spread over the ancient world, and their influence reached far into the Christian era.

Their record for miraculous cures was partly based on their location. The temples were established on beautifully landscaped pastoral slopes, and the climate was usually salubrious. More important, the hopelessly ill were weeded out during a preliminary check-up. This bolstered the temple's reputation for "cures."

Once past this initial examination, the patients were taken on a tour of the halls, where impressive images of Aesculapius and other gods were on exhibit. Then one by one the group filed down tottering ladders to subterranean baths. Here the patients were scrubbed and cleansed, inside and out. According to reports, some of them underwent a "foodless diet" for about 15 days. When ready for treatment they were given special white linen vestments, supposed to be especially conducive to dreams. And dreams were the mainstay of Aesculapian therapy.

When the temples were small, this dream-therapy was conducted around a statue of Aesculapius. The patients rested on the floor, and hoped that the god would reveal his healing recipes during the night. But as the temples grew, special porticos were built and equipped with couches (the patients often supplied their own mattresses). Once bedded in these outside dormitories, the sufferers were put at ease, sometimes by surreptitious doses of sedatives like poppyseed and hemlock. An aromatic (perhaps narcotic) smoke drifted forth from inside the temple . . .

Children implore Aesculapius for a cure of sick father. Holy serpent guards sacrifices placed on altar.

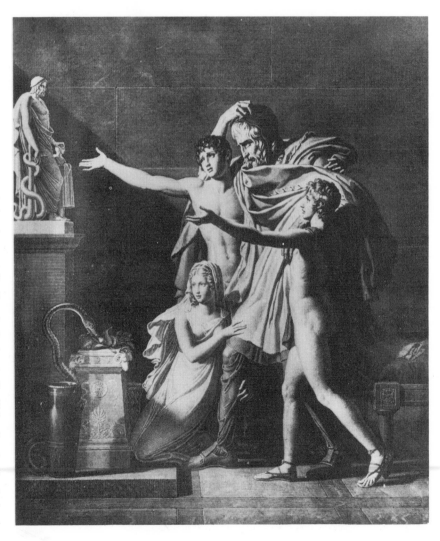

DREAM AND GET WELL

The priest-physicians tried to induce dreams in which Aesculapius would reveal the cure to the patients.

A solemn pageant appeared before the drowsy eyes of the sufferers. To make sure that they "saw" Aesculapius, a tall priest donned the god's mask. Just before dawn, he made the rounds of the dormitories, accompanied by tiptoeing assistants. Ventriloquism may have been used to impress the patients with revelations coming from nowhere. There is no conclusive evidence that hypnotism was employed. Oddly enough, substitute dreamers were allowed to appear in the temple to take the place of patients who were unable to appear themselves. One Laconian woman, Arata, suffered from dropsy; she sent her mother to the sanctuary to receive the god's message. As the rites were performed, her mother had a vision: Aesculapius cut off her daughter's head, let the water drain from the neck, then replaced the head. When the mother returned, Arata was cured.

These incubation ceremonies were made more mysterious by the use of holy snakes. With the aid of heat and soft flute music, tame reptiles were coaxed to lick the patients' wounds, from ulcerated toes to swollen eyes (dogs were trained to do the same). To help relations between reptiles and patients, popona, a kind of "snake-biscuit," was placed on sale. The patients bought it, and fed it to the serpents.

Such emotion-charged ceremonies were abetted by rational therapy. Patients were bathed, massaged or treated with soothing ointments. Surgery was sometimes attempted. And above all, fresh air and recreational activities (the theatre at Epidaurus seated 12,000) helped to insure some kind of relief. The patient could at least leave the establishment refreshed and strengthened in his faith. In the light of modern psychotherapy, the Aesculapion compares favorably with the sanitarium or rest home.

Originally, the temples were sustained by gifts from the pilgrims. When the establishments expanded, outright fees became necessary. The priests could "revoke the cure" if the pilgrims tried to avoid payment.

Patient (left) is brought to holy tree in temple yard by male nurses. One bearer attempts to attract snake while patient implores it to lick his wounds. Bearers also helped care for patients, held them during operations. (Relief in Ny Carlsburg Clyptothek, Stockholm.)

Incubation sleep (below) depicted on relief of Aesculapian temple. The healing god (left) appears to the dreamer, "making him whole." Serpent, supervised by priest, climbs into patient's bed and licks his wounds. Note tablet used for clinical record.

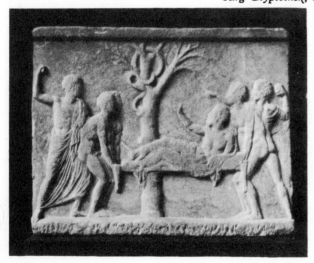
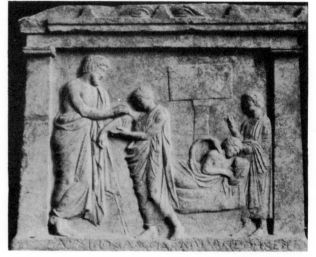

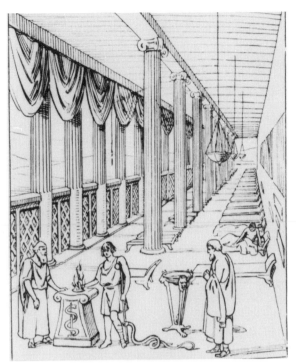

Portico at Epidaurus. Patients slept on couches to receive dream-message from Aesculapius.

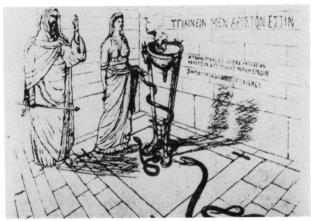

Entrance hall of temple at Cos. Walls display testimonials.

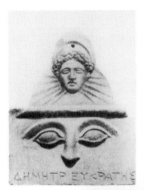
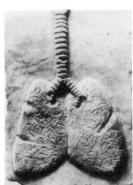

Votive offerings (above) are crude tokens of eye and lung cures. These reliefs show what Greeks knew of human anatomy.

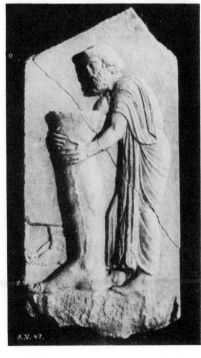

Patient with varicose vein offers replica of leg to Aesculapian temple priests who have helped him to recover (right).

One masked "Aesculapius" is reported to have forgotten himself by shouting at his patient: "Thou art healed. Now pay the fee." Bills were based on ability to pay. A grateful boy, for instance, offered 10 dice to the gods for his cure, while Phalysius of Naupactus gave 2000 gold coins (about $10,000) for the restoration of his sight. Time payments, stretched over a year, were arranged for the father of a boy cured of dumbness. Other pilgrims paid their way with precious-metal replicas of their restored organs or limbs. Such gifts give us a faint idea of the anatomical knowledge of the period. Their receipt was proudly and faithfully recorded by the superintending priest.

The votive offerings found in the temple ruins at Epidaurus and Athens are replete with dramatic case histories in which the patients described their cures in great detail. Their testimonials were placed in the entrance hall, to impress the newly arrived sufferers with the temple's successful record. Most of these histories were medical fairy tales, but they served as part of the therapy. The priests reading them to the illiterate crowds exaggerated each kernel of truth to catch the credulous and win over the doubters.

GREEKS LINK HUMANS TO LAW OF UNIVERSE

In the sixth century B.C., the Greek medical scene compared favorably with the view from a high mountain top on a misty day. At first, only a few peaks emerged from the wall of fog below. Then the fog lifted, and the sun shone down upon a fairly perceptible landscape. There were still many shrouded patches, but the Ionian medico-philosophers shed new light on the intellectual landscape. They pronounced that the universe was governed by laws, and that these laws also applied to the human body.

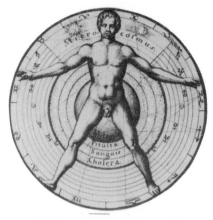

World (Macrocosm) and man (microcosm) both subject to rule of spheres.

PYTHAGORAS: NUMBERS

Pythagoras was the most original of the Ionian philosphers. He expounded the theory that numbers were the ruling principle of the universe. Thus, the stars moved through the firmament at fixed distances, and their harmony corresponded to the tonal intervals on a musical scale. The human body was also arranged according to musico-mathematical rules, and a sick man was simply out of harmony with himself and the universe. All the doctor had to do, therefore, was tune him up again, so that he felt "fit as a fiddle."

Sickness itself, Pythagoras discovered, was subject to an arithmetical progression, and from this concept Hippocrates later devised the idea of "critical days" for all disease. The mathematical clarity prevailing in some of his ideas did not keep Pythagoras from founding a mystic sect pledged to celibacy and strict dietetic rules. Members of the circle were not permitted to laugh for fear of upsetting the proper balance of mind and body.

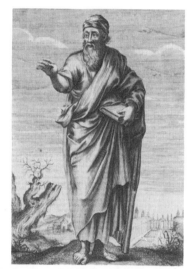

Pythagoras founded school of physician-naturalists (Crotona, Italy, 529 B.C.).

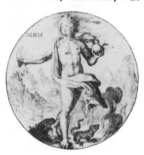

Fire

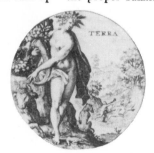

Earth

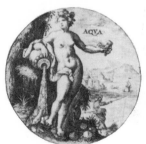

Water

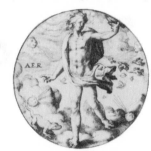

Air

20

DEMOCRITUS: ATOMS

If the theories of Pythagoras seemed coldly mathematical, Democritus (c. 460-365 B.C.) worked out a more complex and dynamic concept of man and universe. He believed that the world was composed of atoms, and that all events could be ascribed to the continual regrouping of these invisible and indestructible globules. There was a kind of mad scramble, he said, in which atoms of similar size would line up with one another, purely by chance, to form new matter. Later on, Epicurus (342-270 B.C.) borrowed this theory and applied it to medicine. He thought the human body composed of atoms and pores (the space between atoms). Health prevailed while the atoms moved about, but faulty circulation meant sickness, especially if it occurred in the intestines. The physician's problem, obviously, was to keep the pores clean and the atoms moving.

Democritus was no physician, but he wrote avidly on anatomy, epidemics, prognostics and diet. Like the other Ionian philosophers he approached medicine rationally, convinced that diseases as all other happenings in the universe — were subject to definite laws.

Democritus (460-365 B.C.) held: to keep healthy; keep pores clean, atoms moving.

EMPEDOCLES: ELEMENTS

A student of Pythagoras, Empedocles, was greatly influenced by the theory of numbers. The number four was especially significant, he said, since the world was composed of four elements: fire, earth, water and air. Each element had the definite quality of hot, cold, moist and dry, respectively, and these elements recurred in the body as the four basic fluids. According to Empedocles and his followers, blood was hot; phlegm, cold; black bile, moist; and yellow bile, dry. Disease was the imbalance of these four humours.

To restore health, the physician attempted to counteract this imbalance. Thus, signs of a cold (excessive phlegm) called for a hot remedy. Fever (surplus of blood) called for a cold one, like cucumber seeds (hence, "cool as a cucumber.") Through such teachings, Empedocles laid the foundation for the humoral system which prevailed for the next 2000 years.

Among his disciples Empedocles enjoyed the reputation of a god. To preserve this legend, he mysteriously disappeared "taken away to Olympus."

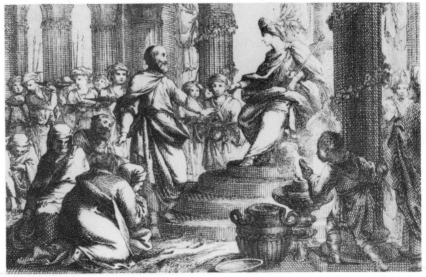

Democedes, honored at Persian court. A member of the Ionian school, he excelled in practical medicine—reset Darius' ankle, relieved his queen of a boil on her breast—later became highly paid municipal physician.

HIPPOCRATES

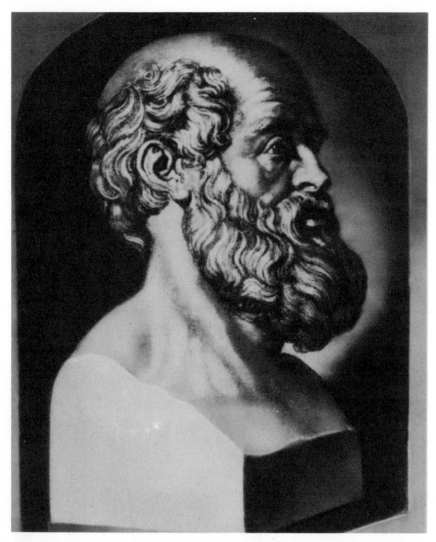

The Father of Medicine: No authentic portraits of Hippocrates exist. Yet the statues that have come down to us under his name give us an idea of what the ancient Greeks considered the image of a great and good physician.

But if the details of his life are compressible, a whole library has already been written around the massive texts called *Corpus Hippocraticum*. This collection of notes and jottings was compiled more than a century after Hippocrates' death. At that time, a book-loving Pharaoh, Ptolomy Soter (323-285), commissioned his Egyptian scholars to prepare a complete, authentic edition of the famous doctor. The over-zealous scholars collected every piece of writing with a Hippocratic label on it that they could find. Consequently, medical historians are still locked in philological battle: of the 70-odd pieces which made up the original *Corpus*, less than 20 have been definitely credited to Hippocrates. Whether or not he inspired the rest, the fact remains that the collection presents an excellent picture of Greek medical practice. If the perspective seems at times a bit faulty, these texts are still unsurpassed in depth, color and vitality.

Thus, the name "Hippocrates" stands for a number of significant ideas and practices; it symbolizes all that is great and lasting in medicine.

If a "Who's Who" were compiled for ancient Greece, the entry under Hippocrates would be surprisingly short. The only facts known about the life of the greatest of physicians seem to be these: Hippocrates was born c. 460 B.C. on the Greek Island of Cos; he was of small stature; traveled widely and died in Larissa c. 377 B.C. It might be added that in his time Cos was famous as a health resort and later on as the site of an Aesculapian temple. This, and the fact that his father (probably other forebears) practiced the art, helps to explain some of his tenets. The profession was hereditary in Greece so Hippocrates undoubtedly became his father's apprentice at an early age. He grew up in a medical atmosphere.

Though the Hippocratic oath falls under this cluster of ideas, it is now frequently stated that Hippocrates did not write it. Moreover, careful textual analysis has revealed that the oath was devised, not for the profession as a whole, but for a medical family guild, the Asclepiads, to which Hippocrates undoubtedly belonged. Knowledge was passed down in this group from father to son. This helps to explain the oath's proviso that the student must support his teacher. Hippocrates' reputation in the Middle Ages accounts for the oath's acceptance as a code of ethics for the entire profession.

In the treatise "On Epidemics" can be found a short passage which perhaps expresses clearer than the "oath" the essence of Hippocratic thinking. Here Hippocrates emphasizes that the medical art consists of three main factors: "the disease, the patient and the physician." This seems obvious today, but before Hippocrates disease was a divine infliction, the physician was a mere delegate of the gods, and the patient could only recover through faith. Healing rites were mystic and theurgic, and disease lay in the foggy province of temple priests. If therapy was sometimes rational, "medicine" was a jumbled collection of fact and fancy.

But Hippocrates saw disease as a natural process, one which developed in logical steps, like the acts of a Greek play. Moreover, he saw the patient as an individual whose constitution would react to disease in its own way. This revolutionary concept was neglected for centuries, but it has taken on increased importance in modern times.

As for the doctor, Hippocrates viewed him as a man of science instead of a priest. The Hippocratic physician observed disease, classified it and predicted its course. He practiced in accordance with the laws of science — as far as science then existed — and felt himself bound by the ethical precepts of his profession.

While Hippocrates freed internal medicine from the bonds of superstition, he found, in surgery, an established body of rational methods. With athletic contests so essential to Greek culture, the treatment of fractures and dislocations was highly developed. In this field, Hippocrates recognized that broken parts must be aligned for normal mending. Traction had to be applied to both ends of a fracture, then released, gradually, as the parts fitted together. As always, he urged the doctor to look beyond the local fracture to the patient's total reaction. Mobilization was recommended at an early stage, since "exercise strengthens and inactivity wastes." Today, this maxim is still followed in the doctor's attempt to avoid "atrophy of disuse."

Hippocrates is said to have stopped plague by lighting fires in Athens' streets. London doctors harking back to Hippocratic folklore tried same method during great plague of 1665.

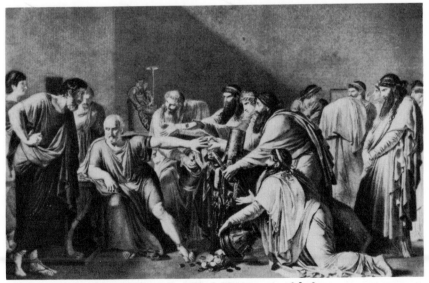

Artaxerxes, according to legend, offered Hippocrates fabulous sums to come to Persia. Hippocrates declined indignantly to aid "the foes of Greece."

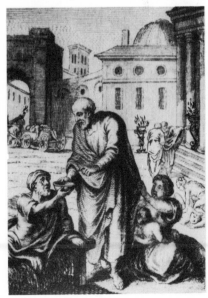

MEN OF HONOUR

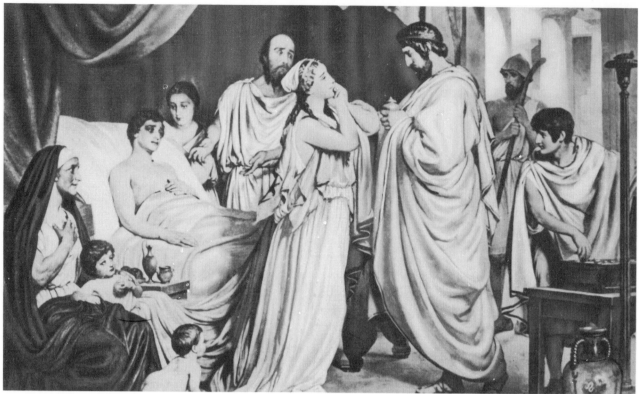

At the bedside of a sick youth Hippocrates reassures worried mother. (Mural by Rosenfelder in University of Koenigsberg.)

"Some patients, though conscious that their condition is perilous, recover their health simply through their contentment with the goodness of the physician."
—Hippocrates

The teachings of Hippocrates have shaped the course of medicine, and so has the example which he set as a man. The relations between Hippocrates and his patients were dictated by human rather than religious concepts. The doctor's duties toward the sick and toward society were eloquently defined in the writings that have come down to us under the name of this great physician.

The basic theme of these writings is simple: that only a man of character can be a good doctor. "Let his disposition be that of a man of honor," wrote Hippocrates, "let him behave to all honorable men in a friendly and easy spirit." And let him conduct himself with a spirit of serenity.

As for the art of medicine itself, doctors were born, said Hippocrates, rather than made: "A natural talent is required, for when nature opposes, everything else is in vain, but when natural disposition leads the way . . . instruction in the art follows." Such ideals precluded any undue emphasis on fees. Though Hippocrates never denied the doctor's right to earn an honest living, he appealed mainly to the physician's love of his fellow man, whether rich or poor. This appeal to honor, to charity, has ennobled the profession, even in its darkest hours. It pervades and uplifts all of Hippocrates' technical writings, especially his famous idea of medicine as a tripart relationship between patient, disease and doctor.

PATIENT

A Vibrant Whole

After Silenus had helped himself to some cheese before bedtime, he awoke the next day with painful indigestion. But Proclops, his friend, who had eaten an equal portion suffered no ill effects. Since the cheese had affected each man in a different way, Hippocrates reasoned that Silenus, the man, was sick, and not Silenus' stomach.

As it happened, Silenus had spent a strenuous day at the gymnasium. He was tired and overheated when he ate the cheese. Thus, a surplus of "fire" had upset his humoral balance. To correct this, Hippocrates advised Silenus to avoid strenuous exercises, or to cool off before eating. If he did not, serious trouble might ensue.

Hippocrates knew that the course of any disease was determined, to a great extent, by the patient's environment and way of life. He knew, further, that a "discordant" organ could upset the whole person. "To heal even an eye," he contended, "one must heal the head, and indeed, the whole body."

DISEASE

Governed by Rules

The Ionian philosopher Pythagoras had held that a plan underlay all the happenings in the universe. The stars moved on a prescribed course, he said, and similarly the reactions in the human body occurred in a definite sequence. Hippocrates applied this philosophy to medicine, and concluded that there was nothing "sacred" or mysterious about sickness but that each had its discernible pattern.

He tried to discover rules which applied to all diseases, and evolved the theory that there are three stages — acridity, coction and solution — common to every illness. In the preliminary stage, an irritation appears; when it ripens, the body "grapples" with it; if the body wins, the disease is eliminated; if it loses, the patient dies.

Hippocrates also observed and recorded the critical signs and stages of specific diseases. He established rules by which the doctor would know what to expect, and what to do at the right moment. This, he argued, would help the patient and impress his family.

DOCTOR

Nature's Helper

Hippocrates' discoveries led him to extoll what he called the *vis medicatrix naturae*, the healing power of nature. According to this principle, nature creates adequate countermeasures enabling the human body to combat disease. The doctor's aim, therefore, is to release and reinforce the body's innate powers of recovery. He is nature's helper, not its master.

To help nature, the doctor must know the disease, its course and possible outcome. To obtain a clear picture of the affliction he must taste his patient's urine, listen to his lungs, and check his breathing, color and other outward signs. Beyond that he has to understand the patient as an individual. This is in many cases more a matter of intuition than textbook learning. Even the modern physician who has at his disposal superb diagnostic instruments, still needs the gift of Hippocratic discernment.

Hippocrates had only scanty knowledge of anatomy yet his principles for treatment of fractures were sound (below).

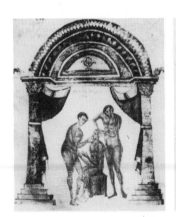
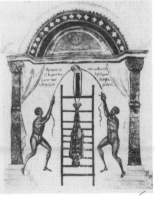
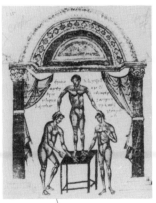
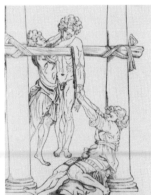

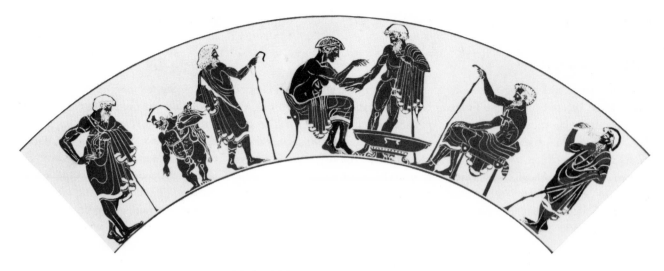

GREEK DOCTORS
VIE FOR PATIENTS

It would be a grave error to deduce, from the charms of the Venus of Milo, that all Greek women were beautiful. At the time of Hippocrates, great sculptors like Phidias, Polycletus and Myron were depicting ideal types, rather than specific statesmen, athletes or goddesses. They were trying to picture the world as it should be, to express it in cold if classic repose, but this was a far cry from human frailty and the daily toil of Greek life.

In the same way, the ideals of Hippocrates and those of the average Greek doctor could hardly coincide. Hippocrates' precepts did not take into account all the economic and social problems of the day, though the humble practitioner was forced, as always, to deal with such problems at first hand. It would be an error, therefore, to label the physician of 450 to 350 B.C. as strictly Hippocratic.

Though the Greek doctor had been honored since Homeric times, he took his place professionally with the artisans. He worked with his hands, like the shoemaker or potter. To become a doctor, all he needed was a few patients and a shingle. No one cared much about his training. Performance counted, but even here ethics was only a slight barrier against fraud or incompetence. As Hippocrates put it: "There is no punishment connected with the practice of medicine except disgrace; and that does not hurt those who are accustomed to it." To acquire a decent medical background, the young Greek candidate attached himself to a practitioner and accompanied him on his rounds. (According to Plato, Hippocrates taught medicine in this way, and received a tuition fee from his students.) After this training, the young doctor stepped out into a medical free-for-all.

Above: A busy day in a Greek Jatreion, (polyclinic), at the time of Hippocrates. The doctor raises his hand to cut a patient's vein. A large basin stands ready for the spouting blood. Other patients, characterized by walking sticks, watch the operation. The man at the right, perhaps the nervous type, holds up an aromatic herb, just as a swooning lady would use smelling salts. At left, dwarf welcomes new patient.

There were few permanent offices in those days. The doctor was obliged to travel from town to town in search of patients. He offered his services in the open market-place, or in a nearby village dwelling. Medical activities were evidently considered free shows.

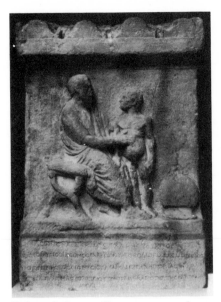

Enlarged liver afflicts patient, doctor examines it. Hippocrates warned that hardening was a "grave matter."

Competitors in the crowd might heckle, or attempt to win the patient over to their own medical dens. Obviously, the doctor's lot was far from ideal. Even Hippocrates was aware of some of these pitfalls. To impress the public, he told the doctor to perfect himself in the arts of diagnosis and prognosis. If he could tell his patients what ailed them, how they felt, and what symptoms came next, he was likely to gain new followers. If he could do all this without asking too many questions, the public would gain confidence in his medical acumen.

Hippocrates also gave some pointers to the city doctor with a permanent office. His rooms should be equipped with chairs of equal height, he said, and with spotlessly clean napkins and sheets. The light should be good, but not glaring on the patient's eyes. Apparently, the great physician would have been an advocate of the ubiquitous Venetian blind, were he alive today.

Various Greek cities seem to have recognized, dimly, the doctor's role as a social servant. They created the post of city medical officer in order to obtain advice on epidemics and other questions of public health. Some of the towns also established public "jatreia," on the order of the modern polyclinic. In Delphi, a special tax was raised to maintain the local

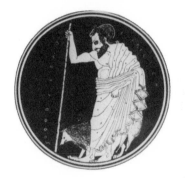

Greco-Jewish doctor.

dispensaries. The public health officers were probably responsible for giving medical care to the poor. They were elected by the assemblies, and usually proved quite competent. Democedes, for instance, was a famous court physician before he accepted bids to serve as the medical officer in various Greek towns. Other doctors, like Evenor of Athens, proved valiant in times of epidemics. The assembly awarded him a crown of green olive (3rd century B.C.), "for the goodwill he showed to the people of Athens." Another medical officer, Menocrites, received a permanent seat of honor for the yearly athletic games.

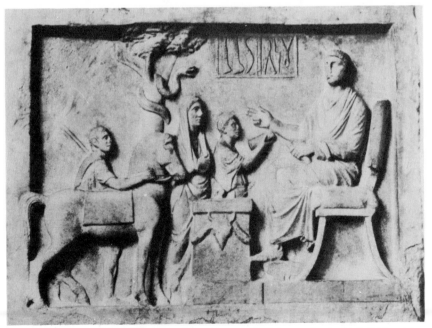

Greek doctor is idolized by grateful patients. Serpent and surgical instruments point to blend of religious and rational elements in Greek medical practice.

27

ARISTOTLE EXPLORES MAN-BEAST-PLANTS

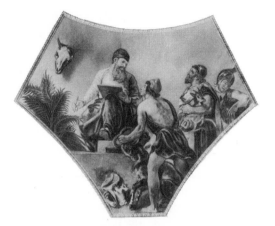

Aristotle receives specimen collected during trips of Alexander the Great.

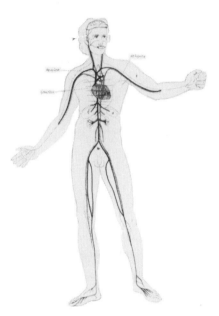

Aristotle's sketchy idea of the inner man. He thought the heart was the body's nerve center, and held that it could never become diseased. This retarded cardiac research for centuries.

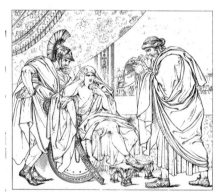

Alexander had complete confidence in his physician Philip. He handed Philip a letter that accused the doctor of intent to poison him, then trustingly drank Philip's medicine (after B. West).

Aside from Hippocrates, Aristotle (384-322 B.C.) perhaps exerted the most marked influence on medicine. While this influence was not always beneficial, he did establish medicine as a part of the biological sciences. This he achieved through a simple equation: He pronounced man an animal. By making man a part of his system of all animate nature, Aristotle established a bridge between biology and medicine.

Up to this time Greek knowledge consisted of an agglomeration of facts with little relation to each other. Aristotle organized them into a system with a logical understructure. In his writing we can discover the basic idea of evolution. Darwin called him the world's greatest natural scientist — all others seemed "mere schoolboys" in contrast. Yet many of his ideas on the animal body, revered through the ages as gospel, were completely wrong. A man who tried to press all living things into neat cubbyholes was likely to make mistakes.

Without dissecting the human body, Aristotle speculated about the heart and concluded that it was the body's nerve-center and the organ of thinking. In the brain itself he saw only a bloodless mass of two elements, earth and water, with the regulation of the heart as its main function. If Aristotle did advance biology, he hamstrung it at the same time by his emphasis on logical thinking rather than observation. One of his fatal misconceptions was the idea of "spontaneous generation." He believed in creatures generated by dunghills, or by a hardening of the dew. This idea prevailed until the 19th century when Pasteur exposed its absurdity.

Because he tutored young Alexander of Macedonia, Aristotle profited greatly when his world-conquering pupil opened the door to the East. Though Aristotle was at odds with Alexander on politics and philosophy, the king saw to it that his teacher

28

was supplied with a wealth of new specimens of exotic plants and animals. For medicine, Alexander's expedition to India had great importance.

The King's staff organized a department of natural science which collected not only specimens of every kind of natural life but drew up reports on unusual herbs and their use in medicine and cosmetics. Fusing practices and ideas contributed by Babylon, Syria, India and Israel, medicine took on the characteristics of Hellenism. It became world wide in scope. Rich but amorphous it eventually lost the singleness of purpose, the rational unity that had made it great in Hippocratic days.

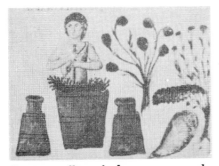

Peasant collects herbs to cure snake bite as taught in poem by Nicander.

When Aristotle retired to Chalcis in 323 B.C., he turned over his private university, the Lyceum, to Theophrastus, his friend and pupil. Botany was the new teacher's main field of research. In his *Inquiry into Plants* he created a monumental canon of medical botany. From it we learn that the ancients had an inkling of anesthesia; "Dittany is a plant especially useful for labor in women. People say that it makes labor easy or stops pain altogether."

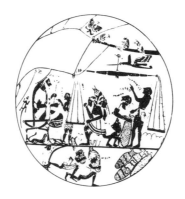

ROYAL DRUG EXPORTER

The possession of an important drug monopoly had brought prosperity to the Greek island of Cyrene since the 6th century B.C. One of the greatest Greek masterpieces of vase painting shows Arkeselias II, King of Cyrene, as he directs personally the loading of bales of this substance, silphos. The silphos trade, was carried on all over the ancient world. The plant appeared as an identifying symbol on all Cyrenean coins, and buyers paid heavily to obtain it for use as a spice or medicine.

FIRST IMMUNOLOGIST

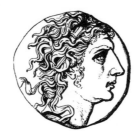

Mithridates Eupator, King of Pontus (132-63 B.C.), unwittingly helped to

Nicander, a versatile Greek doctor, poet and herbalist wrote a poem (c. 215 B.C.) that for ages enjoyed as much fame as Homer's Odyssey. The verses sang not of gods and heroes but of snake bite — and what to do about it.

The title of this snake-bite epic, "Theriaca," became the name of a universal antidote, theriac, a fantastic mixture of odd ingredients. According to its proponents, theriac could be used either for or against anything — a marvelous combination of both antidote and cure-all.

Nero's court physician, Andromachus, improved on the recipe and claimed that 64 substances went into his special version.

Theriac became a mainstay of all pharmacy shops. When Claude Bernard, the famed 19th century physiologist, was a drugstore apprentice, the pharmacist told him to dump all the leftovers and unsalable drugs into a big jar and mix everything up thoroughly. Farmers bought this conglomeration and were highly incensed when the supply of "theriac" ran out.

establish the principle of immunology. The king lived in perpetual fear that his foes would kill him. Anxious to discover a substance to counteract their deadly potions, he tested poisonous drugs on criminals — then gulped some of these substances himself in ever-increasing quantities. He found, that taken in this manner, they had no ill effect. Thus Mithridates, discovering a way to make man poisonproof, attained immortality as the world's first immunologist.

29

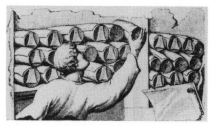

Library founded by Ptolomies became depository of Greek medical literature.

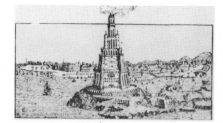

Alexandria, founded in 332 B.C. effected fusion of cultures of East and West.

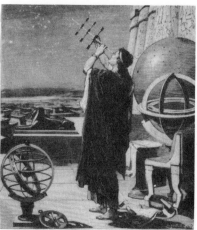

Hipparchus, Alexandrian scientist, applied geometry to exploration of heavens.

ALEXANDRIA
NEW CAPITAL OF MEDICINE

One year before his death in 323, B.C., Alexander the Great visited his new imperial capital on the Delta of the Nile. Alexandria rose at the strategic crossroads of Asia, Europe and Africa. With her great boulevards, gymnasia, hippodromes and shops and her fine harbor that dominated trade between East and West, Alexandria became the great new center of the ancient world.

Under Ptolemy Soter (323-285 B. C.), a vast headquarters for research and teaching, "The Museum," developed on Alexandria's outskirts. Here Euclid worked out his geometric ideas, Hipparchos founded astronomy and Archimedes applied the lever of his genius to mechanics. The greatest glory of this new city of some 600,000 was its 700,000 scroll library, where the Ptolemies kept many copyists busy editing the Hippocratic collection.

The great mathematicians and mechanics like Archimedes accelerated medicine's trend toward accurate observation and measurement. The Egyptian tradition of embalming helped Alexandrian pioneers in anatomy. It enabled them to obtain material to explore the inner workings of the body, which Hippocrates had neglected. The great Alexandrian school of medicine influenced the training of doctors for centuries to come.

For the young doctor of antiquity the simple secret for success was the announcement that he had studied in Alexandria. Patients throughout the ancient world recognized that the Alexandrian doctor had a more systematic training than any of his predecessors.

Alexandria attracted the best scientific and medical talent. It developed big doctors, if not great ones, and apparently competition among physicians was keen.

To assess the development of medicine in Alexandria is difficult because we must depend entirely on the writings of the leaders and adherents of the various schools. To take such writings as evidence of the true state of practice is a pitfall that has ensnared many medical historians. Un-

doubtedly, however, medical culture in this period grew broader than in any previous one.

In the urban setting in which the Alexandrian doctor practiced, a certain amount of ostentation became a necessity. Only if a doctor acquired prowess in a special field, or developed a theory that appealed to the public could he gain distinction.

Unfortunately theory and ostentation became more important for the Alexandrian physician than knowledge. The doctors splintered into separate sects, each eager to use suffering humanity as the guinea pig for its pet theories.

After a short flourishing of experimental medicine, disputes replaced bedside observations. Dogmatists, empiricists, methodists and pneumatists split off from the mainstream of Hippocratic learning. They developed systems that spun out as artfully as spiderwebs — and were just about as solid. To evolve the basic truth in any of these teachings, more practical research was needed.

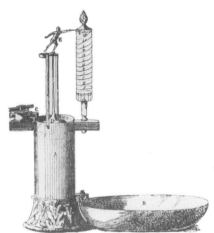

Waterclock enabled doctors to measure patient's pulsebeat more accurately.

Herophilus, one of the leaders of the Alexandrian School, was still able to maintain the proper balance between theory, experiment and practice. Not content with the physician's traditional task, he sought to learn more about the human body by exploring it through dissection. Like Erasistratus, another successful practitioner, he spent a great deal of time in the dissecting room. According to Tertullian, these fanatical anatomists opened the bodies of 600 living criminals to observe nature at work. While such wholesale slaughter is improbable, Herophilus conducted experiments that refuted Aristotle by

Seeking to cure King Seleukos Nicator's son Antiochus of his deep melancholy, Erasistratus put his finger on the prince's wrist as the ladies of the court passed. The pulse of young Antiochus grew quick when his stepmother Stratonice appeared. Diagnosing the case as love, Erasistratus persuaded the king to divorce his wife and let his son marry her.

showing that intelligence did center in the brain, not the heart and brilliantly traced the course of the blood through the arteries and veins.

More important to practical medicine, however, were his experiments on the pulse beat. He used primitive water clocks, which Alexandrian scientists had developed, to classify the pulse of his patients.

Erasistratus spearheaded another movement in Alexandrian medicine. "Why bother with the whole patient when only his kidney hurts? We know little about the functioning of the

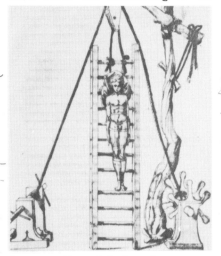

Levers, pulleys of Archimedes were utilized in Alexandrian orthopedics.

kidney," Erasistratus argued, "but we don't need to know much. So let us use local therapy for local complaints and get to work on the patient where it hurts him." It was this sort of reasoning that made Erasistratus open the abdomen of a man with hepatic disorder to apply his medicine at the critical point. This became known as Methodism — with the stress on the method of cure, not the cause of disease.

As an ardent anatomist and experimenter, Erasistratus ranked with Herophilus as a leader in the profession. On their medical philosophy they differed widely.

In contrast Herophilus was called a Hippocratic doctor. He pronounced that the patient, not local symptoms alone, should be the proper subject of all good medicine. Since he adhered strictly to the corpus Hippocraticum he headed the school of Dogmatists. Erasistratus opposed such teachings but he was not averse to utilize his opponent's research on the pulse. This enabled him, according to Plutarch, to diagnose the sickness of a king's son as what we would call today a "case of erotic repression" (below).

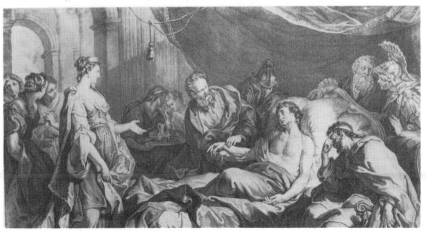

31

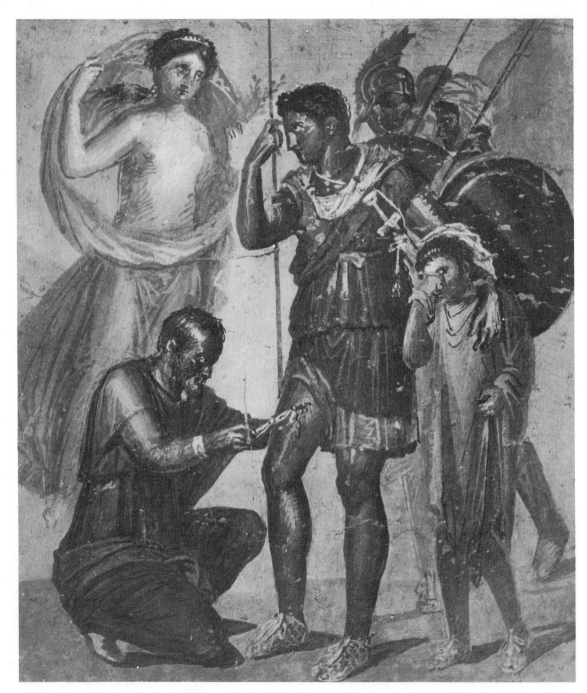

When an arrow pierced Aeneas' leg, in the battle before Troy, Venus appeared with a shining vase filled with dittany and other analgesics to soothe the hero's pain. Pompeian wall painting, first century A.D.

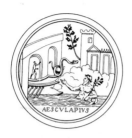

AESCULAPIUS COMES TO ROME

After the decline of Greek power, Rome absorbed Alexander's empire and became the political master of the ancient world. Spiritually, however, Greece remained the leader. With her art and science, the vanquished conquered the conqueror. In Roman medicine, too, most of what was good and lasting came from Greece and Alexandria. This dependency is clearly borne out by the legend of Aesculapius' landing in Italy.

In 293 B.C., as Livy reports it, a plague raged in Rome. When the domestic deities failed to help, the Sibylline books were opened. On their advice a mission was sent to Epidaurus, the important seat of the Aesculapian cult. When the ship returned to the Tiber with the ambassadors, the Aesculapian serpent that had boarded the vessel in Epidaurus, escaped and swam to a little island in mid-river. The plague disappeared and the island became the seat of Aesculapian worship in Italy. Asclepios became Aesculapius, and the influx of Greek doctors into Rome began.

From the outset the Romans felt inferior to the Greek refugee doctors, even to those who had flocked to Rome before Greece lost her independence. Altogether — the medical men arriving in the eternal city from Alexandria and the Greek mainland received a rather chilling welcome. It took them some time to gain acceptance. In the process medicine was watered down from the original Grecian ideal to the more practical demands of the Romans.

Below: The Temple the Romans erected on the island in the Tiber where the Aesculapian snake had landed. This was later transformed into a hospital for sick slaves. Emperor Claudius decreed that those who recovered were to be released from bondage and allowed to enter the City of Rome as free men.

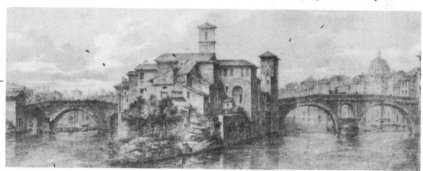

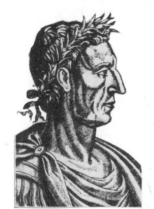

In Cato the Elder, a foe of all Greek learning, the doctors found an antagonist who labeled them as charlatans. Cato indignantly called the Greek physicians foreign "rabble" and forbade his family to employ their services. To cure disease, Cato claimed only one remedy was needed. "Cabbage juice," he declared, "is good for everything . . . If there is any bruise it will break it up, and if any ulcer or cancer appears on the breast . . . mashed cabbage will heal it." Nobody on his vast estate could escape his treatments. Through this therapy he caused the death of his wife and a son. But Cato, upright unto absurdity, would rather let his family die than call a foreign physician.

33

CAESAR WELCOMES DOCTORS

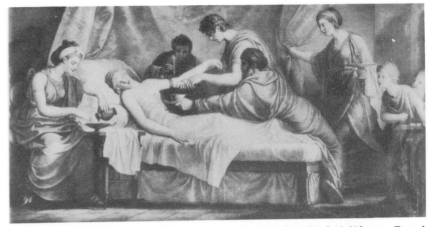

Young doctor at bedside of Roman girl. (Mural in Faculté de Médecine, Paris.)

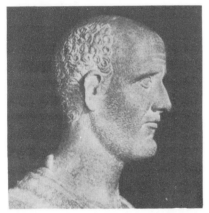

Asclepiades of Prusa gained safe foothold for Greek medicine in Rome. He believed in speedy, pleasant cures.

Greek doctors continued to pour into Rome, and gradually broke down the prejudice against them. To be sure, some of the Eastern physicians turned out to be quacks, but others, like Asclepiades of Prusa, were excellent physicians. As a matter of fact, the arrival of Asclepiades, in 91 B. C., brought about the first official acceptance of the medical profession in Rome.

Asclepiades had been thoroughly trained at Athens, Alexandria and other medical centers. He was also blessed with a dynamic and affable personality. These attributes helped him to win the patronage of such rich and important Romans as Cicero and Crassus the triumvir. Moreover, his forms of therapy contributed a great deal to his success. Instead of forcing patients to swallow foul concoctions, he prescribed pleasant hygienic and dietetic remedies: baths, massages, walks, runs, rides and special wine diets. Such measures, he told his patients, would re-agitate their "sluggish atoms." And to Asclepiades, the disturbance of the body's atom-circulation was the essence of disease.

Since these therapies were mild, they could be energetically applied. Asclepiades believed that the doctor was a man of action, and not a mere bystander or "helper of nature," as Hippocrates had held. Thus, he always suggested two or three remedies to his patients, and promised them a speedy, safe and agreeable cure (his credo was "cito, tute et jucunde"). No wonder that he became the most famous, and the richest and most fashionable doctor in Rome. He also set his theories down in a great many books. In the light of recent reappraisal, these works were of great importance in the development of atomistic medicine.

In his day, Asclepiades was considered "self-assured" by some, and "utterly conceited" by others. At

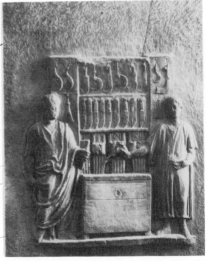

In cutlery shops Roman surgeons bought sparkling instruments. In Galen's opinion, they were rarely used.

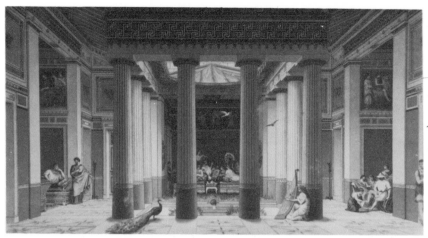

Luxurious urban living increased debilities, brought greater need for doctors.

After Caesar's death, the cause of medicine was further advanced by Antonius Musa, a disciple of Asclepiades. The Emperor Augustus had suffered from an obstinate rheumatic complaint. When hot compresses and hot baths failed to relieve the pain, Musa, a Greek freedman, was called to the imperial bedside. He boldly reversed the therapy, and tried cold douches and ample doses of cabbage juice instead. The Emperor recovered, and promptly awarded Musa with the gold ring of knighthood. Augustus also erected a statue in the physician's

one time he broke up a funeral procession by bringing the "corpse" back to life. The members of the dead man's family, deprived of their inheritance, were outraged; envious colleagues laughed it off as a trick; but the people praised his "superhuman" ability. Meanwhile, Asclepiades, who had probably noticed that the "dead man" was merely in a coma, made no strenuous effort to hide his prowess.

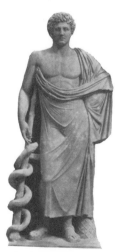

Augustus had Musa, his physician sculptured as Aesculapius in gratitude for emperor's recovery from rheumatism.

The favorable impression which Asclepiades and his followers had made upon the people soon bore tangible fruit for the doctors at large. In 46 B.C., Caesar granted Roman citizenship to all practitioners of medicine.

In the same year, Rome suffered from famine and all foreigners were expelled. But the Greek doctors were encouraged to stay, and even received gratuities.

Respect for the medical art had grown in proportion to the need for good doctors. With the increase in the urban population came much luxury, and conversely, much squalor. Moreover, Caesar's military ventures had drained the supply of competent physicians. To ease the shortage, Caesar cleverly exploited medical friend and foe alike. Even the great Marcus Terentius Varro (117-26 B.C.), was won over to the dictator's side. Varro was an early exponent of the germ theory. His *Rerum Rusticarum* contains these lines: "Small creatures, invisible to the eye, fill the atmosphere, and breathed through the nose cause dangerous diseases."

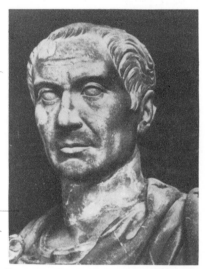

Caesar took medical profession under his wing; he needed doctors, both at home and on far flung battlefields.

honor. To show his appreciation of the medical arts he issued a decree which exempted all doctors from taxes (10 A.D.).

Musa acquired a flourishing practice among such intellectual and political leaders as Maecenas, Virgil and Horace. But most important of all, he succeeded in raising the prestige and social standing of the whole medical profession.

35

COMPILERS AND COMPOUNDERS

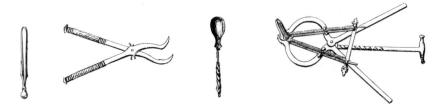

Instruments used by Roman surgeons found in Pompei. At right, vaginal speculum.

The suggestion to become a doctor probably would have mortally insulted a young Roman patrician seeking a career. Rome's political and intellectual leaders had accepted doctors, such as Asclepiades and Musa. But the profession still bore the stigma of social inferiority. A true Roman left the dispensing of pills and other work with one's hands, to the foreigners, slaves and freedmen. This attitude explains why native Romans made few contributions to medicine and why the one great Roman

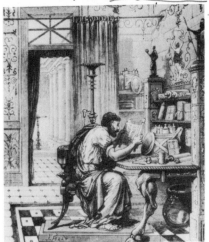

book on medicine — *De Re Medicina* by A. Cornelius Celsus — did not come from the pen of a doctor.

Celsus compiled this large-scale cyclopedia as a "Medical Home Companion" for the rich landowner and he wrote it in an impeccable Latin.

In his book, Celsus gives a systematic survey of medicine and lays down the principles of good surgery. Highly practical like most Romans, he found surgery particularly appealing. Though tonsils were plucked out by the fingers, other operations, such as lithotomy, hernia and tapping in cases of dropsy, called for a variety of surgical instruments. These included lancets, cauteries and trephines, all lucidly described in *De Re Medicina*.

Celsus was strictly a "desk doctor" who did his only operating with his pen in rehashing a library of Grecian medical writers. He did apply much common sense to medical procedures. Like a modern physician, he advocated a good balance between experience and medical theories — a radical idea in his day when doctors denied that medicine needed any theoretical basis.

Pliny, like Celsus, had the free-born Roman's low opinion of doctors. "It is at the expense of our perils that they learn," Pliny said. " . . . They experiment by putting us to death." He considered any Roman who took up this "lucrative" calling a renegade.

While commenting so bitterly on physicians in his *Natural History*, Pliny became in spite of himself a chronicler of medical history. He compiled his medical notes, he declared, only because doctors had already taken too much of his money.

A voracious reader, Pliny had a gift for organization and gained a reputation as one of the most learned men of antiquity. But he was more erudite than wise. He collected facts avidly and miscellaneously, facts about plants, animals, races, — virtually every living thing. Though he served his country as a provincial administrator, minister of finance and fleet admiral, he still found time to write on natural history. It is well known that he finally became the victim of his own curiosity. In 79 A. D., he climbed toward Vesuvius to observe a strange fume and was caught in a major eruption. Though Pliny opposed doctors, he preserved much medical lore and was probably not original enough to either hinder or hasten the forward march of medicine.

In imperial Rome the sale of drugs deteriorated into a racket. So much adulterated medicine was sold that "pharmaci" connoted "poison makers." In addition, fakers, abortionists and sure cure healers of intimate ills, compounded their concoctions with the aid of tortoise blood, crocodile dung and other worthless ingredients.

The fancier the name and the higher the price of a remedy, the more people seemed to believe in its efficacy. For instance, a rich man whose slave Galen had cured of a dangerous tumor asked for the recipe. When the Roman discovered that the ingredients were cheap, he demanded something fancier — "not that simple stuff for beggars." Reliable physicians like Galen did not trust the pharmacists to prepare medicaments but mixed the pure raw materials right before the patient's eye.

Roman practitioners carried the equivalent of a modern doctor's bag with medicine boxes and vessels artistically decorated with ivory inlay representing Aesculapius and Hygeia.

On the whole, Roman materia medica may have killed more patients than the prevalent diseases. Yet there was one man whose prescriptions offered reliable guidance to the doctors and

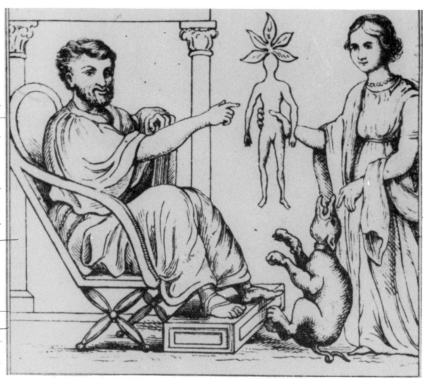

Dioscorides (fl. 1st c. A.D.) receives mandrake plant from goddess of discovery. A dog was used to pull the mandrake from the ground. Its juice served as an aphrodysiac.

the sick. Just as Webster today signifies good spelling, so the name of Dioscorides for centuries meant sound medical botany.

Dioscorides collected plants, animal and mineral substances during his wide travels as a surgeon in Nero's army. In addition, he experimented with their pharmacal properties. Of the 600 plants faithfully described in his herbal, about 100 are still mentioned in the modern pharmacopoeia. Among these is opium, a first with Dioscorides. In a practical arrangement, he classed the remedies according to the troubles they cured.

Below: Roman drug establishment; left to right: sale — storage — mixing — pressing of oils. Pompeian mural.

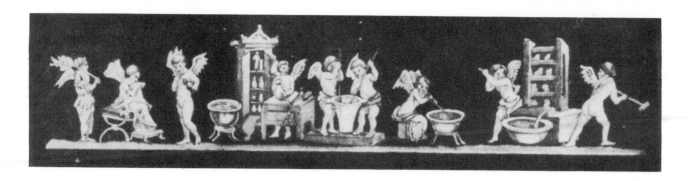

ROME GIVES TO THE WORLD: ARMY MEDICINE

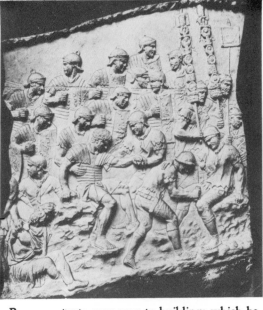

Army surgeons (right) treating the wounded. For emergencies Roman soldiers carried first aid kits with bandages. Emperor Trajan is reported to have torn his tunic into strips when bandages ran short in battle.

To the development of medical care the Romans made one epochal contribution. They introduced "first aid on the battlefield."

The army surgeon was a "must" for military expeditions operating vast distances from home. In the Roman military jargon, each cohort (420 men) was accompanied by one to four doctors with a high ranking surgeon supervising each legion, or ten cohorts.

While Rome was the first nation of antiquity to assume some responsibility for the common soldier injured in battle, it was not mercy but Roman efficiency that would not permit the needless loss of life so far from the home front. Nevertheless this was a far cry from the Heroic Age which wept over the wounds of its Grecian kings and generals but left the stricken G. I.s of the day to the vultures and beasts of prey.

Once efficient first aid was developed it became necessary to organize convalescent procedures. Travel time alone forbade sending the injured home for nursing. The solution was the original portable hospital, a series of tents, arranged somewhat like our "corridor system," set up spaciously to provide fresh air, yet close enough to permit effective administration. Eventually tents gave way to buildings which became permanent convalescent camps situated at strategic points.

Remains of these early veterans hospitals have been found along the Danube and the Rhine, and other life lines in the Roman military sphere. These "valetudinaria," or infirmaries, had not only wards but recreation areas, the ever present Roman bath, pharmacies and accommodations for officials taking rest cures.

It was the military, however, and not the medical man who had charge of hospital administration. Aurelian's decree, issued about 270 A.D., shows the draconic strictness prevailing in these institutions.

"Let each soldier be cured gratuitously by the physician . . . Let them conduct themselves quietly in the hospitals . . . and he who would cause strife, let him be lashed."

These valetudinaria must have run with timetable efficiency. Yet another factor of great moment, concern with the patient's mental state was lacking.

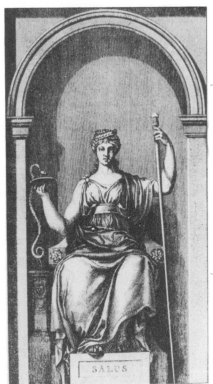

Salus, Roman Goddess, personified prosperity and public hygiene.

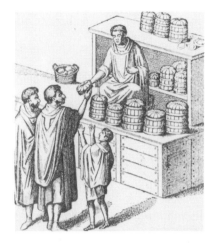

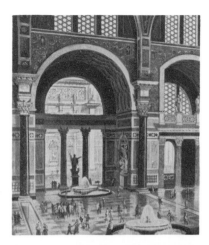

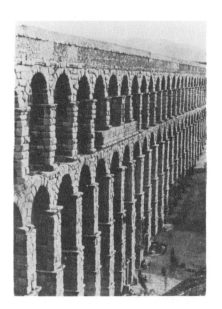

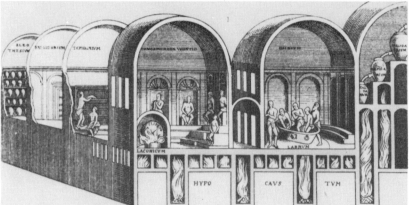

Sweat bath — heated by flame in double wall — first use of "radiant heating."

PUBLIC HYGIENE

The practical genius of the Romans, unproductive in abstract science, expressed itself admirably in administration and in engineering feats, hardly surpassed to this day. Both these talents accelerated the progress of medicine. If the Jews were the first to codify the laws of public hygiene, the Romans applied them on a large scale throughout their sprawling empire.

With characteristic mechanical inventiveness, Rome built aqueducts, instituted flood control, insisted on solid construction for both houses and streets — all measures designed by those in power to preserve the health of the citizens. Medicine in Rome acquired an almost modern outlook through its concern with urban welfare.

It was the medical men's insistence on clean drinking water, unadulterated foods, that effected control of epidemics, however primitive, and so made city living possible.

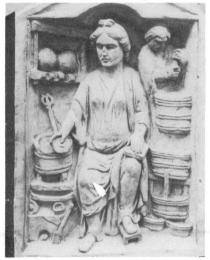

Woman pharmacist (soapmaker ?) works with prescription book on her lap.

39

QUACKS OVERRUN ROME

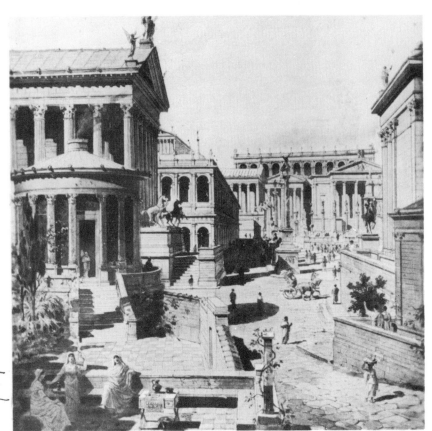

By 100 A.D. the medical scene appeared vastly different from Rome's early days: there were too many doctors in Rome — too many quacks, specialists and conflicting schools of medicine. The change seemed almost miraculous. There had been no physicians in the early Republic. Then Cato, the austere aristocrat, had fought to keep Rome doctorless; under his influence, laws were passed to stem the flow of refugee physicians from

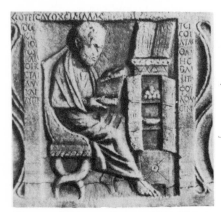

Roman doctor in front of his library. Christian sarcophagus, 5th century.

Greece and Alexandria. But in the first century B.C., the floodgates were suddenly thrown open, and "doctorless" Rome became a thriving medical center.

Augustus' tax-exemption edict had much to do with this rapid transformation. It was easy to join the medical ranks and thereby avoid taxes. As in Greece, all the aspirant had to do was call himself a doctor, and — he was a doctor! There were no licensing laws until 200 A.D., no state supervision, and no educational requirements. Consequently, droves of quacks entered the profession. Specialists showed up everywhere. Rival schools clashed. Students obtained speedy "degrees" from Thessalus of Tralles, Nero's own quack physician. A weaver's son,

Thessalus had arrived in Rome boasting loudly that he could turn anyone into a doctor within six months' time. According to Pliny, "he attracted numerous students of the lowest ranks." Hippocrates he called "a pitiful ignoramus," and he called himself, in his epitaph: "The conqueror of all physicians."

Paradoxically, Thessalus was progressive in his emphasis on bedside instruction. He took his students along on his rounds. Martial has satirized the practice as follows:

I called you, Dr. Symmachus, for a slight indisposition.
You brought your hundred students as befits a real clinician;
With hands all chilled by winter's blasts they practiced their palpation:
The fever that I did not have is now a conflagration.

40

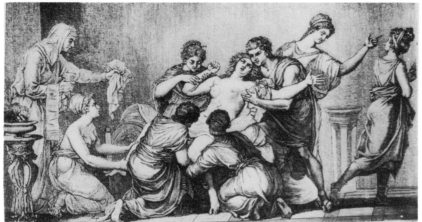

Childbirth scene in a Roman house. Soranus (ca. 100 A.D.) recommended obstetric chair with two women standing in back, one kneeling in front.

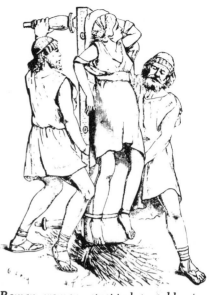

Roman woman, strapped to table, is rudely shaken to accelerate birth.

PREGNANT WOMEN NEGLECTED

There were two kinds of patients whom the ancient physicians always avoided: the near-dead, and the childbearing woman. In the former case, they were simply exercising prudence, but childbirth was out of bounds for a number of reasons. There were problems of morals and modesty to consider, and problems of social position: in Greece and in the East, women were confined to the domestic sphere. Finally, there was the hurdle of colossal ignorance about childbirth. So the maternity chamber was left largely to the midwives, though the doctors were at times ready with advice on difficult cases.

But modesty, morals and social position underwent drastic changes in Imperial Rome. Women were no longer confined to the home. In fact, they claimed their full share of the debaucheries of that dissolute period. Sexual freedom was common in every rank of society. The brothels which sprang up all over Rome were frequented by all classes. Even Messalina, the wife of Emperor Claudius, was said to have stood at her door in a yellow wig, her bare breasts decorated with golden nipples, offering "love to all comers."

In the wake of this dissipation came the usual increase in gynecological troubles. Abortion was widely practiced by shady woman doctors. Speculation on the perfect contraceptive ran high. And women, pregnant by chance or choice, demanded some sort of benefit from the newly acquired medical knowledge. Consequently, there were significant stirrings in the fields of obstetrics and gynecology. And the most important spokesman for the new science was Soranus.

Soranus was one of the great ancient doctors. Trained in Alexandria, he practiced in Rome for forty years (98-138 A. D.). His treatise on gynecology served as an excellent antidote against the prevailing superstitions. It was sound and comprehensive with regard to pregnancy, and almost modern in its approach to contraception and abortion. Hippocrates had once suggested that if pregnancy had to be ended for medical reasons, the woman should "jump vehemently flinging her legs against the buttocks." But Soranus, in open disgust, said that conception should be prevented in such cases. To this end, he suggested pessaries made of wool drenched in fatty substances, or in other mixtures.

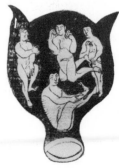

Soranus' idea of children in womb. Moschion illustration, 6th century A. D.

41

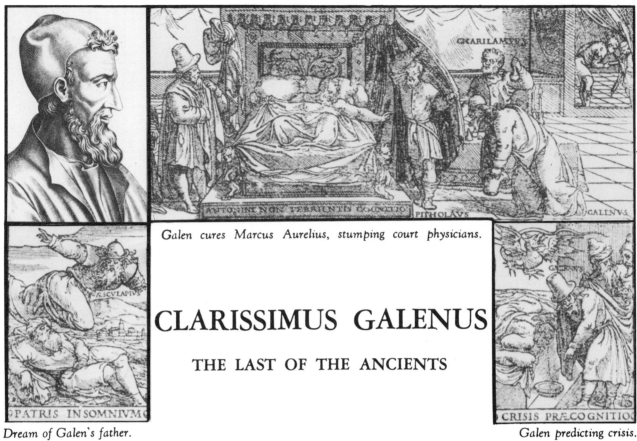

Galen cures Marcus Aurelius, stumping court physicians.

Dream of Galen's father.

Galen predicting crisis.

CLARISSIMUS GALENUS

THE LAST OF THE ANCIENTS

Like the brilliant sunset just before the earth plunges into darkness, Clarissimus Galenus of Pergamon gave ancient medicine a spectacular grand finale just before the civilized world faded away into the dark ages. He wrote more than 300 books and brilliantly fused into one unified system the themes and ideas that had been agitating doctors since pre-Hippocratic days. Surviving from his vast works are the remains of 118 books now condensed into 20 tightly printed volumes.

Galen is said to have kept 12 scribes busy recording his brilliant anatomical observations, case histories, polemics and autobiographical fragments. They represent a vast reservoir of ideas in which the unwary reader can easily drown. Aside from the medical aspects of his work, his writings do give us a remarkably clear picture of his life and times (c. 130-200 A.D.). They reveal a highly educated and gifted physician of overtowering stature. In brilliance and influence he surpassed even Hippocrates but lacked his depth, selflessness and serenity.

Like most great Roman doctors, Galen was of Greek origin. When he was born in the city of Pergamon in Asia Minor, his father, a prominent and prosperous architect, named him Galenos — signifying the continuous, ordered rolling of the waves. Galen's father Nicon, tortured by a temperamental, shrewish wife, hoped that his son could achieve a life more peaceful than his own.

One night in 147 A.D. Aesculapius appeared to Nicon in a dream and told him to have his son take up the healing arts. Galen made haste to please his father. The temple halls of the Aesculapion in his native Pergamon offered the medical student much clinical material. They were filled with the sick who had come to seek cure by incubation sleep.

Inspired no doubt by these scenes Galen thirsted to acquire more medical knowledge. He studied in Smyrna, and by the time he was 21, had become a well trained doctor. He also had written a textbook on the uterus for midwives, a work on ophthalmology and three books on pulmonary disease and its treatment. But like a true philosopher, he concluded that he knew nothing. To increase his knowledge, he made a tour of all the major medical centers of the world. For nine years he traveled and studied in Corinth, Phoenicia, Palestine, Crete, Alexandria and other places of medical interest. Soon he acquired a background in medicine that none of his colleagues could surpass.

Returning to his native Pergamon at the age of 28, Galen became medical supervisor of the gladiatorial amphitheater. Since he believed that a doctor without knowledge of anatomy had no more value than an architect without a plan, he supplemented his work in the arena with experiments on animals. Because human bodies were not available he dissected animals of every kind, even a hippopotamus and an elephant. What he found as an investigating scientist, he described and analyzed with the brilliantly trained intellect of a philosopher.

Naturally, a restless mind like Galen could not be content for long in provincial Pergamon. In 162 A.D. at the age of 32 he went to Rome. The bustling metropolis fascinated him but its medical life seemed in a sad state. According to Galen's sarcastic report, faction-torn doctors, aligned in numerous medical schools, practically overran the town. They comprised all shades, from mountebanks and poison mixers to eminent court physicians. Fees ran from 29 cents a visit to the equivalent of $2000 for a consultation by one of the medical coryphaei. A continuous war raged between empirics, dogmatists, eclectics and the adherents of other schools.

Ethically, the profession stood at low ebb. The sick became so befuddled with all the different cures prescribed that they shopped around trying to find a doctor who would strike their fancy. Galen compared his colleagues to robbers practicing in Rome, while their equals worked up in the hills. He decried the fashionable doctor's growing political influence as he wheedled his way into the graces of the mighty. "The greatest flatterer, not he who is the most skilled in the art, receives all advantages and finds all doors open," he complained.

The Methodists drew Galen's hottest fire. Thessalus, a rank proponent of this school, had asked for only six months to educate a doctor. This enraged Galen. He pointed out that he himself had studied medicine for almost twice as many years. A speaker of great power, Galen continually stood up in the medical meetings to debunk the theories of his foes. Ironically, the doctors came to blows in the Temple of Peace. It served as Rome's "Academy of Medicine," a research and discussion center which boasted of a splendid library.

In the meantime Galen's practice grew, and his diagnostic insight gained him many patients among the mighty. His life's ambition seemed to be fullfilled in 174 A.D. It was in this year that Marcus Aurelius returned from a campaign against the Germans. One night Galen was called to the imperial palace: The emperor was ailing.

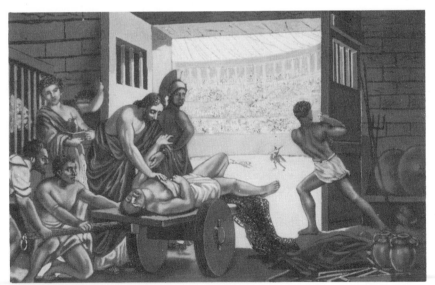

After his grand tour, Galen became official doctor of gladiatorial amphitheatre in his native Pergamon. Bloody spectacles proved for him a medical bonanza. Romans shied away from dissection but cheerfully exposed the living to butchery.

43

GALEN: Continued

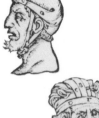

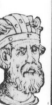

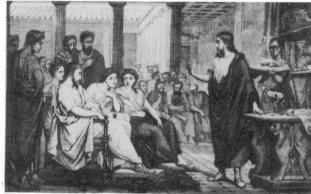

The court doctors who had accompanied Marcus Aurelius on his campaign appeared to be in a quandary about the imperial "fever." Marcus Aurelius asked Galen to feel his pulse, but the latter said he had no point of comparison. By questioning the attendants and appraising the situation shrewdly, Galen diagnosed the Emperor's trouble as an upset stomach. He prescribed an ancient version of our hot-water bottle — a wool bandage impregnated with warm spikenard to go about the belly. Such medication worked wonders — especially since the Emperor agreed with the diagnosis.

"Yes, that is it — it is exactly as thou sayest . . . I feel that cold food is disagreeing with me," the Emperor repeated thrice.

From this time on, "the Emperor never stopped praising me as a philosopher and a physician not hidebound by rules," Galen bragged in his case history.

Honoured by the Emperor, Galen found himself eagerly sought as a consultant. He cured the wife of the consul Boethus of her melancholy and received 400 gold pieces as his fee. In addition he took care of patients who wrote to him for advice from Gaul, Spain and Syria. He prescribed the cures and sent out remedies, painstakingly assembling the medicines himself. For doctors who relied on druggists, "those dealers in adulterated wares" he had nothing but contempt.

Galen devised artful bandaging methods (above left) which were used for centuries.

Perhaps the most interesting case that came Galen's way was that of a Persian sophist, who complained of a numbness in his fourth and fifth fingers. Galen checked on the patient's history and finally traced the trouble to a neural injury of the backbone. He

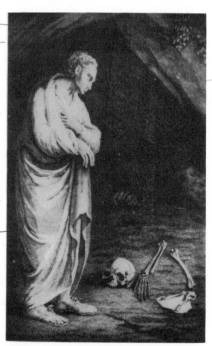

Galen taking on the Christian faith — a legendary assumption. His writings seemed to suggest belief in one god.

Galen (above) is said to have lectured on anatomy before Marcus Aurelius and the empress Faustina. He welcomed the laity to his demonstrations, claiming that its judgment was often sounder than that of the doctors. He shrewdly observed that "common sense" is a misnomer, since it is far from common.

then treated the patient's brachial plexus and effected a cure.

Many of Galen's anatomical findings, such as his discovery that aphasia could be produced experimentally by cutting the laryngeal nerve showed amazing insight. He wrote many books on anatomy, but performed altogether only one dissection on a human, the corpse of a drowned man. Despite his authoritative discussion of other anatomical "facts," he derived most of them by way of analogy from his dissections of pigs and monkeys.

Galen dominated medical thought far into the 16th century. Even in 1559 the College of Physicians in London requested one of its members, Dr. John Geynes to retract his statement that Galen's works contained errors. The doctor knew what was good for him and submitted an apology. He banned forever the dangerous thought that the great Galen could be wrong!

44

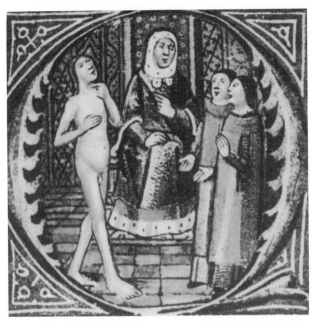

LECTURE ON CONGESTION OF THE THROAT

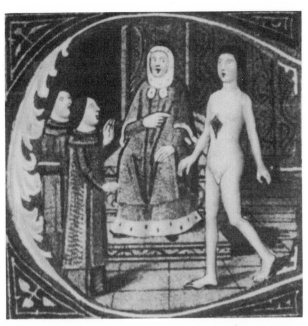

WORKINGS OF THE HEART EXPLAINED

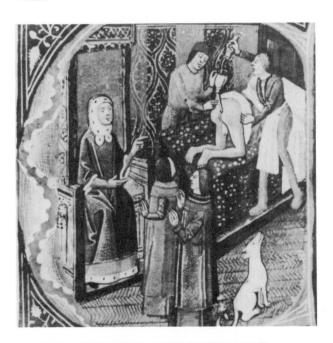

GIVING OF ENEMA DEMONSTRATED

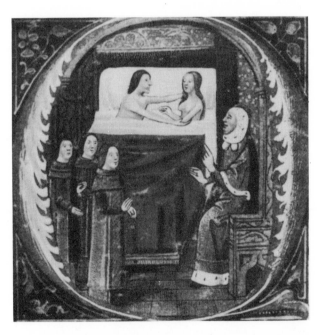

SEX EDUCATION WITH AID OF DUMMIES

Initials from Dresden Galen manuscript (15th century). Whether a medieval doctor was faced with a case of throat irritation, an ulcerated leg or a prolapsed womb, the "Prince of Physicians" was likely to provide a ready answer. Also, the monotheistic philosophy permeating Galen's writings made them acceptable to Christians and Arabs.

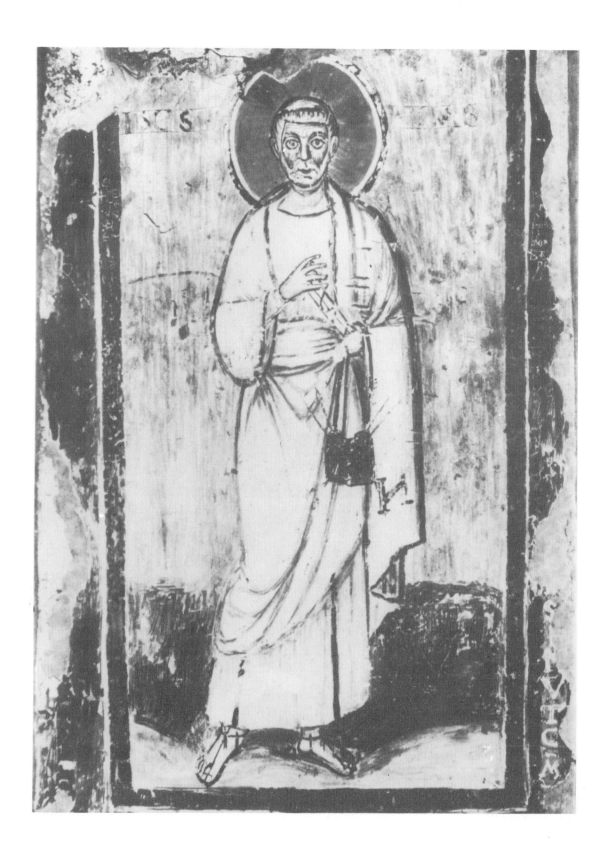

THE CHURCH PRESCRIBES FAITH

A mood of doom descended over the ancient world in the period following Galen's death. Rome's decline, long imminent and predicted, became a reality. Barbarian hordes overran the Empire. Frightful pestilences decimated its cities. The people were torn from their moorings, helpless in the face of defeat, terror and plague.

Philosophy and the old gods, beacon lights once, had by this time become meaningless. Greek and Roman religions had never provided much sustenance for the human spirit and, in this worn-out and cynical age, men could no longer seek guidance from their empty and ritualistic practices.

Into this world the Christian faith entered with its new gospel. Its message of salvation and brotherly love seemed to hold out renewed hope to a crushed humanity. It was this emotionalism which changed drastically the direction of all medical endeavor. Since pagan medicine had been unable to deal with large-scale, war-borne pestilences, confidence in the physician was undermined. The tenet of Christ-

St. Luke the Beloved Physician. (left) He holds a case with medical instruments (7th century catacomb mural).

ian healing once more revealed the deeply human function of medicine, but in doing so it overemphasized healing by faith and neglected what was sound in the teachings of ancient medicine.

Christ's message to a suffering humanity proclaimed worldly medicine unnecessary. Christ himself was the supreme healer, the saviour of body and soul. Faith in him, in his disciples, and in the gospel would heal the sick, the maimed, and the suffering. "Is any sick among you?" asks the Epistle of James. "Let him call for the elders of the Church, and let them pray over him . . . the Lord shall raise him up."

Implicit faith in divine mercy made inquiry into the causes of disease unnecessary and even culpable. The doctor who cured patients by rational methods of his own devising actually meddled sinfully with God's designs. In the view of the early Christian Church the employment of drugs implied a lack of faith, and medicine itself was a godless science. In the fervent religious temper of the times, it was only natural that scientific medicine should suffer.

All the mystic methods of faith healing, the laying on of the hand, the use of amulettes and exorcism received official sanction. The Church provided its halls with couches, reminiscent of Aesculapian dormitories. The sick slept in churchyards in the hope that they would be miraculously healed. All were welcomed, in the infinite pity extended to the suffering, a fact that accelerated the spread of the new religion.

The Christian physicians gave a broad humanitarian outlook to medicine. Rich or poor, sinner or virtuous, no matter of what race or class, all received selfless assistance. There was no disease, however contagious, or noxious, that the early Christians did not try to alleviate through the gentle ministry of hope.

Since pity and brotherly love were held as the highest moral virtues, those who helped the sick earned the blessings of salvation, which God had reserved for the meek and the humble.

This philosophy freed the sick from the odium of inferiority. However decrepit a body might be, it was but a wretched mantle of the soul — and the soul was pure before God.

47

CHRIST, THE HEALER

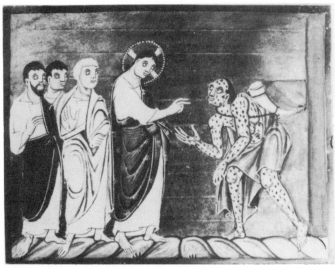

Leper cured by Christ. (Evangelarium of Otto III, 1000 A.D.)

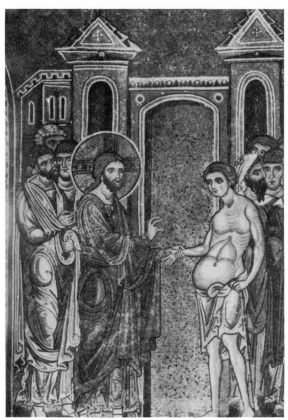

Dropsy relieved by Christ. (Mosaic in Monreale.)

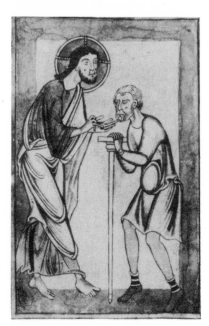

Christ restores blind man's sight.

"To preach the kingdom of God and to heal the sick" was what the followers of Christ went out into the world to do. The Apostles and Christian priests became doctors. The way already had been marked by the healing miracles of Christ.

With the psychic elements of disease and its cures known to modern medicine, not all of Christ's deeds of healing are a mystery. A compassionate, forceful personality understandably acted as a tonic on impressionable souls. Jesus made wonderful use of a prescription, more potent than is generally realized: the kind word.

When Jesus recognized the blind man of Jericho as his brother, the afflicted eyelids, whose condition had been aggravated by humiliating neglect and ill treatment, sprang open. Christ had lifted the man's spirits and enforced his will to be well. In the same way the man with the withered hand received the incentive to move it.

Numerous, too, are the cases of mental disorder cured by Christ. Many of the unfortunates were believed possessed by demons. Their fellow men had ostracized them or laughed off their complaints. Christ knew the suffering of these crushed souls.

Jesus cured the man of Gerasenes, (below), "who had devils a long time" by a form of psychiatry that had to wait almost 2,000 years to be generally accepted. This sufferer's condition had been aggravated by the cruelty of his fellowmen. Driven out of the city he had been compelled "to dwell in tombs." Christ looked at this pitiful creature as an ill person and treated him kindly. This change broke the chains of mental disorder and appeared to the onlookers as a miraculous cure.

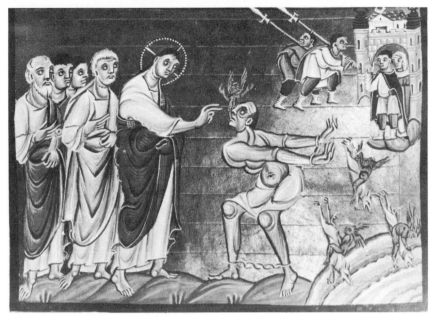

THE GOOD SAMARITAN

The story of the Good Samaritan (below) embodies all the elements of Christian medicine. The Samaritan's ready administration of "first aid" was the fulfillment of a Christian duty: to help those in need whether they were rich or poor, regardless of their race and creed. To this parable told by Christ, St. Luke added a number of medical touches, which prove him distinctly a physician well versed in wound treatment as practiced in his time. The use of wine for the soothing of wounds was recommended by Hippocrates and later by Galen, an early recognition of the antiseptic quality of alcohol. Experience also taught the ancients that wounds bathed in oil would heal better. The coating would serve to protect the wound from what we now know to be external contamination.

The doctor speaks in the Gospel of St. Luke. The most cultured of the Evangelists was known as St. Luke the "beloved physician," and Christ's deeds were described by him with literary skill and medical insight.

The many accounts of miraculous healing are told in St. Luke more fully than in any other gospel, with understanding and in a language that only a doctor would use. Unlike other writers of his time St. Luke characterized the man afflicted with dropsy not as "one with evil spirits in his abdomen" but one suffering from hydropikos, a term used nowhere else in the New Testament, but familiar enough to a student of Hippocrates.

Where other Evangelists referred to cases of "lameness," St. Luke, adding significant clinical history, described the man as congenitally lame ("from the womb of his mother"). Throughout his text, he tried to convey the concise clinical significance of the miracles and was careful to make fine distinctions, as between atrophy, the withered hand, and apoplexy, the sudden stroke.

It was, however, in spirit more than in terminology that Luke approached the modern physician. Sympathy for the suffering fills the pages of his gospel. He had a keen understanding of women's frailties, and knew the relation of sickness to mental anguish.

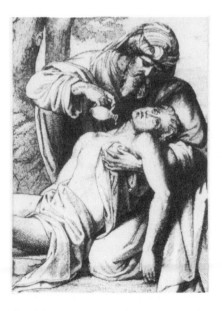

Good Samaritan treated wound expertly. 49

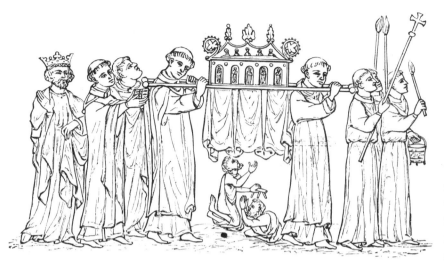

Cripples in hope of recovery touch relics of deceased saint.

MONASTIC

Cassiodorus (490-585?) served for many years as chancellor of Theodoric, the Ostrogoth ruler of Rome. He influenced the King to preserve the existing medical system and to encourage its growth by protective legislation.

When Cassiodorus retired from active statesmanship to the monastery he had founded in his native domain of Squillace, he took along his vast collection of classical writings. The Church had hesitated to accept ancient medicine, but Cassiodorus praised its merit with frankness. "Study the Hippocratic books on herbs and healing methods, which I have brought together in my library and have bequeathed to you," he commanded the monks. Cassiodorus deserves a niche in our book for being the first to recommend the study of medical pictures in cases where knowledge or inclination

As the Church took a firm hold on medicine, the secular doctor found himself pushed into the background. Yet, lay physicians did not disappear completely. The courts of the Frankish and Germanic kings continued to employ doctors who had at least a semblance of medical learning. Their status, however, was not an enviable one. When Queen Austragild contracted the plague, she requested as a last favor that her husband, Guntram of the Burgundians — "a good and God-fearing prince" — have her attending physician executed immediately after her death. The next morning the bereaved husband performed the desired ceremony. Thus, the spirits of the "angelic queen and the inefficient physician took a synchronous and, it is to be hoped, peaceful flight into the unknown together" (Dana).

For the populace at large, faith healing offered the chief hope of cure. Gregory of Tours threatened to class as a heretic any sick person who visited the local physician. A pilgrimage to St. Martin's shrine, he advised, would cure all ills. For dysentery, all a pilgrim needed was a pinch of dust from the saint's tomb. Inflammation of the tongue? Just lick the railing of St. Martin's sanctuary.

Uncounted Christian "cures" of this sort have led to the belief that the Middle Ages were a period of hopeless retrogression for medicine. However, this verdict is not completely right. While scientific pursuits were in a state of coma, the traditions of ancient rational medicine lingered on.

After a period of adamant opposition to the writings of Galen and Hippocrates, the Church gradually began to look more favorably at Greek and Roman medicine. Though little was done to further scientific inquiry, the basic medical ideas developed by Greece and passed on to the world by Rome rested safely in monastic library vaults. The survival of these ideas must be credited to two statesmen of the Church, Cassiodorus and St. Benedict.

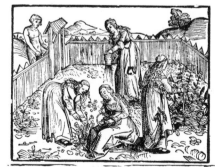

Gardens of Benedictine abbey of Reichenau were unequaled in herbal wealth.

MEDICINE

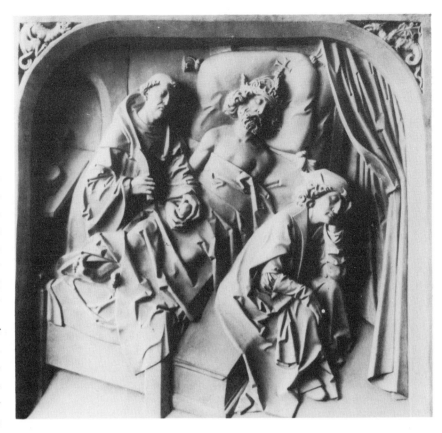

to read the text was wanting. "If the language of the Greeks is unknown to you, study the herb book of Dioscorides . . . who has depicted the herbs of the field with astonishing accuracy." It was Cassiodorus who made the monasteries asylums of ancient learning and effected its transfer to more enlightened times.

The second benefactor, Benedict of Nursia (480-543), created the Benedictine Order and thus started a truly organized Christian interest in medicine. When he founded the monastery of Monte Cassino in 529 A.D., he made care of the sick a cardinal monastic function. He introduced an entirely new concept of Christian duty. Instead of passive devotion and asceticism he prescribed for his brethren useful pursuits such as reading, copying manuscripts, the care of herb gardens, and the study of medicine.

When in 1022 the German Emperor Henry II visited Monte Cassino he suffered a bladderstone attack. It is not improbable that the royal patient was put to sleep with a soporific and then operated on, (see above relief from Bamberg Cathedral). The world however heard of the event as a miracle: While the emperor lay suffering in the monastery he fell asleep. St. Benedict appeared to him with a medical iron. He cut open the patient's body. "When you awake," St. Benedict said, "you will hold in your hands three stones." Henry II awoke free of pain and found the stones as promised.

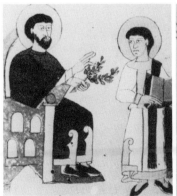
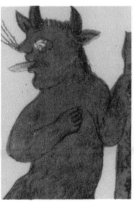
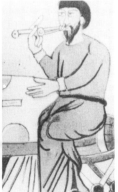

Another monastery that excelled in medical pursuits was the Benedictine Abbey of Fulda. It flourished under its abbot, Rabanus Maurus (775-856), whose profusely illustrated Encyclopedia (left) shows entries such as "Herbs," "Devil," "Eating."

51

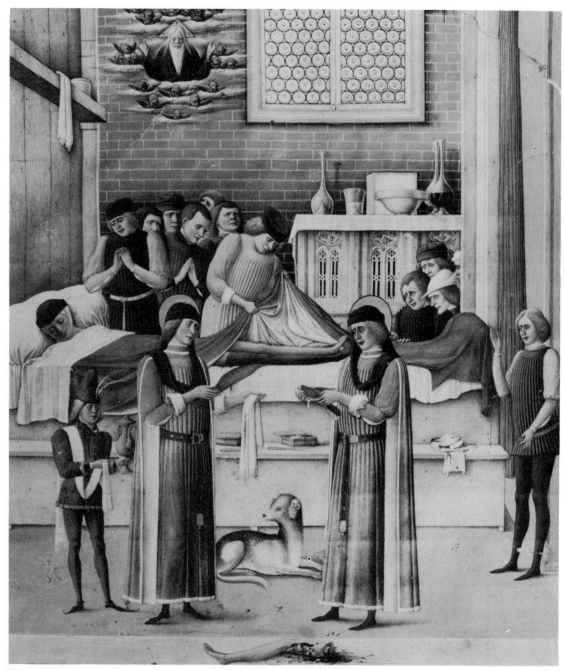

The miracle of Saint Cosmas and Damian. Miniature painting, (School of Bellini). A man with a cancerous leg fell asleep while praying for recovery in the Church of Cosmas and Damian in Rome. In his dreams the saintly surgeons Cosmas and Damian appeared to him. They looked at his leg but seemed hesitant to amputate. At this moment the body of a Moor was brought into the church for burial. So, the holy pair decided to amputate the diseased leg of the sleeping patient and replace it with the sound one of the Moor. The patient awoke and found his leg healed, although black in color. Joyfully he told his dream to everyone. When the Moor's grave was opened the bystanders noted that his body showed one white leg.

THE SICK PRAY TO SAINTS
WHO ARE FELLOW SUFFERERS

A bond between the early Christian martyrs and the people at large lay in the suffering which they shared. During their holy ordeals, the martyrs had been subjected to torture of the most infernal kind. Their limbs had been maimed, their eyes stabbed, their teeth knocked out. As saints they later assumed patronage over those parts of the body that had been molested in their own martyrdom. St. Erasmus, i. e., had his intestines torn out. This made him the protector against intestinal trouble. A red hot helmet had been put on the head of St. Just — headache sufferers pleaded for his assistance. For similar reasons other saints assumed patronage over parts of the body.

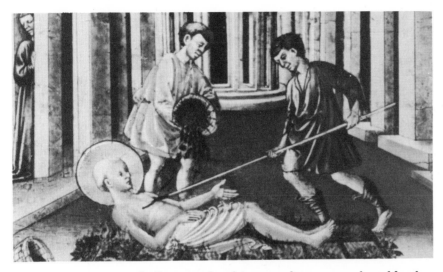

St. Lawrence forced in 249 to lie on a grate heated by glowing coal became the patron saint of backache sufferers.

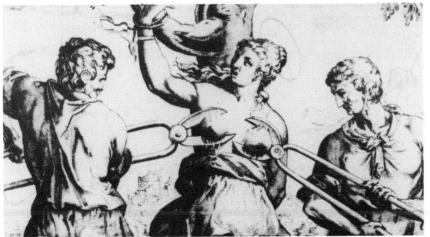

St. Agatha, deprived of her breasts in anti-Christian outbreak helped nursing mothers, cured pectoral pain.

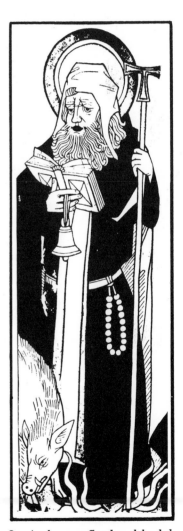

St. Anthony suffered and healed ergotism, "St. Anthony's Fire."

53

HOSPITALS

"MONASTIC MEDICINE'S CHIEF GLORY"

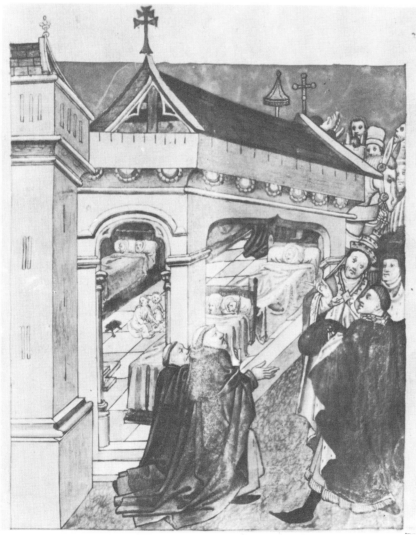

Church dignitaries take worldly potentate on hospital inspection tour. Note modern looking tile floor. On the whole, hygienic conditions were poor. Lack of social services compelled sick mothers to take their children along to the hospital.

If Christian strictures hampered the forward march of scientific medicine, the early Church contributed to social medicine in two important ways. First, the clerics created sanctuaries for the wayfarer. The Christian hospitia were modelled after the Roman valetudinaria. In these havens the monks and nuns took it upon themselves to nurse, feed and clothe the homeless. Leprosaria and permanent homes for the old, sick or poor were established along similar lines. Most of these hospices offered nursing care — but no medical aid. They represented hospitals without doctors.

In addition, the Middle Ages saw the rise of the monastic infirmaries. Here the modern hospital had its true origin and to its growth the doctors contributed greatly.

When in 820, Rabanus Maurus drew up the blueprints for the Abbey of Fulda, he added a special wing for sick brothers, a lazaretto for those with contagious diseases, and an apartment for a bona fide monastic doctor. Abbot Gozbert did likewise while building St. Galle (816-837), and soon the procedure became standard. Gozbert also mapped out the traditional medicinal garden outside the hospital.

When the monk-physicians had gained enough experience, sick and needy laymen came to the infirmaries for medical aid, and the wards were gradually filled to overflowing.

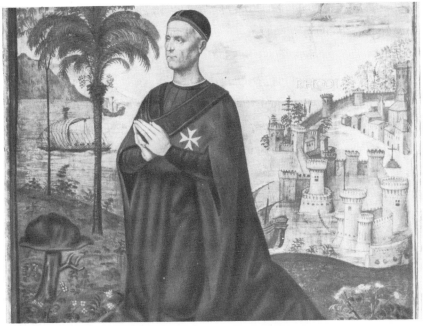

A knight of Rhodes. This order gave a military note to hospital organization, stressed cleanliness and strict schedule. After evacuation of their Jerusalem establishment, "Hospitallers" moved their headquarters to Cyprus, afterwards to Rhodes (1310). The eight-pointed cross signifies the eight virtues to which knights were pledged.

The monks had attempted, at first, to visit the sick in neighboring towns, but the Church complained that such activities led to the neglect of spiritual duties. In the infirmaries, however, the monk physician was able to treat the poor. The Church sustained these polyclinics and hospitals until the decline of feudal power cut off funds for medical care.

Actually, the monastic hold on medicine was not uncontested. By the eleventh century the secular School at Salerno had challenged clerical dominance. Before this, Jewish doctors had held important court posts, and quacks had thrived on medieval ignorance. The Church itself sometimes had recognized empirics, called *medici laici* or "idioti." Thus, as the

cities rose, the monasteries were quick to ally themselves with the growing number of distinguished lay physicians. An English chronicle cites the honorarium that should be paid to a lay doctor, attached to an abbey: "one loaf of bread, one gyst of best beer, 40 shillings per annum, and on fish or flesh days to be served as one of our monks."

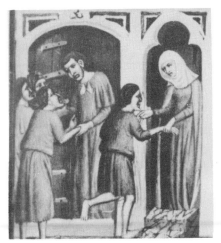

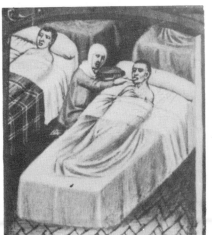

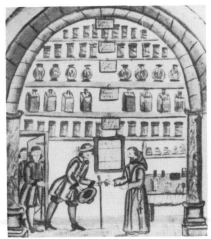

Needy wayfarers receive assistance. Medieval hospitia were not medical institutions but refuges of the poor, and the sick.

Modern doctor-staffed hospitals had their origin in monastic infirmaries with their wards, apothecary shops.

55

Chapter 5   Moslem Medicine

LIGHT FROM THE EAST

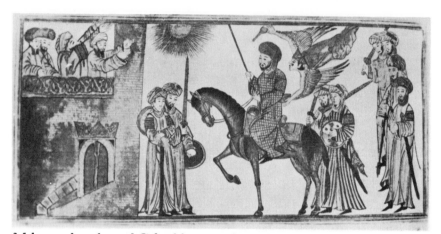

Mohammed, with angel Gabriel hovering above. The great prophet's precepts contained many rules of health: one meal a day, one bath a week, love once a month.

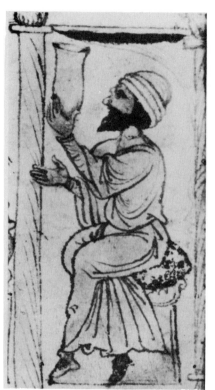

Arab physician could remain seated in presence of caliphs and other dignitaries.

Within one generation, the prophet Mohammed (c. 569-632 A.D.) brought unity to the scattered tribes of Arabia. Then, in the century after his death, turbaned horsemen fanned out across three continents. In the name of Allah, they struck through Jerusalem and the Middle East, through Syria and Persia to the banks of the Indus. In the West, they swept up into Spain, towards all of Europe, until Charles Martell stopped them at Poitiers in 732. Then the great empire split into caliphates, with Bagdad and Cordova as the eastern and western capitals. While Europe was shrouded in medieval darkness, these cities became twin centers of civilization.

Like the Romans, the Arab conquerors respected the superior cultures of the subjected peoples. They were particularly impressed by the school of medicine at Gondisapor, Persia, which was founded in the sixth century by the Nestorians, a group of displaced Christians. The patriarch Nestorius had been banished from Constantinople in 431 for heretic opinions on the nature of Christ. He and his followers migrated to the Syrian town of Edessa where they used their knowledge of Greek medicine to advantage. The city was soon hailed as a "second Athens."

When the Church continued to persecute them, the Nestorians fled to Persia, where they were welcomed by Chosroes the Blessed. Chosroes, an enlightened monarch, had brought Jewish, Hindu, Syrian and Persian physicians together at Gondisapor. When the Nestorians brought Greek lore to the city it became the medical center of all Asia.

In the 7th century, when the Arabs swept into Persia, they took Greek manuscripts from the school at Gondisapor, and from the libraries of every province. Then the medical wisdom of Hippocrates and Galen traveled by camel and ship to Bagdad, Nishapur, Samarcand, Cairo and Cordova. Here the parchments were retranslated from Persian into Arabic, and the "barbaric" Moslems became purveyors of classic medicine.

If the Arabian language served as the new vehicle for medicine, most "Arabian" doctors were Persians, Jews, Greeks, Christians or Byzantines. The members of the Bakhtischû family were Nestorian Christians. They were prominent in medicine for about three centuries. George (Jurjus) Bakhtischû headed the school and hospital at Gondisapor in the 8th century. He also directed the translation of Greek classics into Arabic for al-Mansur, the caliph of Bagdad, who hired him in 764. Later, his grandson Gabriel Bakhtischû, also a skilled physician carried on the medical work at Gondi-sapor. When the medical experts at the court of Harun al-Raschid were puzzled, the famous caliph called for young Bakhtischû to cure him. To test the physician's knowledge, he once presented the doctor with a glass con-taining the urine of "one of the caliph's

favorites." "What shall we feed the patient?" al-Raschid asked, and Bak-tishû promptly suggested — barley. The "patient" was a donkey.

Bakhtischû must have cured Harun al-Raschid, for the caliph lived to hear the tales of *A Thousand and One Nights*, and to found the Academy of Bagdad, where Greek manuscripts were studied and translated. Like other Moslem leaders, Harun al-Raschid placed a heavy premium upon these parchments. When he conquered the Byzantines, Greek lore was his "most coveted booty."

This hunger for manuscripts was graphically illustrated by the case of the Nestorian translator, Hunain ibn Ishâq (809-875), called Johan-nitius. Hunain was a great philologist; his extensive translations became stand-ard texts, and his methods of revision, comparison and research were de-

cidedly modern. Consequently, when-ever he finished a bulky tome, he brought it to Caliph al-Mamun, who placed it on a scale, then paid the scholar its weight in gold. People said Hunain used heavy paper for his translations, and wrote them out in large, bold letters.

Hunain was also a physician of in-tegrity. When he first came to court, the caliph offered him riches for an unobtrusive poison to use on his enemies. Hunain refused to comply, and spent the next year in prison. At the end of the year, the caliph asked for the drug once more. This time the alternative was death, but Hunain replied that his profession commanded him to help mankind. Thereupon the caliph confessed, "Thy laws are sublime," and made Hunain his court physician.

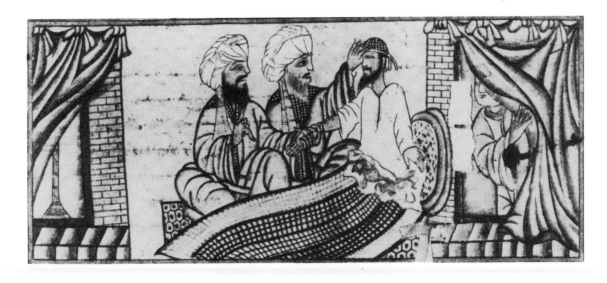

Arab doctors feel fevered brow, take pulse, "the messenger who does not lie."
As for fees: "Ask thy reward while the sickness is at its height."

RHAZES

BEDSIDE CLINICIAN

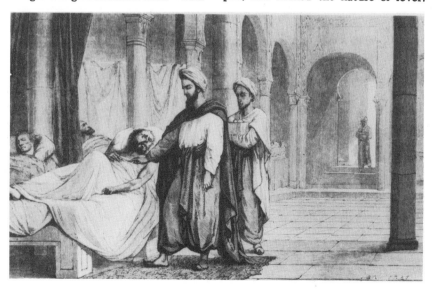

Paved streets, exquisite minarets, hospitals and great physicians, at Bagdad, Cairo and Cordova.

The Golden Age of Arab medicine extended roughly from 850 to 1050 A. D. By that time the great work of translation had been completed, and the new knowledge had sifted down to the practitioners. Then the ingenious Arabs developed algebra and the numeral system; they catalogued the stars, established the first pharmacies, fostered chemistry and discovered a host of new drugs. At Bagdad, and later at Cairo and Cordova, great hospitals and academies were established. Cordova alone, with a million people, boasted paved streets, public lamps, a thousand baths, exquisite minarets, schools for children, and the greatest library since Alexandria. From these cities there emerged great doctors.

Rhazes (841-926), called the Experienced, came to Bagdad from northeast Persia. Until he was 40, he sang, philosophized, and played the lute. Then he took up medicine. He journeyed through Jerusalem and Africa to Cordova, practicing his newfound art, and gathering information from "women and herbalists." When he returned to Bagdad, he was asked to select a good site for the new hospital. He hung up fresh meat in different parts of the city, then chose the site where the meat showed the least signs of putrefaction.

Rhazes was the greatest bedside clinician of his day, and pupils voyaged from all over the empire to hear his lectures. The public, he told them, liked to "shop around" for a pleasant cure. But only the quacks had pleasant cures, so the doctor "must often endure poverty." The patient should stick to one good physician, he said, or he would end by "distrusting them all." Rhazes taught his students a long list of cures. He also showed them the difference between measles and smallpox, and defined the nature of fever.

Rhazes emphasized bedside observation, (as in ward right). Bagdad hospitals provided music, story-telling, readings from the Koran, running water, convalescence rooms and barred cells for the insane. All sick received care, whether natives or strangers and small sums were paid to them on their departure to sustain them during period of rehabilitation.

AVICENNA

TEXTBOOK-WRITER

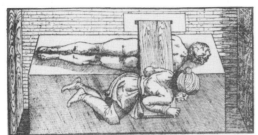

Hefty Avicenna straightens a crooked spine.

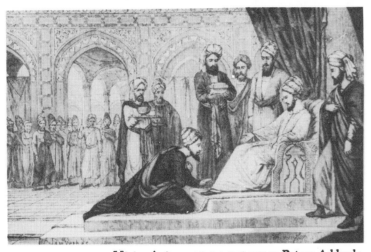

Vizier Avicenna pays respects to Prince Addaula.

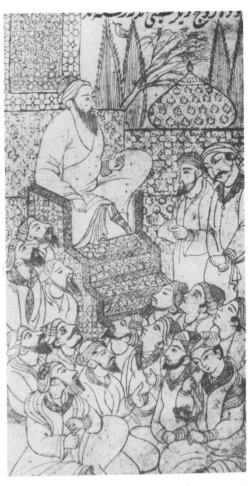

Verbose Avicenna (above) discussed weighty problems such as: why hair grows not on the nose; why breasts grow not on the belly; why the stomach lies not behind the mouth, and last but not least why calves are not on the front of the legs. For urine retention cases, he recommended placing a flea in patient's urinal passage. (Persian miniature, Meyerhof Collection, Cairo.)

Avicenna, the Persian (980-1037), was a drunkard, a wanderer, and a brilliant physician. At ten he knew the Koran by heart; at 17 he had mastered philosophy, natural history, poetry, mathematics, law and medicine. A year later he cured a Samanid king, and gained access to the royal archives. Then he moved on, restlessly, from court to court, in favor and out. At Hamadan, he became prime minister for curing the colic of Shams Addaula. When angry subjects demanded Avicenna's head, the emir banished him to save his life. He was called back shortly, however, to cure more colic.

Avicenna's supreme achievement was his *Canon of Medicine*, perhaps the most influential textbook ever written. Its million words, both foolish and wise, were absorbed for six centuries thereafter by the medical schools of Asia and Europe. Here Avicenna showed an amazing knowledge of symptoms and pharmacology.

It is disputable whether he was right when listing love in his Canon under mental diseases.

At 57, Avicenna died from a combination of wine, women, and overwork. To read Avicenna today is distinctly a heroic task.

CURE

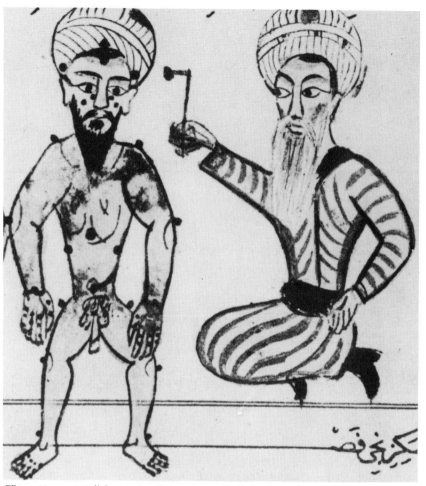

The cautery was "the national instrument" of Arabia after Albucasis revived it. The doctor, above, brands lepers' sores.

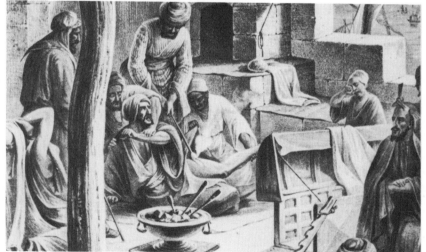

In two major fields of medicine, gynecology and surgery, the Arab doctors were decidedly incompetent. Moslem modesty kept them away from female patients, while the proscriptions of Allah against cutting human flesh, dead or alive, made dissection or surgery virtually impossible. At the same time, the surgeon was ostracized in western Europe. The cleric physician refused to shed blood, and by 1163 the Council of Tours had resolved that surgery should be abandoned by schools, and by all decent physicians. Anatomy languished, and surgery might have lapsed entirely, but for the work of Albucasis, an Arab physician born in Spain.

Albucasis (died c. 1013) rescued the surgical craft by reviving the white hot cautery. He taught his students to treat over 50 diseases by fire. This preference, plus Allah's strictures, made the cautery a national instrument in Arabia. Wounds were seared, cancers removed and abscessed sores reopened by the famous branding iron. But flesh-cutting was limited to probing wounds, extracting barbs, or clipping tonsils and polyps. For such operations, Albucasis invented new instruments.

Even the midwives profited from the genius of Albucasis. Up to this time most of the Arabian doctors had

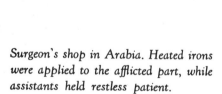

Surgeon's shop in Arabia. Heated irons were applied to the afflicted part, while assistants held restless patient.

BY FIRE

merely theorized on the problems of childbirth. When they did attend a woman patient, a heavy curtain hung between them to prevent any direct examination. But Albucasis, like Soranus before him, had some good advice for the midwives behind the muslin curtain. To ease childbirth, he described what is known today as Walcher's position, in which the woman in labor lies with her hips at the edge of a table, while her legs dangle. He also pictured advanced obstetrical instruments in his famous text on surgery; forceps with crossed blades, and dilators with screw action. Whether the midwives used them is problematical. Guy de Chauliac, the 14th century restorer of surgery, lifted a good many of these instruments right from Albucasis' text.

Albucasis also passed along original methods for cutting stone and supporting female pubic arches. The resourceful physician even pioneered in dentistry. He is said to have performed corrective operations for ugly, irregular teeth.

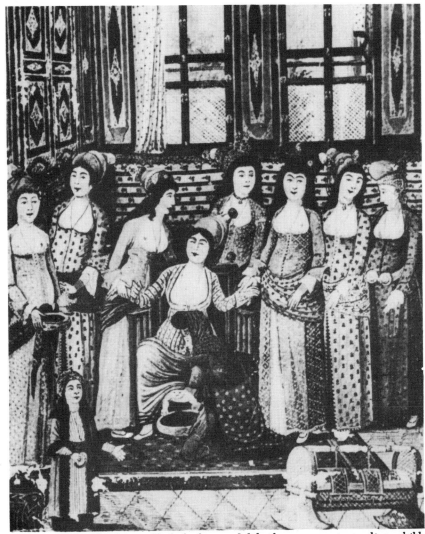

Childbirth in Turkish home. Midwife extracts protruding child.

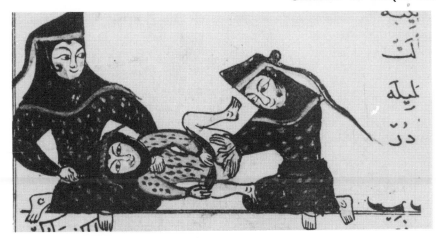

Arab midwives, coached by doctors, are said to have performed lithotomies and treated prolapsed uteri (left).

THE ARABIAN DRUGGIST

The modern drug store, minus the soda fountain, owes its origin to the Arabs. If their medical lore was largely second-hand, the Moslems showed much originality as apothecaries and herbalists. They gave the sick new and wondrous medicaments: alcohol, cassia, senna, manna, arsenic, ambria, camphor, balsam and borax. Wandering savants, like Rhazes and Avicenna, were sure the earth contained specific plants to remedy all ills. They combed the empire for these new substances, and garnered long lists of roots, herbs, seeds and resins from Egypt, Africa and Spain, from India and Persia. Abu Mansur reported that Persia alone offered more active drugs than "all six other parts of the world together."

If the new drugs proved bitter to the palate, the ingenious Arabs devised chemical and mechanical methods to make them sweet. The candy-coated pill, the pellet wrapped in silver foil, a forerunner of the ubiquitous cellophane, were first employed by Avicenna and his colleagues, who always strove to keep their patients cheerful. To this end, Arab pharmacists mixed rosewater with medicines as well as perfume. They invented tinctures, confections and syrups, pomades, plasters and ointments to ease the physician's task. Today's synthetic chemistry stems from their extensive sublimations.

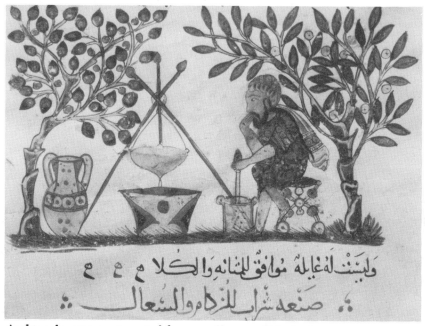

Arabian druggist in open air laboratory filters medicinal wine.

Before the advent of Arab medicine, drug preparation was part of the doctor's job. However, with growing lists of remedies, the Arabs were forced to specialize. Soon pharmacology branched out as a separate medical province, and the apothecary was recognized as a reputable craftsman. His high standing was translated into laws and precepts, which quickly filtered into Europe from Spain and other Arab lands.

A typical apothecary's code that shows Arab influence has been salvaged from the 12th century. Issued at Arles, in Southern France, it called for a clear-cut separation of doctors and druggists. The apothecaries were to keep out of medical affairs, while the doctors were forbidden to own or hold interest in pharmacies. The Arabian provinces set up specific controls to prevent the sale of poisons and harmful drugs, and their pharmacists were pledged to follow the directives of licensed physicians. Such regulations quickened the emergence of the professional pharmacist — although they did not altogether eliminate shady drug shops.

- - - THE FIRST DRUG STORE

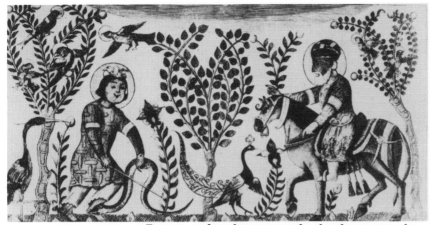

For serpent bite doctor prescribes handy curative plant.

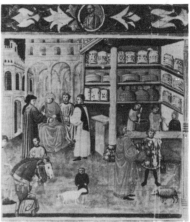

Avicenna in Arab corner pharmacy.

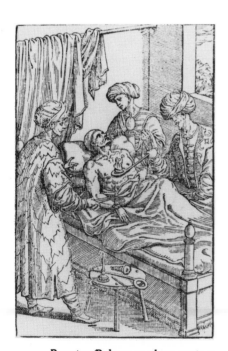

Burning Balsam to cheer patient.

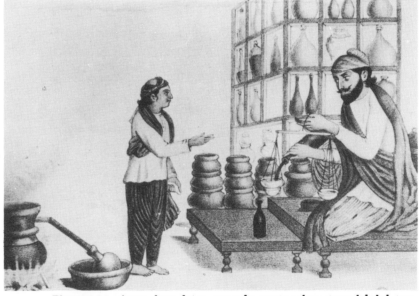

Pharmacist, Attar, kept drugs secret by storing them in unlabeled jars.

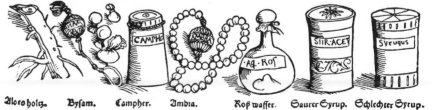

European medicines based on Arab pharmacopoeia: Balsam, camphor, rosewater.

ARABS AND JEWS

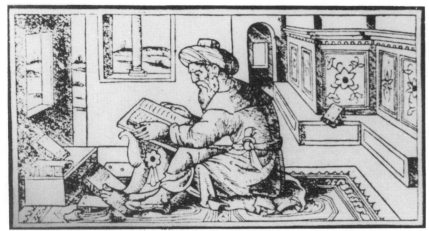

Avenzoar scans Galen for bedside tips.

Bezoar stone legend was first propounded by Avenzoar. Such stones, he said, were large "hardened tears" shed by stags; they served as antidotes for poison. As legend grew, stones became cureals and amulets which were sold widely during plague, and could even be rented by the day.

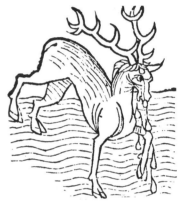

Until the mid-18th century, bezoars were listed as an official remedy in London pharmacopoeia.

The medical leader of the western caliphate was Avenzoar of Seville (1113-1162). As a practical bedside observer, he dismissed Avicenna's *Canon* as a "mere waste of paper," and turned to Galen instead, or to Paulus of Aegina. Consequently, he was able to recognize cancer when he saw it in stomach or gullet and became famous as the first proponent of the nutrient enema. When a courtier's throat suffered occlusion, Avenzoar fastened a goat's bladder to a tube, and injected milk, eggs and gruel through the rectum into the patient's gut.

Avenzoar was on excellent terms with his pupil, Averroes of Cordova (1126-1198), called "The Commentator" for his brilliant interpretation of Aristotle. Averroes is said to have missed but two nights of study in his life: one when his father died, and the other when he married.

While Avenzoar and Averroes were good friends — Arabian doctors as a rule watched each other jealously. Disagreements were at times settled by duel-by-poison. In such duels each doctor was expected to take his opponent's poison, then find a quick antidote. Two court physicians once tried it: The first doctor's draught was fierce enough to "melt black stone," but his rival parried with an antidote. Then the second doctor picked a rose, mumbled an incantation, and asked his antagonist to sniff the flower. The first doctor complied, and protmply fell dead. Fright had killed him, for the rose was only a rose.

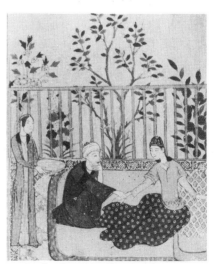

Arab doctor takes lady's pulse.

ALLIED IN MEDICINE

Moses Maimonides was equally famed as a Jewish scholar and physician. He was born in Cordova where he studied the healer's art under Averroes. However, his family soon moved to Morocco, then to Jerusalem and Cairo, to avoid persecution as "apostate" Moslems.

When his father and brother died, Maimonides was forced to earn his living by medicine, "the strange woman whom I first took into my house as handmaid to the Torah." Later on, he became court physician to Saladin, the enlightened Moslem sultan who recaptured Jerusalem in 1187. Maimonides strove learnedly to make Aristotle and Galen gibe with Mosaic Law. The Jewish sage was highly esteemed not only by his own people but also by the Arabs.

As a rule the Jews lived peacefully among the Arabs and achieved a fuller life than the Jews in Christian lands. The Arabs respected their linguistic abilities. The caliphs made use of it by assigning them to translate medical classics into Hebrew and Latin. Jewish doctors brought these translations to Central Europe exercising an accelerating influence on medicine. Many of them attained renown as court physicians and even the Popes made use of their services.

When Maimonides died in 1204 there was a general outburst of grief and Jews and Moslems joined in lamenting him for three days.

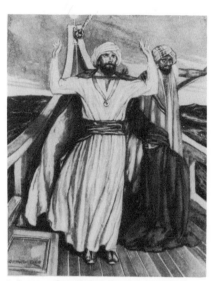

Maimonides fled Morocco in 1165 to escape religious persecution. He wrote dietetic rule book for Saladin.

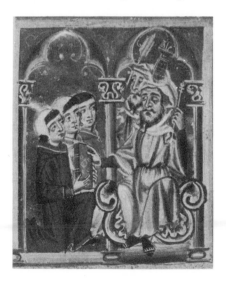

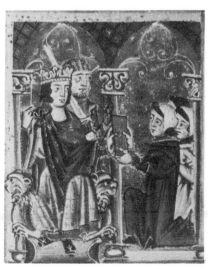

Jewish scholars (left) receive Arab medical manuscript, deliver Latin translation to Christian king (right). This marks end of the ironic route Greek knowledge had traveled: Nestorian Christians, rejected by their own Church, brought Greek texts to Persia in 6th century; Arabs took them from Persia, returned them to Europe with the aid of Jewish linguists. Translations: from Greek into Persian, from Persian into Arabic, from Arabic back into Latin and Greek.

MEDICINE MOVES WEST

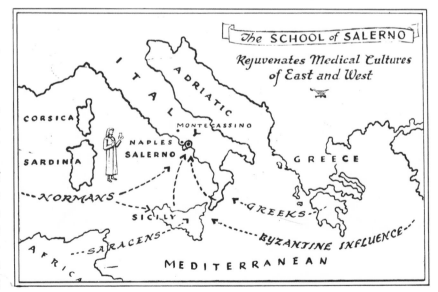

Constantinus Africanus gave Greek classics back to the West.

In the 11th century, the town of Salerno came to be known simply as *civitas hippocratica*. Here men and women, clerics and laymen, natives and foreigners began to practice a brand of medicine that was surprisingly rational.

Salerno's school for the training of doctors had emerged around the year 900. Nobody knew how the school was first established. According to a credible legend, it was founded by four doctors: a Greek, a Jew, an Arab and a Christian, who all desired a training school in which young physicians could pursue medicine, unhampered by clerical supervision or the study of musty books.

In a way, the legend sticks close to the known facts. The air around the Gulf of Naples always had been salubrious enough to attract patients in search of recovery. The neighboring order of Benedictine monks was duty bound to cultivate medicine and the sciences, and a small colony of Jewish physicians had lived around Salerno since Roman times. Also the Arabs across the water dominated the medical field, and the Longobards, who settled there in 568 A.D., had somehow preserved the medical teachings of old Byzantium. Whatever the causes, the new School of Salerno wrested leadership from the Arabs.

Actually, the Crusades had much to do with the reorientation of medicine. Arab medicine had already reached Sicily, the busy trading center which the Saracens conquered in 878. When the Normans took over Sicily and Southern Italy, through infiltration and open conquest, they merely catalyzed the latent cultural fusion between Arabic, Jewish, Greek and Latin elements. Thus, Salerno, the hub of the new Norman rule, soon became a cultural melting pot. During the Crusades, traffic shuttled through the city between East and West. Wounded noblemen landed there for rest cures, or for consultation with physicians, and there was a constant flow of famous patients. By the middle of the 11th century Salerno was well established, and the most productive epoch in medieval medicine had begun.

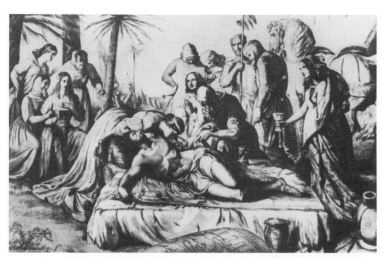

Robert, Duke of Normandy, shown sleeping, while gallant Sybilla, grandniece of Robert Guiscard, sucks poison from his wound. As the legend goes, she saved the Duke, and later became his wife. Robert of Normandy who had returned to Salerno for medical advice had stayed too long away from home and thereby lost his right to the English crown.

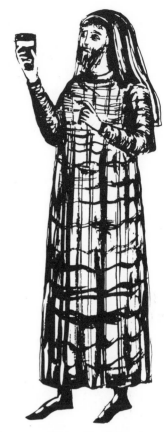

Hippocrates (in medieval dress) inspired doctors of Salerno to concentrate once more upon patients, bedside observation.

Constantinus taught briefly at Salerno, then retired to the monastery of Monte Cassino to translate Arabic texts on medicine, or Arabic translations of Greek texts, into Latin. His work included a few short tracts of Hippocrates and Galen, and *The Perfect Book of the Art of Medicine* by Haly Abbas. The Salernitans seized upon the new learning, for these were the first rational textbooks on medicine to reach Europe in 500 years. New tracts on anatomy and surgery appeared, based on Constantinus. Salerno entered its golden age.

At first, the influence of the Arabian texts was a beneficial one. Later on as their subtleties and speculation became more dominant, they undermined the sound, simple methods of the Salernitan doctors. The new flood of Arabic learning brought back the wisdom of antiquity, but it also contained the seeds of medical decadence.

The earlier Salernitan doctors had gradually abandoned medieval superstition for Hippocratic simplicity. Attention centered on the patient, his diet and mode of life, and theories were formulated through reliance on common sense and observation. Then, with the appearance of Constantinus Africanus around 1070, the pace of medical advance quickened noticeably.

A cure for gout (right). Mathew d'Agello, the Norman chancellor of Sicily, is seated in his private chamber, where a servant has just cut off the head of an Arab prisoner. The blood drains into a large basin, in which the chancellor dips his feet to get rid of gout. The picture first appeared with a propaganda poem by an Italian patriot, Petrus of Eboli, who hated the Norman intruders.

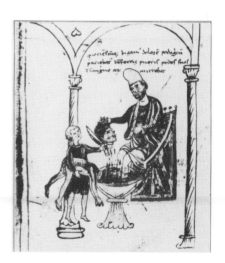

67

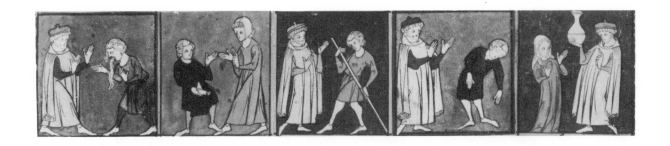

SALERNO'S SCHOOL FOR DOCTORS

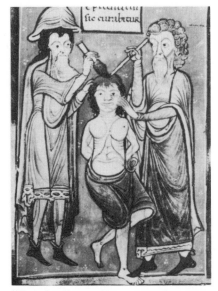

"Branding" an epileptic man by scorching his head with hot irons. This method of "counter irritation" was used for many diseases, each one requiring a different pattern of branding points.

The doctors of Salerno blazed trails as both practitioners and educators. Like the Greeks, they saw that patients were human, that disease was a natural phenomenon and that common sense therapies might help to cure it. The doctor was now called "physicus," or physician, rather than "medicus." The change in terminology emphasized his integration with natural science above and beyond mere medical skill.

The School of Salerno did much to spread this new concept. Salerno was actually the first secular institution of higher learning in the west. It had a lay faculty and an extensive curriculum. Anatomy was taught, based on Galen and Haly Abbas, with pigs for dissection instead of human cadavers. Students assisted at the bedside, and were present during actual operations.

Salerno even boasted of having on its faculty a number of women professors. Dame Trotula was credited with holding the chair of gynecology. She was acclaimed as a teacher, midwife, and a professor's wife. Charles Singer,

the renowned English medical historian, looks skeptically at these appellations. The two Salernitan texts on woman's disease: Trotula Minor and Trotula Major, were in his estimation written by one Trotulus. The subject matter, however, created the mental image of a woman as its author, and Trotulus was replaced in medieval texts by Trotula.

Salerno was not a diploma mill. Roger II of Sicily and Frederick II issued decrees which bound the students to three years' work in the humanities, five years' specialized training and a final stringent examination before the faculty and the Royal Commissioner (1224). The lucky candidate received a ring, a laurel wreath, a book and the kiss of peace. Then, after a year's work with an attested physician, the graduate could hang out his own shingle.

To uphold this new won status the young doctor was required, first, to avoid trouble with the Church by seeing that his patient confessed. Next, he was told to win the patient's confidence. A Salernitan tract tells how this was to be achieved: "When the doctor enters the dwelling of his patient, he should greet with kindly, modest demeanor those who are present, and then seating himself near the sick man, accept the drink which is offered him, and praise in a few words the beauty of the neighborhood, the situation of the house, and the generosity of the family . . ."

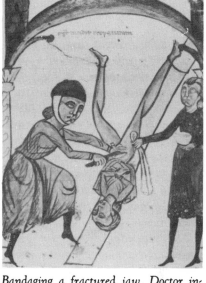

Inclined operating table, with patient's head lower than pelvis, was well known to Salernitans. Reintroduced by Trendelenburg in 1881, it is now used for many surgical operations.

AND SURGEONS

Surgery also became, for a time, an acknowledged discipline in the new secular atmosphere. On the whole, the clerical doctor had refused to bloody his hands, and the craft was left to barbers and amateurs. Now Roger Frugardi of Salerno wrote the first western book on surgery (1170), a classical text later made sound and concise by his student, Roland of Parma (see illustrations, right).

The treatise indicated that Roger could cut well, that he could clot bleeding with mummy powder, or finely cut hair of the hare. Sponges wet with narcotics were held before the patient's nose in a crude attempt at anesthesia. Torn intestines were sewn together over an elderwood tube, or an animal's trachea.

For goiter in its early stages, Roger recommended the oral administration of seaweed ashes, which amounts to a rough form of iodine therapy. Unfortunately, he also thought the formation of pus was a necessary adjunct to wound healing. This theory of "laudable pus" prevailed for centuries.

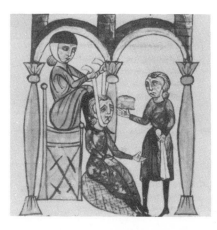

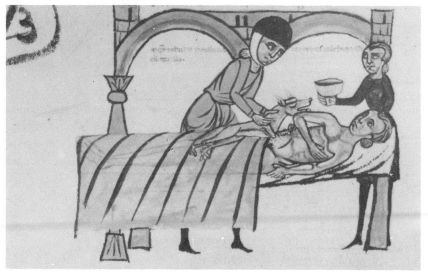

Bandaging a fractured jaw. Doctor insures tight fit by raising bandage ends and stepping down on the patient's shoulders. Bandages were hardened with flour-and-egg mixture (left).

Prolapsed intestines were treated by applying the warmth of a dying animal to the patient's wound. Dogs or cats were slit open before application (below).

69

THE ART OF SENSIBLE LIVING

Dont's from Hortus Sanitatis.

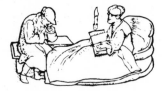

Don't read in bed.

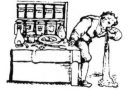

Don't drink too much.

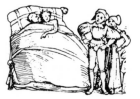

Don't love too much.

Don't strain too much.

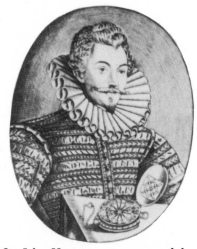

Sir John Harington, poet, compiled an English regimen for Queen Elizabeth.

After the School of Salerno had been firmly established, its professors teamed up to write a simple, readable textbook of hygiene. Little did they know that they had produced the most popular medical book ever written: the *Regimen Sanitatis Salernitanum.* This compact handbook contained about 362 rules of health for daily life, all of them couched in easy jingles of the "apple a day" variety.

The faculty's surprise best seller quickly spread across Europe. (24 manuscript editions are still in existence.) As time went on doctors added new verses to each publication, and rival schools came out with imitative texts. With the invention of printing, cheap popular versions appeared. By 1852, the book had run to almost 300 editions, in many languages and its verses had snowballed to about 3500.

Thus, the *Regimen* became a kind of folk epic, a guidebook for the home containing the medical experience of an entire continent. The Salernitan stamp of simplicity and closeness to daily life insured its popular appeal. The jingles were easy to memorize; they left no doubt about what to do or what to avoid. There were specific herbal remedies for gout, phlegm or ague, and relatively sound advice about diet, sleep, sex, drink and diversion. In later editions, when the more ponderous scholars fell victim to the seductive charm of the book, some lengthy rhapsodies appeared on climate and disease, the four humours, venesection and uroscopy. Such verses provided the profession with indispensable precepts, and thousands of physicians committed them to memory. In this way, the *Regimen* finally became "the backbone of all practical medical literature" up to the 18th century. Salernitan wisdom is heeded even today, in the medical folklore of Europe and America.

AGAINST TOOTHACHE

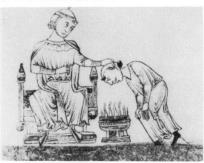

"If in your teeth you hap to be tormented
Burn Frankincense (a gum not evil scented)
And in a tunnel to the tooth that's hollow,
Convey the smoke thereof, and ease shall follow."

Regimen Sanitatis

SALERNITAN WISDOM

If thou to health and vigor wouldst attain
Shun weighty cares—all anger deem profane
From heavy suppers and much wine abstain.

Use three physicians still—first Dr. Diet
Next Dr. Merryman, third Dr. Quiet.

Great suppers will the stomach's peace impair
Wouldst lightly rest—curtail thine evening fare.

Shun idle slumber nor delay
The urgent calls of nature to obey.

Nor trivial count it after pompous fare
To rise from table and to take the air.

Let doctors call in clothing fine arrayed
With sparkling jewels on their hands displayed
For when well dressed and looking over nice
They may presume to charge a higher price. *

But as all practice shows, no doctor can
Make life anew, though he may stretch its span. *

(* Later addition to Salernitan text.)

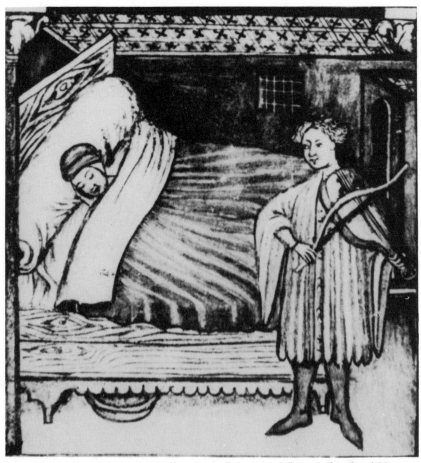

Quiet sleep induced by fiddler. From Regimen of Cerruti family of Verona.

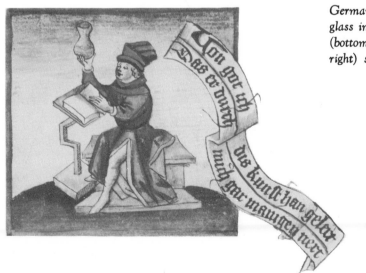

German versions of Regimen. Doctor raises traditional urine glass in Heinrich von Lauffenberg's 15th century manuscript (bottom left). Early 16th century printed edition (bottom right) shows Strasburg lady in tub.

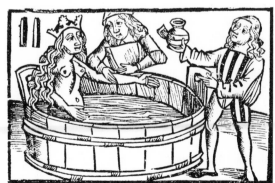

71

"FOUR TEMPERAMENTS RULE MANKIND WHOLLY"

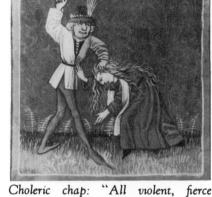

Choleric chap: "All violent, fierce and full of fire."

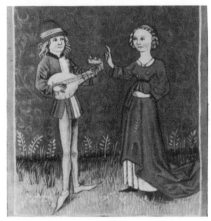

Melancholy man: "A heavy looke, a spirit little daring."

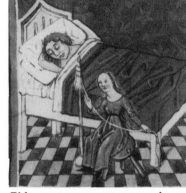

Phlegmatic type: given much to "rest and sloth."

Sanguine fellow: loves "mirth and musick, wine and women."

Through Salerno, a host of Greek medical ideas came trooping into Europe. At the head of the parade marched the doctrine of four humours, which quickly became the most powerful and pervasive concept in medieval medicine. Empedocles had laid its foundation 600 years before Christ, by teaching that the world, the macroscosm consisted of four elements: fire, water, earth and air. Hippocrates and Galen had applied this theory to man. They taught that man was a microcosm composed of four "humours," which resembled the elements: blood (fire), phlegm (earth), black bile (water)

and yellow bile (air). If these humours were properly mingled, health prevailed; if the balance was upset, sickness followed, and it was the physician's problem to restore the equilibrium.

The Salernitan doctors added a final touch: humoral balance, they said, fell into four categories too: in every person, one humor dominated the others to form a new balance, and further, this dominant humour determined a person's physical and emotional characteristics — his temperament. Thus, the sanguine fellow, "inclining to be fat, and prone to

laughter," was surcharged with hot, moist blood; the phlegmatic person, squarish and given "to rest and sloth," was dulled by cold phlegm; a choleric chap, "On little cause to anger great inclined," had hot yellow bile for his dominant humour; and finally, cold, dry black bile depressed the melancholy man, making him pensive, peevish and "ever solitary."

The theory of body fluids remained unchallenged until 1858, when Virchow published his *Cellular Pathology.* He replaced "fluidism" by "solidism," which regarded the cell as the body's cardinal entity.

72

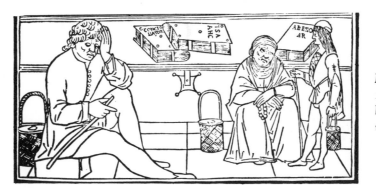

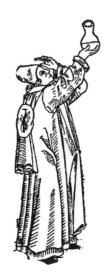

The urine glass served as a convenient window for observing the humours at work. As the theory ran, any "surplus" or abnormal change in the humours could be detected in the urine. Consequently, the practice of uroscopy became standard, and the urine glass, like the stethoscope today, took on a symbolical function as the very keystone of diagnosis. This function had its psychological aspects, of course. The doctors used it with an air of unfathomable wisdom to impress their patients. As Arnold of Villanova (1235-1311) puts it: "If you don't find anything in the urine, but the patient insists on suffering of headache, tell him that it is an obstruction of the liver — just continue to speak of obstruction — a word they don't understand, but one that sounds important."

But the Salernitan doctors were seldom nonplussed; they developed a fine eye for urine, and detected 18 different colors in it. The Breslau Codex of Salernitan medicine devotes about 40 tightly packed pages to instructions on the appraisal of sediment, odor and weight, with tips for strategy against maverick humours.

Isaac Judaeus suggested that the urine glass be divided into four even parts, each corresponding to a region of the body. If the top layer of liquid seemed turbid, there was head trouble to contend with, and so on down to the bottom of both glass and torso.

These "symptoms" gave the doctor a handy index to disease and treatment, especially when coupled with a detailed knowledge of the patient's blood, phlegm and temperament.

The next step was to restore humoral balance, and for this diet was commonly employed. Thus, a patient with fever received "cold" foods, like the onion, while a patient with surplus phlegm (cold) was treated with "hot" foods, like pepper, which "burned." Medicines were straitjacketed in similar fashion, as hot or cold, wet or dry. It was all very simple, and at bottom, simply foolish.

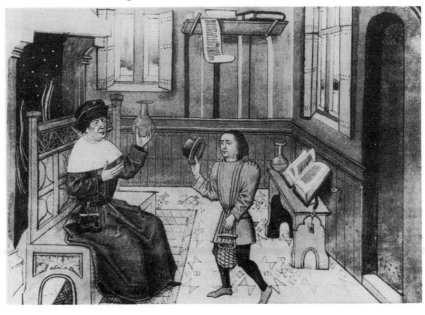

Water-casting was often impersonal. Here servant brings patient's urine for "lab" analysis.

73

"BLOODLETTING . .

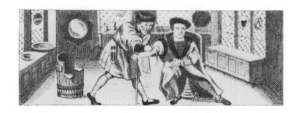

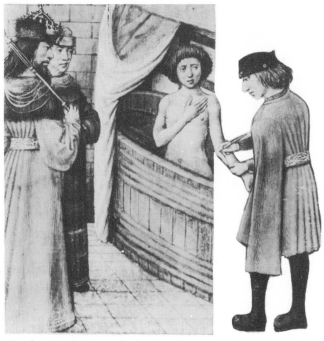

King's son bled in bath by short-robed barber.
Doctor, on King's left, directs operation.

Phlebotomy was by far the most expedient way to rid the body of "peccant" or excess humours which caused ill health. According to medieval thought, the four humours were intermingled, or possibly linked together by tubes; thus, if one was withdrawn, the excess humour would be drained off in the process, and humoral balance restored. The idea seemed to make sense, and since blood was always accessible, doctor and laymen alike rejoiced at bleeding the body at every opportunity.

In the spring and fall, bloodletting was *de rigueur*, since the body, like the modern automobile requiring a change of oil, had to attune the humours to new climatic conditions. For everyday pathological states, like

lovesickness and melancholy, it was decidedly helpful. As the Salernitan *Regimen* rhymed it: "Bleeding soothes rage, bringing joy to the sad, And saves all lovesick swains from going mad." It worked the same cure for those flirtatious ladies who wished to forget lovers and remember husbands. It even worked for the monks who were periodically bled to keep their minds from mundane thoughts. And centuries later, Madame de Maintenon, the consort of Louis XIV, was phlebotomized twice weekly to keep from blushing at the naughty stories told at court.

Though doctors developed the theory behind bloodletting, barbers performed the actual operation — a task too menial for the doctor. It was the

first professional wedge, however, advancing the barbers to barber-surgeons, then to full-fledged chyrurgeons.

The first big question, of course, was where to bleed: on the side of the disease, as Hippocrates said, or on the opposite side? The Arabs adhered to the latter system, arguing that "reverse" or revulsive bloodletting brought better balance, while the Hippocratic method only weakened the patient. The "same-siders," or derivative bleeders, held that the patient's pain was relieved by their method. In the 17th century a dispute about these theories reached absurd heights.

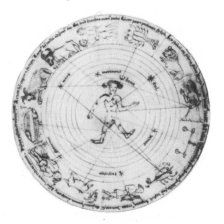

Chart shows when and where to bleed.

74

.. IS THE BEGINNING OF HEALTH"

The next problem was when to bleed, and here astrology came to the fore. The constellation Cancer, for instance, governed the human breast, and bleeding in this region could only be performed when the stellar picture of Cancer was in the ascendancy. The time of day, the season, the position of the moon were also taken into account, along with the patient's temperament. Since many barbers were unable to read, astral charts were prepared which pictured all governing factors, and indicated about 30 points of incision. These diagrams were among the first pamphlets ever to appear in printed form. A few of them actually admonished the physician to use blood specimens for diagnosis; to observe the color, odor, density and foam of blood, and to do the same with sputum.

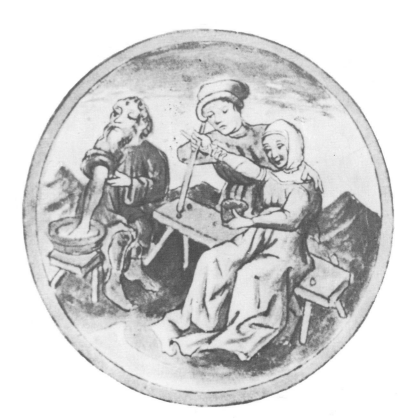

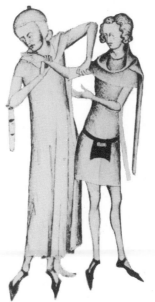

Each spring brachial phlebotomy was performed. Patient (above) clasps wooden stick to swell vein. Man at left soaks skin in warm water to ease forthcoming incision. First barber poles consisted of bloody bandage wrapped around stick to advertise trade.

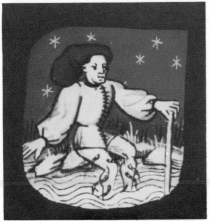

Spring-leeching (Codex Aldobrandini).

Pulse feeling in 1345. Doctor at left explores humeral artery above elbow with left hand, cubital artery at wrist with thumb and fingers of right hand. Even if doctor felt pulse accurately, he was unable to interpret his findings.

75

MEDICINE STYMIED BY LOGIC

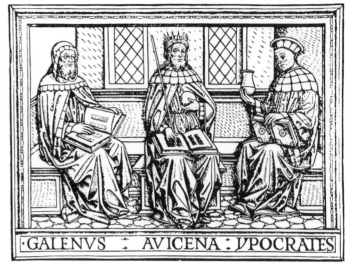

·GALENVS · AVICENA · VPOCRATES·

Masterminds of Medieval Medicine: To know their texts was to be a physician.

When students in the age of scholasticism wanted to find out how many teeth a horse had, they looked up what men like Aristotle or Pliny had to say on the problem. In case they disagreed, brilliant teams locked in a battle of wits and used all tricks of the logical art to arrive at a verdict. The debaters forgot just one thing: to look in the horse's mouth.

The Scholastics believed that any question concerning the universe, heaven, hell or man could be answered by theoretical deduction. The great authorities of the ancient world and the fathers of the Church had already uttered the last word on everything. Science consisted merely in looking into their books and weighing the evidence. Learning became synonymous with logic. The belief persisted that thinking could furnish the answer to any problem — even to that fanciful but typical question of how many angels could sit on the point of a pin.

The growing influence of Aristotle and the Arabic writers since the end of the 12th century sparked this whole movement. The Church had opposed the study of Aristotle up to 1255, when Arabic and Greek translations made his works better known.

Hardly noticeable in early Salerno, Arabic science and philosophy soon gripped the medical imagination as new translations of Averrhoes, Avicenna and Aristotle became available.

The effect of this Arabic-Aristotelian influence on medicine was far from beneficial. The healing art which at Salerno had taken a big step forward toward practical methods once more slipped back into a bookish science. And, of course, that is no science at all.

Medicine thus turned into a mere art of reasoning. On the basis of nothing more than Aristotelian logic, philosophers had no qualms about writing books on medicine. Instead of applying their intellect to the practical evidence of the bedside, the doctors buried their noses in books and busied themselves with commentaries and arguments.

Luckily, however, the seeds of a new medicine did bud forth and soon provided a healthy stimulant for a return to common-sense methods. Surgery played a prominent part in this reformation. More learned than the surgeons, the doctors fell easier prey to the lure of scholastic hyper-intellectualism.

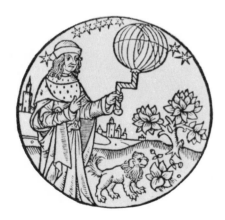

Aristotle in medieval garb. His growing influence made doctors logicians, disinterested in bedside observation.

The surgeons, on the other hand, were craftsmen in the best sense of the word. They found their learning not in books but in the day-to-day struggle with wounds and fractures. The patient's recovery or death put their knowledge to a simple test.

In Bologna a movement gained momentum that was to free medicine from the shackles of scholasticism. The studium generale of Bologna, the cell from which the university grew, boldly affirmed its right to self-government in the face of clerical opposition. Sponsored by a community that had grown affluent through world trade, Bologna's law faculty became the main pivot around which other new schools were grouped.

Theology naturally had a seat here too. But most of the students flocked to Bologna in search of a worldly profession. They wanted to "profess" medicine without having to don the cleric's garb.

The university of Bologna had been organized according to the guild principle, with young men much in prominence. The student was assured of getting his money's worth for his tuition fee, since a professor could not be absent from his lectures for even a day. If a teacher had to leave town he was required to deposit security to insure his return.

Medical instruction had started here early in the 13th century. Distinctly apart from the studium generale, the Medical School was humble in its setting but enjoyed the protection of the powerful law faculty. This gave the university a decidedly secular character. In case of a homicide, f. i. a doctor was called in for an autopsy to turn up possible clues by dis-

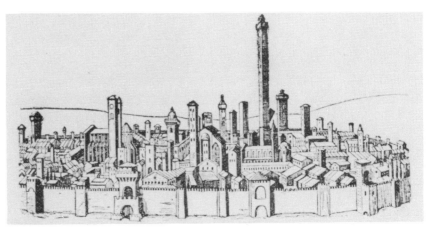

Bologna developed progressive medical teaching based on anatomy.

section. The study of anatomy, in turn, prepared the ground for a flourishing of the surgical craft.

Generally the medieval surgeon, except for the brief Salernitan interlude, rated as the "enfant terrible" of the profession, in the same class as the butcher and the hangman. It was for this reason that, in 1350, the faculty of Paris, forbade its graduates to practice surgery. In Bologna, however, surgery remained a vital part of medicine. Here the atmosphere of comparative freedom spurred the development of fresh surgical talent.

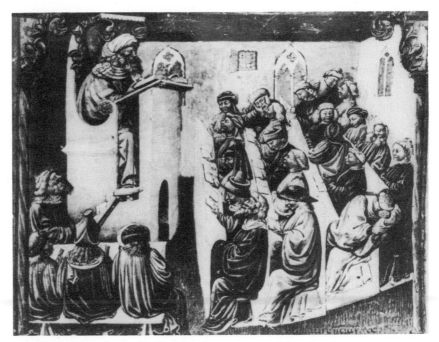

Lecture room in 14th Century Bologna shows laissez-faire attitude of students.

NEW WAYS
TO TREAT WOUNDS

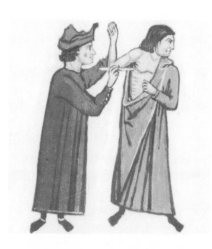

Two doctors, Hugh and Theodoric de Lucca, stood out among the North Italian practitioners of this period.

We have no record of the work of Hugh. Yet through writings of his contemporaries we hear that he refused in 1250 to operate on a nobleman, unless his friends would swear not to hold him responsible should the operation end fatally.

Theodoric (1205-1298), possibly Hugh's son and certainly his pupil, started as a monk and ended as a bishop. His career as a cleric, however, seems not to have impaired his work as a surgeon. His *Chyrurgia* reveals an entirely unconventional approach to surgery. Misguided by the doctrine of Roger of Palermo, surgeons had believed that pus must form in wounds in order to heal. Theodoric vigorously opposed this theory and insisted on absolute cleanliness in all operative procedures.

"Do not impede nature," he admonished his fellow-surgeons, "but let her accomplish agglutinization . . . Keep away from the wound after you have cleansed it thoroughly . . . do not cleanse it with the cautery." Because of its dramatic effects, doctors had widely used this instrument. In the hands of a poorly trained sur-

geon it endangered healthy tissues. Theodoric wanted no part of such methods.

Aside from asepsis, Theodoric recommended anesthesia. He mentions a sponge drenched in hot water containing a mixture of mandrake juice and opium. In cases of difficult surgery the sponge was to be held under the patient's nose. After a little while, "the patient may be cut and will feel nothing as if he were dead."

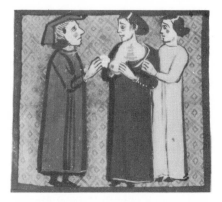

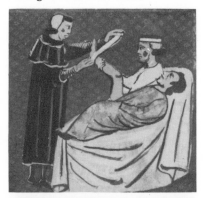

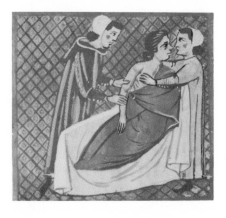

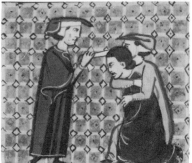

Theoderic de Lucca postulated immaculate cleanliness in all procedures as the basis of surgical success. (14th century miniatures from Theoderic's Surgery in the possession of the University Library of Leyden, Holland.)

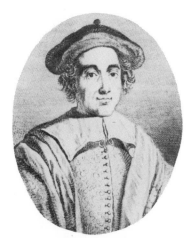

Lanfranc of Milan brought new methods of wound treatment to France.

An Italian surgeon did much to stimulate the rise of the medical arts in 13th century France. Choosing the wrong side in the fight between the Guelfs and the Ghibellines Lanfranc was forced to leave his native Milan. When the exile settled in Paris, he spread the Italian gospel of "healing wounds by first intention" — an expression he introduced. He strove to effect a healing so clean that not a scar could be seen.

The University of Paris rejected him as a teacher because it could not allow any married layman on its strictly clerical faculty. However, in 1295 Lanfranc found ready acceptance in the Confraternity of Surgeons — the Collège de St. Côme. Lanfranc's shrewd pun about doctor's fees sums up his rather worldly attitude toward his patients: "Do all you can for the poor but get all you can from the rich."

Henri de Mondeville shares with Lanfranc the credit for bringing sur-

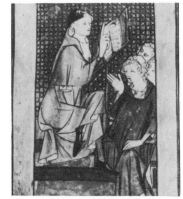

Henri de Mondeville, surgeon-teacher, was cynical about fee collecting.

gery back into the realm of medicine. Like Lanfranc, Mondeville had studied with Theodoric and spread at Montpellier his master's gospel of surgical cleanliness. To enliven his lectures, Henri used 13 anatomical wall charts, reproduced in small scale in a manuscript version of his works. They represent the first known attempt at medico-visual education.

Adept in suturing, Mondeville urged that all wounds be closed speedily to prevent the air from causing pus. (Even 700 years later Lister was still to struggle with this idea.)

Henri had very positive ideas about medical etiquette. "Keep up your patient's spirits by music . . . or by forged letters describing the death of his enemy."

Though the modern doctor cannot go along with such cynical expedients, he may find a basic truth in Mondeville's observation: "Never dine with a patient who is in your debt, but get your dinner at an inn. Otherwise, he will deduct the cost of his hospitality from your fee."

On the payment of medical bills he commented gloomily: "I have never found anyone so rich, or even so honest . . . who was ready to pay what he had promised unless obliged and convicted."

Petrus Hispanus another contemporary crowned his success as a doctor by ascending the papal throne, as John XXI (1276). Born into a doctor's family, he became an accomplished physician. His *Liber de Oculo*, a standard work in its field, won praise for its unusual prescriptions, such as infant's urine as an eyewash. His *Thesaurus Pauperum*, contains among other useful information, a collection of recipes for every known disease. It survived for centuries as an in-dispensable reference book. In it can be found homely hints for first-aid such as: "In hysterical fainting blow pepper and salt up the patient's nose. She will soon come round."

After only seven months of papal glory, John XXI was killed one fine day when the roof collapsed.

John's enemies quickly asserted that when the fatal blow fell the medical pope had been admiring himself in the mirror — "a warning to all those puffed up by their state and dignity."

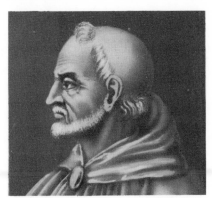

John XXI, doctor and Pope, wrote learnedly on eye care.

INSIDE OUT

ANATOMY ADVANCES

SURGERY RESURGENT

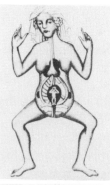

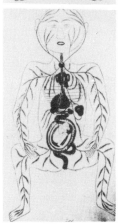

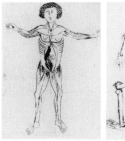
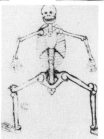

Much as had been done by the great surgeon-teachers of this age, their efforts were bound to remain hamstrung—as long as the basic discipline, anatomy, remained banned from the curricula. During the crusades, the Church had taken a stand against dissection of the human body. While the School of Bologna had been able to circumvent the clerical dictum, the ban had stymied medical progress in most other schools.

Actually, Pope Boniface VIII had issued his famous bull of 1300 against the cutting up of dead bodies with good reason. The crusaders had adopted the practice of boiling their dead comrades, severing the flesh from their bones, and shipping the bones back home, to avoid burial on heathen ground. When the Church put a stop to this barbarous custom, the ban was interpreted to include all human dissection.

But clandestine autopsies were performed in spite of the order. Under the pressure of avid students anatomy

Outdoor class in anatomy at University of Paris. Students exhibit livelier interest in corpse than in professor's preachings from Galen.

was gradually accepted as an academic subject.

Mondino de Luzzi of Bologna (1275?-1327), ranks as the first great anatomy teacher. Though Galen dominated his lectures, he taught anatomy in a systematic way, and gave his students their first glimpse into the body.

As his star pupil, Guy de Chauliac described it: "My master . . . having placed the body on a table . . . gave four discourses over it; the first dealt with the nutritive organs, because they putrefy first; the second, with the spiritual members; the third, with the animal members; the fourth, with the extremities . . . In this way, he teaches anatomy from the bodies of men, monkeys, swine, and other animals, and not from pictures, as did Henri de Mondeville."

Guy de Chauliac had studied in Bologna. Bringing the new gospel of anatomy to France, he put surgery on a more rational basis. Formerly, surgeons had merely cured wounds. De Chauliac raised surgery to its rightful place as an independent department of the medical arts. As an operator, he personified the bold, yet thoughtful surgeon-in-action. As a teacher, he put forth his *Great Surgery*, of 1363, a textbook based on intense anatomi-

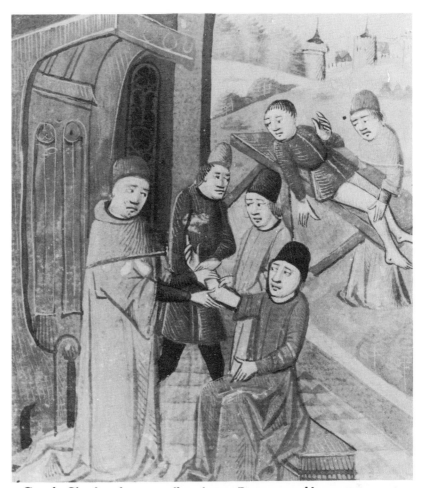

Guy de Chauliac diagnoses elbow lesion. Patient on table awaits operation.

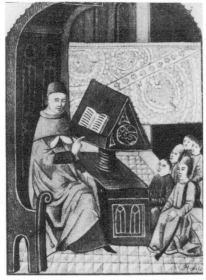

Guy de Chauliac (1300-1368) lecturing.

cal study. The book gained its author worldwide repute and was translated into French, Provencal, English, Italian, Dutch and Hebrew.

His credo showed him as a man of vision and high idealism: "A good surgeon should be acquainted with liberal studies, with medicine, and above all with anatomy; he should be courteous . . . bold in security, cautious in time of danger, circumspect in prognosis, pious and merciful, not greedy of gain, but looking for his fee in moderation, according to the extent of his services."

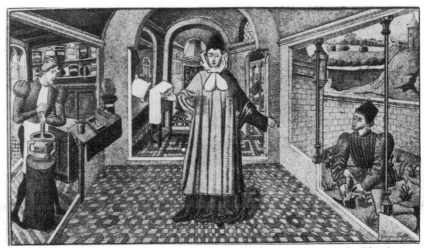

Hospital pharmacists prepare ointment under direction of Guy de Chauliac.

81

WOMAN'S TROUBLE - A.D. 1400

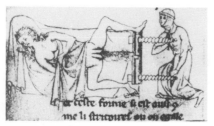

Galen dressed in medieval garb, lectures on woman's disease and anatomy.

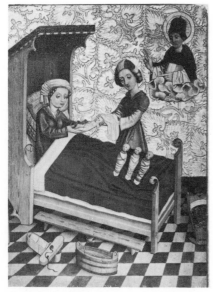

Vaginal dilator first described by Arabs, reappears in 14th century.

During the Middle Ages gynecology was a weedy, neglected patch within the field of medicine. Women were known in those days as "sisters of Eve," and as such, they represented sin incarnate. Their sufferings were shrugged off by legitimate physicians. They considered it beneath their dignity to take action. Thus, Guy de Chauliac, "the Restorer of Surgery" disposed of gynecology with three short paragraphs. The *Breviarium Practicae* (ascribed to Arnold of Villanova) impudently treated the subject along with the natural history of vipers, "since women are for the most part poisonous creatures." If pictorial evidence is any criterion, this gross medical neglect could hardly be blamed on the age-old cult of feminine modesty.

Actually, most medical literature about female disease was too speculative and inaccurate, in medieval times, to be of any real value. Some scholastics held the comfortable belief that menstruation was merely woman's atonement for Eve's original sin, while others explained it as a surplus of the four humours. These latter savants thought that "woman by nature has more blood than man." This brought about the natural month-

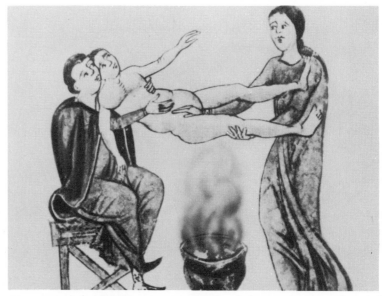

Inter-vaginal fumigation, an ancient form of therapy in cases of genital troubles, was highly recommended by medieval scholars.

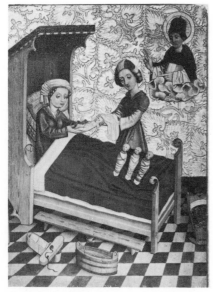

Quadruplets presented to neatly dressed mother. Tyrolean painting. 15th century.

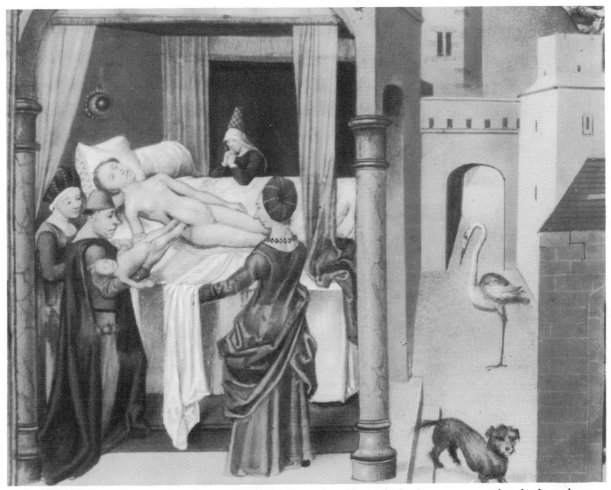

Caesarian operations could not but end fatally for the mother. The methods of extraction were hopelessly crude.

ly outlet. Albertus Magnus, the great Dominican theoretician, deduced from this that women were "hotter" by temperament than men. It was wrong, therefore, he concluded, to forbid them to indulge in regular sexual intercourse.

But among this plethora of nonsense, some few insights were decidedly prescient. The famous prophetess, Hildegard of Bingen, for instance, seems to have had a shrewd inkling of modern organo-therapy; to secure fertility, she suggested that sterile women should dine on the uteri of virgin cows and sheep.

If gynecology was a weedy, neglected patch of medieval medicine, obstetrics, in the modern sense of the word, was the jungle itself, remote and unexplored, and governed largely by God. He had willed that women in labor must be left to their own devices. Childbirth, therefore, was simply unlisted in the medieval book of medicine, and the feudal mother was entrusted to the frequently dirty hands of a dowdy band of midwives. These midwives were hired at times by city governments; they were sworn in legally, and all gynecological questions under the law (such as rape) were remanded to them, rather than to physicians. Though the medieval lying-in chambers often seem neat and comfortable, the midwives themselves had so little practical knowledge, and their training was so inadequate, that the mother's chances for survival from parturition were less than even. The great dangers were puerperal fever and sheer butchery, from clumsy tactics during a difficult accouchment. Even primitive tribes had more advanced manual aids for birth than the medieval midwives.

83

JOHN OF ARDERNE SUGGESTS:

TEST FOR ANAL CANCER

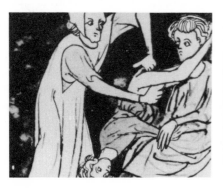

John of Arderne, proctologist.

In England, John of Arderne (1307-1390) performed almost the same service for surgery as did Guy de Chauliac in France. Both men had studied at Montpellier. Arderne stayed on the continent as an army surgeon, and so acquired his first experience in surgery and proctology. Hemorrhoids, anal inflammations and fistulae were occupational diseases in those days, since the knights in armor spent most of their time on horseback. Thus, when Arderne returned to England to take up private practice in 1350, he was well equipped to deal with anal troubles. He developed an ingenious operation for "fistula in ano," and performed it frequently among his princely clientele. (Dr. Ralph Major has calculated that Arderne's fee for an operation would correspond to about $48,000 today.)

Arderne was probably one of the first surgeons to formulate the threat of cancer. "I have never seen any man who recovered from cancer," he wrote, "but I have known many who died of it." He was an excellent diagnostician, and therefore able to distinguish astutely between the somewhat identical symptoms of anal cancer and fistula. In both diseases, the patient is driven to stool and complains of darting pain. Arderne suggested that the surgeon should first insert his finger in the patients' anus. If he detected a normal fistula, he could operate; but if he detected a hard, stony mass ("a tumour of great hardness . . . called bubo from an owl, because that bird lurks in darkness"), the patient had cancer, and the doctor was urged to abstain from any surgery.

"It will only give you disgrace if you operate," said Arderne. Instead, the doctor should mollify the pain through palliative enemata, and advise the family that "there is no cure, and death is at the gates." Arderne was wise enough to know that a surgeon's success often depends on his ability to resist the urge to operate.

In 1376, this pioneer proctologist wrote his famous treatises: *Fistulae in Ano* and *The Use of Rectal Injections*. In these works, he described his equally famous operation for hemorrhoids (see below).

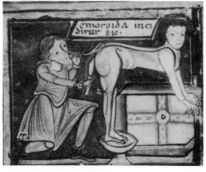

Grave anal problem is appraised at left. Arderne advised against surgery if cancer were detected, but devised operation for hemorrhoids (right). Patient leans on block as doctor hooks down and clips off offending veins. To staunch blood, patient was afterwards seated on hot sponges.

84

In an age of chivalry, Arderne was held in high esteem by many noble families, and frequently served as body physican for the great knights of the day. He practiced among the nobility at Newark and London, and wrote extensive treatises on the general field of surgery. Here again his advice holds good today: "If you must cut, do so boldly." But he also fell victim to the superstitions of the time, and relied on the efficacy of charms and amulets for internal diseases beyond reach of the knife. To cure epilepsy, for instance, he recommended that the patient wear a piece of paper around his neck on which the words "Jasper Balthazar" had been written with the blood of his little finger.

CHAUCER'S "DOCTOUR"

In the Canterbury Tales, Chaucer, Arderne's contemporary, delivered a caustic description of the English practitioner. His "doctour" spouted Aesculapius at all times, and looked to the stars (and the four humours)

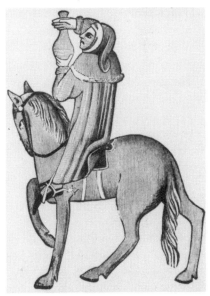

for guidance. This poetic figure has since been identified as Dr. John Gaddesden, whose *Rosa Anglica* drew similar caustic fire from Guy de Chauliac (he called it a "Rose — not too sweet smelling, and made up of children's fables"). But Gaddesden stumbled on the ultra-red light theory five centuries before its time: when Prince John had smallpox, he wrapped him in red cloth, and hung red curtains around bed and sickroom to cure the disease and reduce pockmarks.

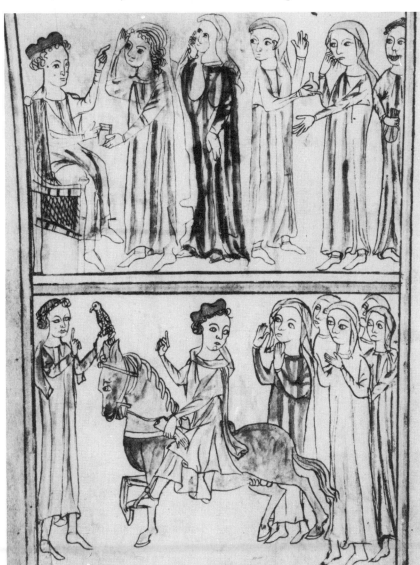

Group of ladies (above) consult English doctor. Assistant at far right holds purse, ready to collect. (below) Doctor departs, acclaimed by grateful patients.

85

DOCTORS COPE WITH NEW HEALTH HAZARDS

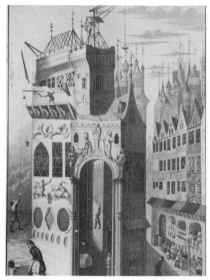

With the revival of trade in the 14th century cities rose in importance, while manor and monastery declined. The merchants had amassed large fortunes, and the population of Europe began its gradual shift to urban centers of wealth. Here the craftsman gained freedom from feudal taxes and churchly restraint. Patrician and merchant bought up his goods and services to furnish homes or embellish wardrobes. Here, too, the abandoned serf sought work or bread, but found instead a new and terrible kind of poverty and filth.

Meanwhile, the new universities fostered the revival of learning; under their supervision, the first trained physicians emerged to shake loose the clerical hold on medicine. They found in the merchant and patrician families a new group of pecunious patients — but there were other classes too, requiring medical care.

The Rise of the City. Craftsmen at left build upper wall. Shops at right sell boots, cloaks, hats. New towns created both wealth and squalor.

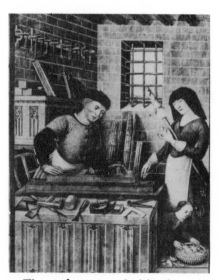

The craftsman worked hard to sustain his newfound prosperity; and for security he joined the ubiquitous guild. These close-knit trade associations furnished food and nursing care for members in distress, and even set funds aside for their funerals.

Patricians ruled the new city-states. Their fortunes grew and brought about a search for beauty and comfort. Money was made and spent, and prosperity spread among the artisans. The doctor, who aligned himself with a rich patrician family also prospered and assumed aristocratic airs.

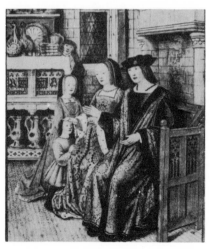

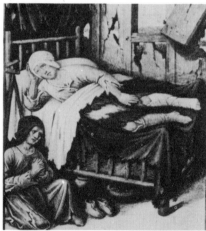

The serfs were now abandoned to utter squalor, with fresh air as their only bounty. The old serf could only pray for delivery from his disconsolate state. The young serfs might try their luck in the city. With no trade to pursue and no field to till, most of them joined the mounting ranks of beggary.

86

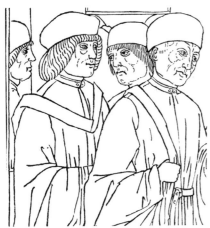

The guilds were town life incarnate in the late Middle Ages. Each of the trades banded together to supervise its members, and the guilds themselves joined to help administer the city government. Even the beggars had their "union," and so did the lay physicians.

By the early 1300's, the doctors' guild in Florence had attained sixth place among the tradesmen, between the silk workers and the skinners. In their struggle for recognition, physicians set new standards: no Florentine could practice medicine, for instance, until he had passed the public examination conducted by consuls of the guild. When the plague of 1348 revealed a doctor shortage, the physician's guild moved up to second place, to attract more practitioners. Standards were again raised in 1349 by a law which forced all doctors to attend courses and periodic dissections at the School of Medicine.

In 1377, the city fathers of Nuremberg revived the ancient practice of hiring a "city doctor" to treat the indigent. A certain Magister Petrus was given a salary, a horse and a supply of farm products to act as "medicus noster." He was expected to stay at his post in time of plague. In 1426, Emperor Sigismund is said to have decreed that each imperial city must hire a town physicus to attend the poor at a salary of 100 guilders a year — "For the high-hattish Masters of Physics give their service free to nobody — wherefore they all will go to hell"

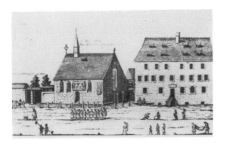

AGING SUCCESSFULLY
. . . MEDIEVAL VERSION

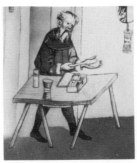

WOUND SURGEON

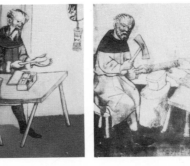

FILE-MAKER

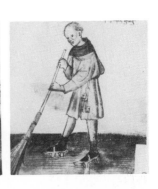

STREET SWEEPER

The idea of social security dates from 1388, when Konrad Mendel founded the "Guild of the Twelve Brothers." This practical merchant knew that middle class artisans, once they grew old, had little to fall back on. Accordingly, he established a home in Nuremberg to give security and happiness to the twelve (for the apostles) craftsmen who could live there worry-free (see home and brothers in above sketch). The brothers had to be honorable citizens of Nuremberg; they could be sick, but not bedridden. Mendel provided them with workshops so they might continue their trades at leisure — a wise solution for geriatric problems even today. There was an adjoining chapel for prayer, but the project was wholly sustained by patrician governors. Here was a clear example of a worldly group which attempted to solve new urban social problems — the former province of the church.

The Mendel foundation lasted for over 500 years, deriving its support from landholdings. As each new brother entered the guild, he sat for a portrait which showed him busily engaged at his trade. These portraits yield invaluable information on crafts in the rising towns.

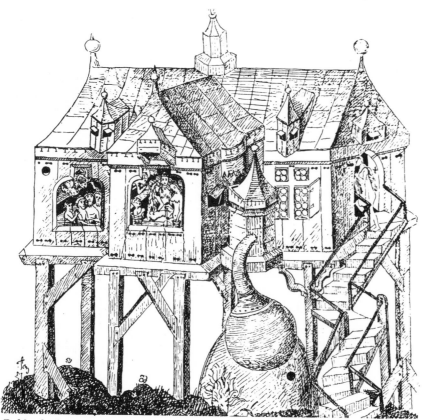

Housewife spills slop on serenaders.

CITY LIFE -
BEWARE OF CONTAGION

City air makes free, the saying went in the late Middle Ages. And free it was indeed, for work or trade — but decidedly malodorous. A great stench rose up from the garbage and filth piled high in city lanes and ditches. When country folk moved into town, their cattle added to the foul confusion. Pigs roamed the streets at will (poor Philip, son of Louis the Fat, was killed, for instance, when his horse shied at a hog in front of the Royal Palace). The newcomers were baffled by the congested living conditions; they camped like gypsies in dark, airless rooms, and tossed their slop and offal through the windows with no regard for passersby.

This total lack of sanitation among the poor affected whole towns and brought on the danger of contagion. The homes and bodies of most patients needed scrubbing before medicine could be effective, but water was then at a premium, and canals for slop had yet to be employed. Then the great plagues struck the congested centers, and compiled their methodical equation between filth and death. As the bodies mounted, the doctors began to formulate new principles of public hygiene and quarantine which led, slowly, to the reform of communal living. In the meantime, the cities attempted half-measures to cope with the hopeless squalor.

Public bathing, an old Roman custom, had been kept alive by the widespread Germanic tradition of river bathing. Now, in the 13th century, the custom was revived, and increasing numbers of public bathhouses appeared in the cities. They were in no way an index of personal cleanliness, however; people of all classes were vermin-ridden; their homes had almost no facilities for washing, and

Public bath with central heating system as depicted by Konrad Kyesser (1405).

public sweat baths simply gave them a chance for comfort and relief. Thus, the withdrawal of bathing privileges was considered a fearful punishment. When Henry IV was excommunicated by the Church, for instance, he was forbidden to take hot baths. Conversely, a guest was always highly honored when offered a bath, and the poor considered money for baths (badgeld) as a great blessing.

Modesty never really existed at a time when whole families huddled together in one bed, uninhibited by nightgowns. So men and women flocked to the public tubs together. They rejoiced in scraping the dirt off itching bodies, and with their ablution came song, drink, dance and debauchery. These mixed frolics resulted in prostitution at the bathhouse, but worse than this, the congregation of all kinds of people in the same tubs proved highly unsanitary. Though the city fathers had built them with good intentions, the baths soon flourished as centers of public contagion.

The main trouble was management. Instead of employing doctors as supervisors, the baths were turned over to the "bathers," a venal group quite willing to admit riffraff to the tubs and adjoining bedrooms. Like the barbers, the bathers also performed bloodletting and minor surgery.

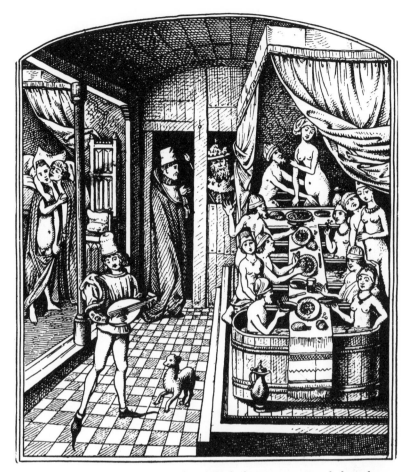

Mixed bath for aristocratic couples. Monk despairs at moral degradation.

By the 14th century, the civic authorities began to restrict the public baths. The plagues had brought out the idea of contagion, and orders were issued against bathing during an epidemic. All victims of contagious diseases were debarred from the public baths till four to eight weeks after recovery. Finally, in the 16th century, syphilis delivered the *coup de grace* to public bathing. The triumphant march of this disease through Europe instilled a collective fear of infection, and communal indoor bathing lost its popularity.

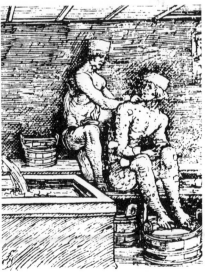

Syphilis led to closing of baths.

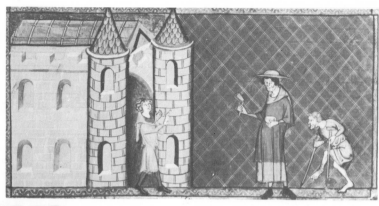

Garbed in traditional costume, leper begs for alms. The afflicted were compelled to wear fur shoes and gloves to prevent spread of disease.

LEPROSY CONQUERED

Medieval man apparently had no real fear of infection; he stepped into the public tub without a second thought. Yet he knew something about contagion as evinced by his efforts to combat leprosy. Isolation of the lepers was strictly enforced.

As early as 583 A.D., the Church had prohibited the free movement of lepers, and had charged its clerics to separate all cases from the flock. The victim of the disease was compelled to wear burial shrouds and to lie in a coffin before the altar. Then earth was strewn on the afflicted and the priest declared him legally dead. From that day on, the leper had to beg alms to support himself.

He also had to carry a pointing stick, to indicate those objects he wanted to buy from itinerant merchants (he was forced to purchase whatever he touched, however inadvertently). His hands were gloved, and fur shoes were placed on his feet to prevent any spread of infection to barefooted wayfarers. Though he entered most towns with impunity, he was often accused of polluting wells and threatened with death.

The Church came to the rescue, however, by founding leprosaria. Matilda, the wife of Henry I, founded several herself, and was famous for washing and kissing the lepers' wounds. By the end of the 13th century, Europe was studded with these leper houses, (there were 2000 in France alone), and the disease soon slackened off. As the 16th century dawned this threat to communal health had been almost completely removed.

Unfortunately, the concept of contagion was confined to leprosy alone. When the plague struck Europe in the 14th century, the medical profession failed to apply the obvious lesson. So the epidemic lashed out across the continent with unchecked fury.

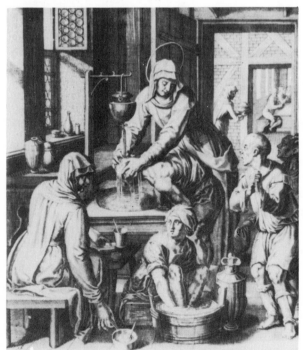

Dressed in telltale garments, he wandered from town to town, clacking a rattle to warn all men of his approach.

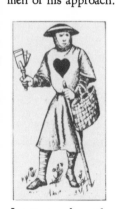

90   *Saintly nuns wash lepers' sores in lazar house.*

Leper sounds rattle

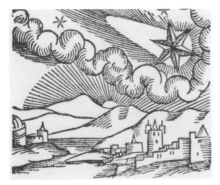

THE BLACK DEATH

The plague which struck Europe in 1347 rang down the curtain on the Middle Ages. Bishop, baron and serf alike were slaughtered by the great equalizer, and the whole feudal structure came tumbling down. Towns and villages were literally wiped off the map. In cities like Florence, Venice and London, over 100,000 inhabitants perished. In Paris and in Avignon, the harvest of death added up to 50,000.

All normal life was paralyzed. "So contagious was the disease," wrote Guy de Chauliac, "that no one could approach or even see a patient without taking the disease. The father did not visit the son, nor the son the father. Charity was dead and hope abandoned." Infants sucked on the breasts of dead mothers, and ghost ships sailed the seas with their crews sprawled motionless along the decks.

The Black Death turned Europe into an abyss of horror; it was probably the most devastating pandemic in world history, and in its wake came crime, unemployment, and further scourges of influenza, scurvy and dancing mania.

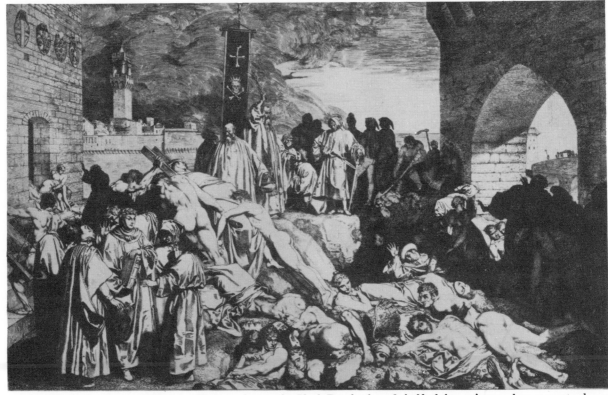

Florence during the Black Death of 1348; half of the city's populace was wiped out.

91

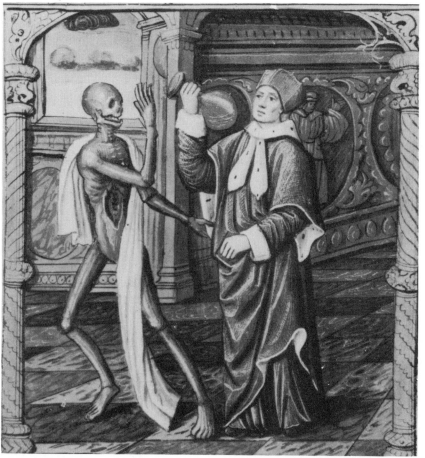

PLAGUE DAZES DOCTORS

In many of the plague-stricken communities, a macabre pantomime was performed, the "Dance of Death." The idea was to exorcise the disease, to outdo death. Strangely enough, even the doctor appeared in the dance, as helpless as Everyman when tugged at by the grinning skeleton.

What could the doctor do to stem the plague? In the words of Guy de Chauliac, who witnessed the epidemic at Avignon, "It was useless and shameful for the physicians, especially because they did not care to visit the sick for fear of becoming themselves afflicted, and if they visited them, they gave nothing, for all afflicted died, except a few, who towards the end, escaped."

Chauliac was one of the few who escaped with a light attack, and even he stuck to his post in Avignon only "in order to avoid infamy." Other physicians fled, and were labeled as cowards; or if they remained, they were accused of murdering patients to acquire their fortunes, or of charging outrageous fees. These accusations were based, no doubt, on an undercurrent of popular resentment: when faced with the horrors of plague, the profession had nothing more concrete to offer than bombast.

The doctors learnedly ascribed the plague to astral influences, to comets whose tails had poisoned the world. Or they remained silent as the populace blamed Jews and lepers for poisoning the wells, and drove off or slaughtered these innocent scapegoats. Then the "polluted" wells were sealed, and the people drank water from the same rivers in which deceased plague victims were being dumped.

Medical remedies were equally preposterous. To clear the plague-ridden air, the learned doctors advised the use of strong odors, since "poison counteracts poison." Patients were urged to stand with an empty stomach over a latrine, and to inhale the stench for hours. The chief medical standby, of course, was phlebotomy; but bleeding simply drained the poor victim of all his strength, and thus hastened his death. According to Chauliac, external swellings could be softened with figs and cooked onions, peeled and mixed with yeast (foreshadowing the use of antibiotics), then opened and treated like ulcers. Plague boils were cupped, scarified, and cauterized. Fires were lighted in the streets to clear the air, and purgatives were widely employed to clear the system, but all such remedies proved futile. About a quarter of the population of Europe was wiped out.

A few sound lessons were driven home, however, during the epidemic. Although Gentile de Foligno died of plague in Perugia, Italy, he left behind a sensible blueprint for medico-municipal action in times of crisis. Such plans were soon adopted. In 1374, Venice became the first city to forbid travellers or merchants who might be infected with plague from entering the town gates. Three years later, the republic of Ragusa, in Dalmatia, established the first quarantine system. Cargoes and sailors from plague-stricken regions were detained for 30, later 40 days on an adjacent island. (The time limit was finally fixed at 40 because all acute diseases, like the biblical flood, were believed to be limited to that duration.) The cargoes were unladen, fumigated and, if necessary, destroyed. Even the sailors were wisely exposed to air and sunshine. In 1383, Marseilles followed suit with a special quarantine station. Throughout Italy, public measures were codified at this time for airing homes, burning clothes and controlling roads and water supplies. This recognition of the need for social protection supplanted the old theological reliance on prayer and resignation.

The concept of communal medicine proved helpful when the plague returned to Europe in the 15th century. This time, the cities recovered more quickly; their political and cultural growth continued without serious interruption, and the science of medicine began to thrive in the new centers of learning.

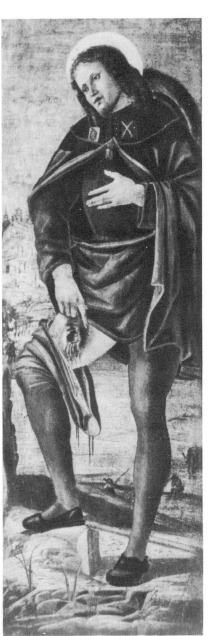

Saint Roch, (above), points to sore contracted while tending plague sufferers. Plague boils appeared on groin and in armpits, accompanied by gangrenes and inflammation of the throat. St. Roch recovered from plague but died wretchedly when imprisoned in Montpellier dungeon.

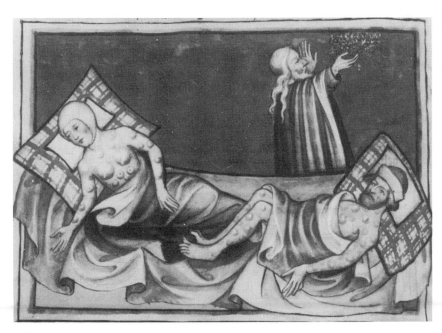

Doctor despairs at two patients covered with plague buboes.

93

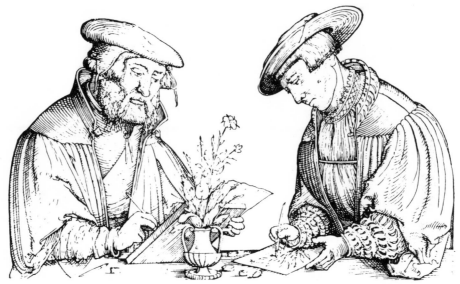

Artists sketch herbs directly from nature to enhance medical texts.

NEW VISTAS FOR MAN AND MEDICINE

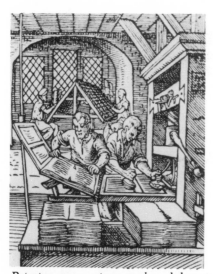

Printing gave wings to knowledge; it sped the dissemination of medical news. This in turn awakened interest in research. Yet improvement of practical medicine was rather slow in coming.

The epidemics of the 14th century, struck damaging blows at urban life, but they could not check the steady advance of civilization. In ravaged Italy, the people recovered with remarkable resilience. They patched their wounds and reshuffled their political and intellectual forces. By the beginning of the 15th century, the peninsula fairly rocked with the power of new ideas. Art, science and medicine burgeoned with undreamed of vitality, and a whole new concept of life was born.

In the Middle Ages, man's earthly trials had been considered as mere preparation for heavenly redemption. Worldly pleasures and concerns seemed sacrilegious, or at best unimportant.

But with the dawn of the Renaissance, this attitude was reversed. Man set himself up once more in the center of the stage and, instead of contemplating Heaven and Hell, he contemplated himself and the universe. Problems of health, science and culture took on new significance; the senses were aroused, and powers of observation were renewed by man's close attention to nature. Taking a cue from the ancient Greeks, man discovered himself.

His desire for knowledge and beauty was inspired by the serene ageless quality of Greek art, and by the wisdom of Greek literature. Consequently, he searched avidly for long-lost works of sculpture, and for

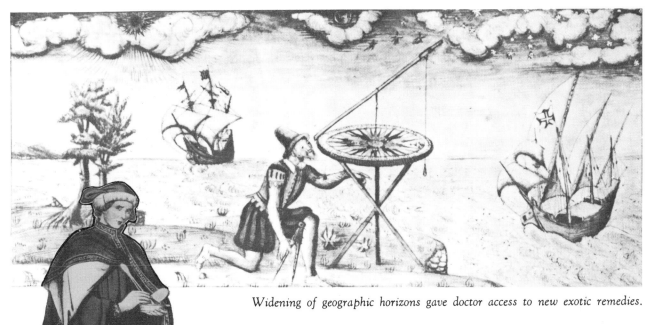

Widening of geographic horizons gave doctor access to new exotic remedies.

Doctors exchanged clerical garb for rich robe of Renaissance academician.

original manuscripts. This latter quest became almost a mania, since the ponderous interpretations and comments of Arab and medieval scholastics had distorted the originals beyond recognition. But aid was received from an unexpected quarter. The Turks took Constantinople in 1453. Greek scholars fled to Italy and there performed the invaluable task of translating and editing the original works for their new hosts. Greek wisdom, medical and otherwise, was at last available to satisfy the growing appetite for knowledge.

The Arabs too had contributed something valid. Their numerals, mathematical learning, algebra and arithmetic, were vital to the shift from qualitative to quantitative methods in science. Measurement began to replace speculation during the Renaissance, or at least there were signs that a flexible system of mathematics would bolster the advance of science in the succeeding century.

This horn of plenty inevitably spilled over directly onto the field of medicine. As man became the very center of human interest, his body was made the subject of ardent research. Artists worked hand-in-hand with doctors in the attempt to explore the body's miracles. They did so out of the same passion for observation and research which made the Renaissance "the Age of the Eye." Instead of imitating hackneyed illustrations of men, animals and plants, the artists looked to nature for inspiration. By the end of the 15th century, the first valid studies of morbid anatomy had been made.

At the same time, geographical expansion reaped a whole new crop of plant-medicines and healing drugs. And the invention of printing gave the medical profession a chance to study precedents and obtain guidance from masters old and new. Once more the artists helped by illustrating medical texts with remarkable skill and accuracy.

At first tradition incarnate, scholastic medicine, did not give way before these assaults of a new naturalism. The medieval dogma was too deeply imbedded in the universities. But by the mid-16th century Vesalius had published his striking text on anatomy, Paré was at work on the battlefield, Paracelsus was shouting from the platform and the walls of medieval medicine at long last began to crumble.

95

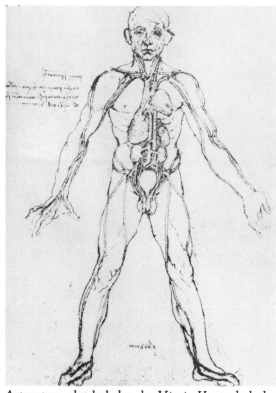

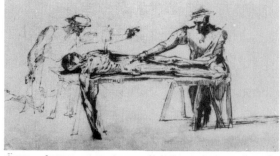

Artists dissect corpse by candlelight to discover "mathematics" of human form (see compass at left).

DA VINCI AND DÜRER

ARTISTS SPEARHEAD MEDICAL ADVANCE

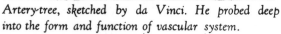

Artery-tree, sketched by da Vinci. He probed deep into the form and function of vascular system.

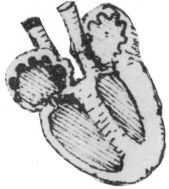

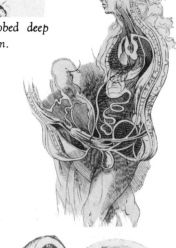

Da Vinci explored hydraulic interaction of heart and blood vessels. It was his opinion that man was only "as old as his arteries." (Above left).

Study of coitus (above right). Leonardo held that female ovum, and seed of male had equal power in generative process.

Uterus during pregnancy: Da Vinci was first to show womb's accurate form.

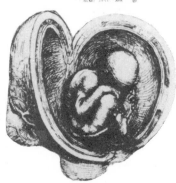

I t was an artist with decided medical leanings who gave the world an astounding example of the Renaissance mind at work. In an effort to correlate art and anatomy Leonardo da Vinci (1452-1519) produced a magnificent series of notes and drawings on the structure and function of the human body.

By candlelight, the great artist dissected over 30 bodies in the Santo Spirito mortuary in Rome. From these dissections, he conceived about 1000 sketches, which he and Marco Antonio della Torre planned to use in a monumental encyclopedia of human anatomy. Unfortunately, his co-worker died and the whole revolutionary project was abandoned. Had the drawings been published, they might have hastened the rate of medical progress.

96

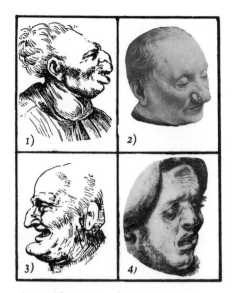

Artists depict age, disease, pain:
1) *Leonardo — man with goiter.*
2) *Ghirlandajo — rhinophyma.*
3) *Leonardo — old man.*
4) *Dürer — man in pain.*

They preceded Vesalius by 40 odd years, but remained unknown until some redrawings appeared in 1796.

Da Vinci had by-passed Galen and started afresh, with the corpse as his only text. He had sketched in great detail and shown an amazing insight into the workings of the heart, lungs, brain, uterus and muscle structure. He injected wax into the organs before dissecting them, and constructed wire cages about lower limbs to examine the play of muscular forces. Da Vinci was the first to study carefully foetal membranes and cerebral nerves; he was the first, as well, to dissect the brain and to describe body muscles and their functions. To explore the structure of the eye-ball, the boiled it in the white of an egg and studied its solidified sections.

Like other artists of his day, da Vinci was determined to depict man,

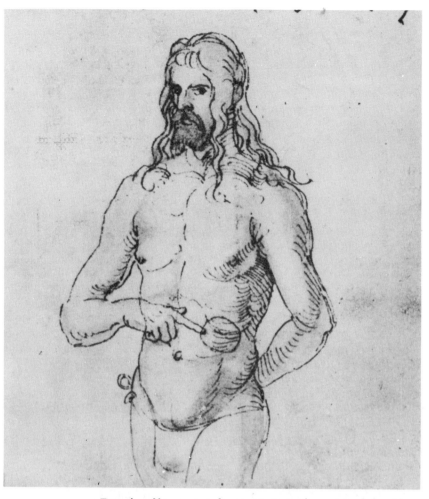

Dürer's self-portrait indicating pain in the region of the spleen.

for better or worse, in all his phases. Accordingly, he followed condemned criminals to the gallows to record their fear-distorted faces. He tried to discover the emotional as well as the physical qualities of man, and here, too, he provided medicine with a basic concept.

Da Vinci and other Renaissance painters portrayed man in sickness and decay; their subjects emerged not as types, but as individuals in pain and anguish. Now the physicians began to observe the effects of disease with similar discernment.

"On the yellow spot where I point my finger, there I have pain."

These are the words Albrecht Dürer scribbled on a self-portrait he sent to his doctor. The artist might have caught a quartan fever when he went to sketch a whale on the Netherlands coast. In this revealing note Dürer pictured effects of his own disease in the region of the spleen. He died in 1528. His friend, Pirckheimer, dubbed in the final sketch verbally: Dürer had "withered like a bundle of dry straw." But his pupils went on to illustrate medical texts.

97

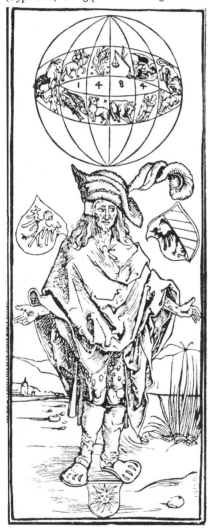

Demon afflicts Job with skin eruption. (Syphilis?) Burgkmair drawing.

SYPHILIS FLOORS EUROPE

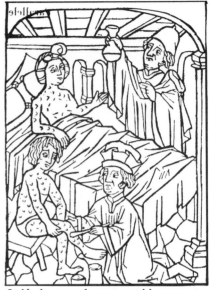

Sickbed scene from pamphlet warning the people of syphilitic infection (1497).

Syphilis has kept in step with western civilization for at least five centuries. According to one chain of evidence, still strongly contested, the pestilence was America's gift to Europe. It struck Naples in 1494, when the city was already rocked by a see-saw battle between French and Spanish troops. Some of the latter had sailed with Columbus. They reputedly had picked up a strange disease in the Indies, which they now passed on to the democratic ladies of Naples. The ladies relayed it in turn to the French when the city changed hands. A year later, the French soldiers were driven off. They returned home, and in three years' time syphilis "plagues" broke out in France, Germany, Switzerland, Holland, Scotland, Hungary and Russia. The great voyagers took it along with them to India, China and Japan, while Jews and Mohammedans, driven from Spain, carried it to North Africa. Thus, syphilis became the calling card of civilized man, who left it at every port he chanced to visit.

Albrecht Dürer drew first pictures of syphilis-type disease, ascribed it to stellar disturbances of 1484, which hover above in zodiac form (left).

Before this epidemic, a mild form of syphilis might have been mistaken in Europe for leprosy, which was known to be contagious. In fact, when the first virulent spread of syphilis began, the people often confused it with leprosy. They knew it to be transferable through contact with the stricken and in its early form syphilis was probably passed on by various types of infection, aside from intercourse.

The origin of the disease seemed obvious, too: the Italians, Turks and English blamed it on the French; the French blamed it on the Italians; the Russians blamed it on the Poles; the Spanish on the Españolas; and the peoples of India and the Japanese blamed it on the Portuguese — all with some justification.

At first physicians tried to dodge the challenge of the new epidemic. They simply refused to examine a disease which began in the "most degrading and ignoble places of the body."

Guaiacum was the "miracle drug" of the Renaissance, the sure-cure which swept through Europe in the wake of syphilis. Guaiac wood came from America, as some said syphilis did. This tallied well with a popular belief: that the Almighty provides the cure of an ailment in the place of its origin. Unfortunately, for the syphilitics, the "holy wood" contained few if any curative properties. This did not prevent its rapid adoption by the medical profession, however, and its amazing if shortlived reputation for curing the dread disease.

In the copper engraving below, from Stradanus' *Nova Reperta*, guaiacum is glorified as the medical triumph of the age. The frame at the left gives a magic flashback to the scene of the infection, a house of prostitution. The patient (at extreme left) is drinking guaiac broth, almost his only nourishment for ten to fourteen days. His physician stands before him, grasping an evergreen rod, the symbol of recovery. On the right, appears a servant who chops off guaiacum wood, to be ground down, weighed and cooked by the near-

by helpers. Guaiac foam was also smeared on the patient's chancres, but his chances of recovery, depended on faith and the meagre benefits of rest. Faith was provided by the Fuggers, an Augsburg trading concern which had cornered the world market on guaiacum. They waged an intensive campaign in behalf of the cure, and even founded a model hospital in Augsburg to administer their product. They also kept prices high, and were suspected to be in league with the members of the medical profession in Germany and other countries.

Guaiacum cure for syphilis. From Stradanus, Nova Reperta — a pictorial tribute to great discoveries of the age.

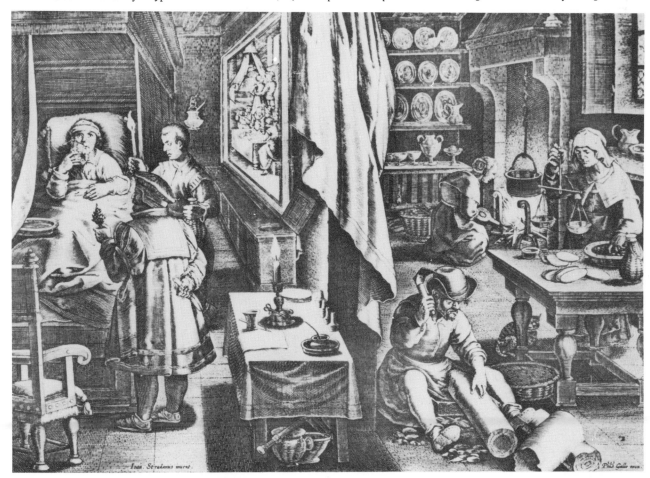

ULRICH VON HUTTEN

A SYPHILIS DIARY

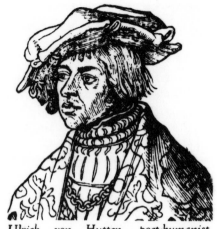

Ulrich von Hutten, poet-humanist (1488-1523) exposed syphilis.

Ulrich von Hutten gauged syphilis as de Quincey later gauged opium: with the care and affection of an indomitable opponent. Hutten contracted the disease in his early twenties, then jotted down a pithy, invaluable report on his sufferings in the years that followed. In those days, syphilis was a "gentleman's disease" and a popular topic. Thus, when Hutten's book was published in 1519, he dedicated it to archbishop Albert of Mayence.

Hutten's physicians first tried to cure him by experimenting with "foreign drugs." They even forbade him to eat peas, since there were "worms therein which had wings" — an early reference to contagium vivum. Then Hutten was abruptly faced with the famous mercury cure. As he described it, his inflamed pustules were anointed with burning mercury salve, though the fluxions had already started to gnaw on the tissues. He was next shoved into a large stove, where he lived for 30 days on a starvation diet. Such stoves were heated with glowing coals, while the patients inside were constantly covered with freshly-warmed towels. Since the chamber was sealed against fresh air, the less stalwart victims either suffocated or died of heart failure during the ordeal.

Hutten came back for ten more mercury cures, though wiser patients preferred to expire from the disease itself. Later, when guaiacum became the rage, the famous humanist hailed its discovery. He considered himself cured (falsely) after 40 days on guaiac juice.

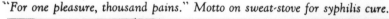

"For one pleasure, thousand pains." Motto on sweat-stove for syphilis cure.

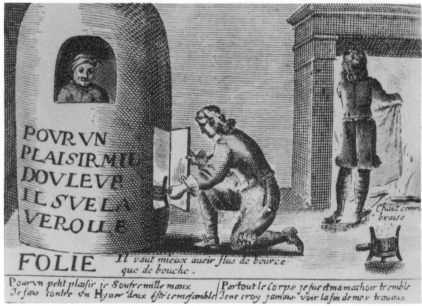

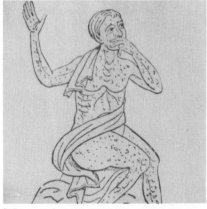

Mercurial poisoning from syphilis cure (above) brings patient's hand to jaw, where stomatosis has eaten away mucous of mouth. Rabelais pitied patients greased with mercury, "their faces sharp as a butcher knife, their teeth rattling like the key-board of a broken down spinet" (Pantagruel II).

FRACASTORIUS

A SYPHILIS POEM

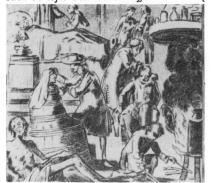

Hieronymus Fracastorius, epidemiologist (1483-1553) named syphilis.

Though Hutten's book was a case history, it described all aspects of the scourge, its background and potential cure. But Ulrich von Hutten wrote like a discerning poet, about "boils that stood out like acorns, from whence issued such filthy stinking matter, that, whosoever came within scent believed himself infected." His pen was moved by compassion.

Syphilis pavilion shows patient at right receiving mercury-salve massage, while lady takes "double-barreled" sweat-bath at left. Bedridden sufferer in back-

ground inhales mercury vapours. Woman in foreground, in last stages of disease, has been given up by doctors: her nose and limbs are eaten away.

Syphillis was named by Hieronymus Fracastorius, a physician, poet, physicist, geologist, astronomer, pathologist, and last but not least, the world's first epidemiologist. In 1530 this nobleman from Verona published a medical poem called *Syphilis, sive Morbus Gallicus.* By so doing, he gave pause to the quibblings of all Europe aimed to pin the blame for syphilis on a particular nation: France, Spain, Italy, or Española. Fracastorius pronounced Syphilus, the mythical shepherd-hero of his poem the first sufferer. The shepherd had offended Apollo and so was punished by the affliction. Thus, from Syphilus (susphilein means swineherd) syphilis was coined, and the 300 alternate appellations of the day gradually fell into disuse. The new label gave unity to the fight against the disease, and the poem itself became as celebrated as the *Regimen* of Salerno.

The poem actually summarized all knowledge about the disease and its treatment, history, facts and fables, and touched on both mercury and guaiacum cures. All this added up to a fresh and concise clinical picture of the great epidemic.

Medicine, after first standing aloof, now took up the challenge. Physicians began a wider use of mercury for syphilis—championing this metallic remedy in defiance of Galen who sponsored the herbal drug tradition. In spite of dangerous after-effects, mercury proved a powerful ally in the fight against the malady of Venus.

Studies in syphilis led Fracastorius to other epidemic diseases. He was the first to recognize typhus fever, and in 1546 he published the famous *De Contagione.* This work offered some amazing inklings of bacteriology — long before the discovery of bacteria. Fracastorius presumed the existence of imperceptible "seeds of disease which multiply rapidly . . .

Acute insight into the nature of syphilis did not keep Fracastorius from the belief that a stellar mixup was the ultimate cause of the disease. Astrology was as real to him as bacteriology to Wassermann, and by the standards of his time, the merit of guaiacum could be proven as irrefutably as that of Salvarsan four hundred years later.

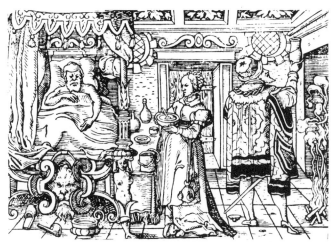

1. "Let's see what the trouble is." Doctor, called by patrician, inspects patient's urine in glow of fire-place.

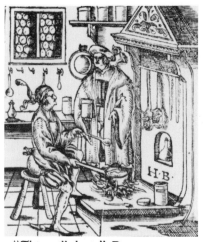

2. "This will do it." Doctor supervises making of drug by apothecary.

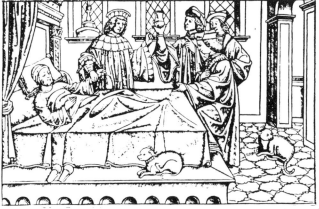

3. "What do you say, gentlemen?" Doctor faced with vexing problem consults colleagues during bedside consilium.

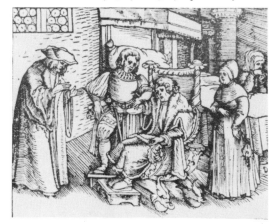

4. Doctor gives learned discourse, while barber does work of bloodletting.

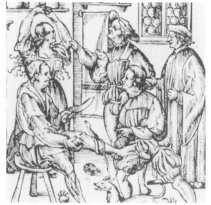

5. "Madame, please quiet down." Doctor consoles patient's wife.

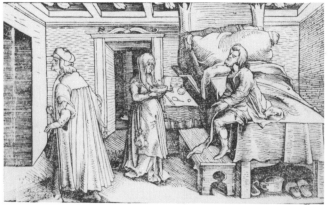

6. "Sorry, I will not handle this case." Doctor walks out on patient who refuses to stay in bed, obey orders.

A DAY WITH THE DOCTORS

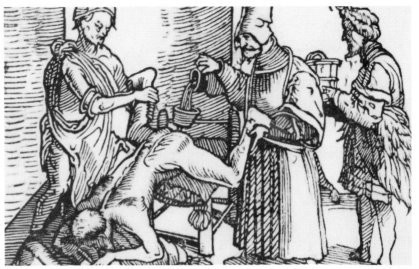

Roving empiric administers enema to patient cringing on cushion.

In an age bursting forth with art, commerce and exploration, the Renaissance doctor barely held his own. True he had acquired some dignity and self-assurance, but his practical knowledge was musty; for diagnosis, he still relied on the urine flask; on the four humours, and on bloodletting, the stock remedy for everything and against anything from plague to dandruff. His practice was now confined, largely to the rich, because it was necessary to make a living. So he hung out his shingle in the city, or attached himself as body physician to a potentate. In the latter case, he appeared each morning in the princely bedchamber to check his master's urine. If he found any sign of trouble, he was more inclined to talk about it than act upon it. But his authority and services were respected, at least while the sickness lasted.

The doctors themselves now achieve a closer solidarity than ever before. They pool their knowledge to hold "Consilia." Printed versions of such sick bed discussions now appear in numerous editions. Recording what was said and done by famed doctors, these casebooks become a valuable antidote against the scholastic tradition. Slowly the patient is alotted space formerly reserved for learned but useless abstractions.

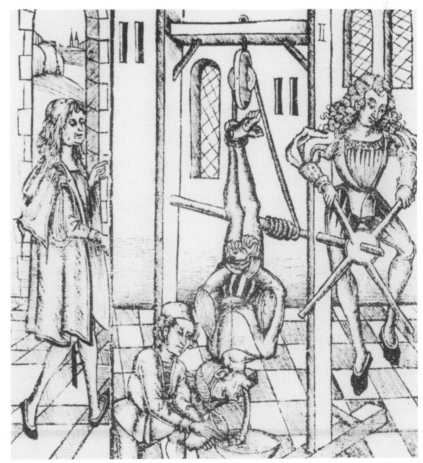

To remove frog from patient's throat surgeon employs pulley attachment.

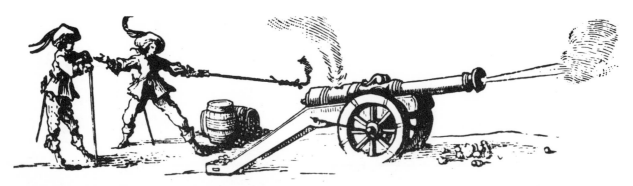

DEEPER WOUNDS - BETTER SURGEONS

By the 16th century, the use of gunpowder had turned battlefields into minor slaughter pits. The cannon, like the atom bomb today, inflicted new kinds of wounds — burns, deep gashes and other mysterious lesions. In range, size, mobility, and firepower, the new weapons grew at a ghastly rate. Wounds grew steadily too, in severity and kind, and wartime became a boomtime for the surgeon.

Though the craft of surgery had flourished in 13th and 14th century Italy and France, surgeons usually had been considered menials. If their patients died, they were likely to be in jeopardy themselves. Surgery became vitally important, however, with the great wars. The usual rush to the bookshelves followed, with few results, since Galen and Hippocrates kept strangely silent about gunshot wounds. So when the surgeon was pressed into service, and asked to patch up wounds for which there were no precedents, he was forced to improvise rather than theorize, to cut with speed and bind or cauterize as best he could. As Würtz, a leading surgeon, phrased it, "Surgery depends more on dexterity than on twaddle."

Dexterity soon followed, and a small band of proficient field surgeons emerged from the bloody campaigns of the early 16th century. They were neither great nor learned physicians, but close contact with the wounded gave them manual skill. They answered the challenge of their times with improved techniques for saving lives. The volunteer field surgeon, Ambroise Paré, reintroduced the ligature, and author-surgeon Hans von Gersdorff applied pressure and styptics to stop heavy bleeding.

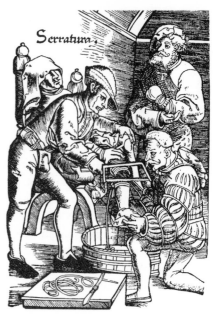

Hans Gersdorff's Feldtbuch der Wundartzney *offered this first picture of an amputation. Surgeon sawed between bandages, wound around limb, then covered stump with bladder of bull or hog. Though anesthetics were available, Gersdorff performed 200 odd amputations without them, for fear of after effects.*

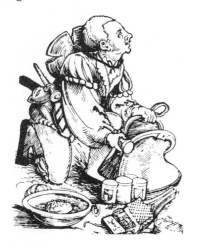

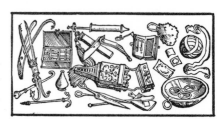

Surgeon's assistant, left, packs doctor's bag with salves and powders. Devices at right were used for fractures, dislocations. After Gersdorff, 1517.

104

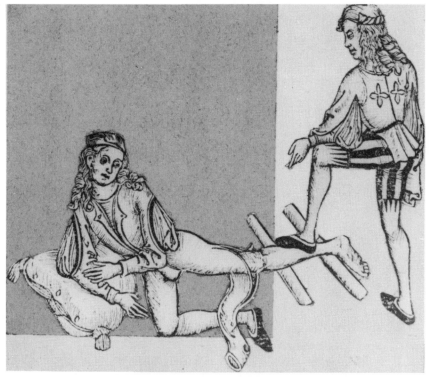

BONE-(UP)-SETTERS

Grinning surgeon rebreaks badly healed leg — shows callous disregard for patient. Illustration from Brunschwig's Book of Chirurgy, 1497, which humbly advocated physician's aid in complex cases. Surgeon's abbreviated costume indicates his mobility, in contrast with lengthy robes worn by physicians.

As the wars spread, men with broken limbs hobbled along the streets of Europe in greater numbers. Their bones had been damaged by cannon shot, which often caused extensive skeletal injuries. To prevent such loss of manpower, army surgeons were forced to revive and improve upon ancient methods of orthopedic surgery.

The Greeks had known about splints, traction, starched bandages and clay casts, but their knowledge had lain dormant during the Middle Ages. In the 14th century, Guy de Chauliac used weights and pulleys and a century later Renaissance doctors joined with mechanists to revive the decisive groundwork done by the ancients in the field of orthopedics.

The new army surgeons produced effective splints for fractures, and invented ingenious traction machines for stretching the affected limbs. Brunschwig, like Hippocrates and Arderne before him removed free bones from compound fractures. Paré reintroduced vertebral operations. By the end of the 16th century, orthopedics was well on its way.

Leg-stretching machine, pictured in Gersdorff's book, was accompanied with rhymes advertising author's dexterity. Patient makes this plea:
When I am stricken hip and thigh
Or wounded grievously do lie
I hope that God will bring to me
Gersdorff's artistic surgery.

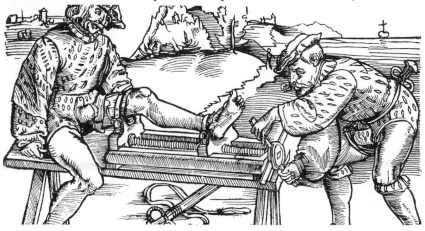

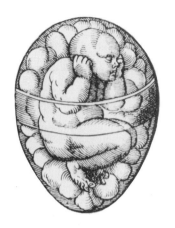

A CHILD
IS BORN
A.D. 1540

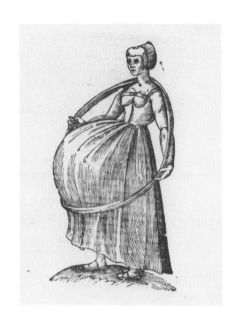

The science of obstetrics was conceived in sweat and begotten with all the groans and labor of childbirth itself. During the Renaissance, for instance, when all forms of medicine showed hopeful signs of advance (not always fulfilled), obstetrics stood still. The belligerent midwives guarded the lying-in-chamber against all medical interference. According to one legend, a physician of Hamburg, Dr. Wirtt, was caught at an accouchement, in 1522, disguised in women's clothes, and was promptly burned at the stake. The story lacks authentication, but it could easily have happened.

Gynecology was still engulfed in medieval darkness. The midwives knew little about parturition, and even less about female anatomy. To bring about labor, the pregnant woman was asked to run up and down stairs, or to shout at the top of her lungs. The midwives might even blow sneezing powder or pepper into her nose. As additional aids to labor, noxious

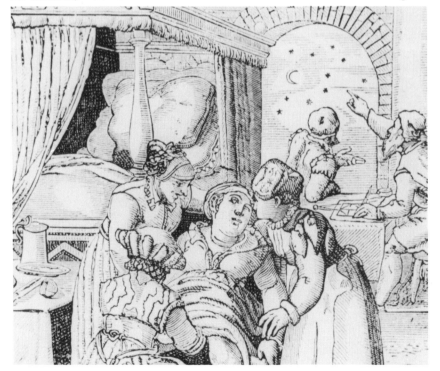

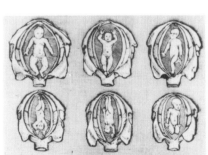

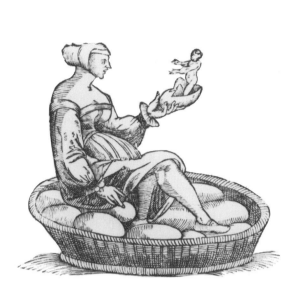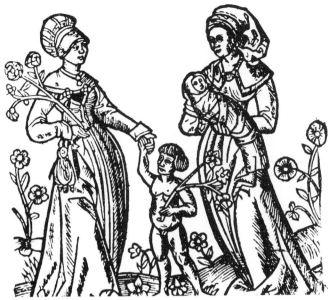

doses were poured down the expectant woman's throat, and her loins were oiled and exercised by rough, dirty hands. The surgeon was called in only when normal birth seemed hopeless; he was allowed to drag the dead child piecemeal from the womb with iron hooks. If the mother died first, attempts were made to save the child. As early as 1280, the Council of Cologne decreed that midwives should pry open the mouth of a woman who died in labor, "so the child would not suffocate."

The pictures on these pages illustrate some of the primitive aspects of Renaissance obstetrics. At bottom left, astrologers keep careful (and discreet) watch on the stars, to determine the child's future. Assisted by three husky midwives, the laboring woman squats on a birthstool, an age-old implement of labor. The embryo (top left) sits, according to medieval (and Renaissance) belief, in an eggshaped uterus, with its face toward the mother's back. Just before birth, the baby was supposed to turn toward the maternal navel. The woman to the right, (in an early maternity dress), eases her burden of multiple embryos with a wooden hoop. Her sister across the page hatches children from eggs. In an age marked by such fabulous beliefs, little that was rational could be expected to happen in the maternity chamber.

The midwife and mother above appeared on the frontispiece of Dr. Eucharius Roesslin's *Rosegarden of Pregnant Women and Midwives*. The book was first published in 1513; it contained no revolutionary ideas, but served, nevertheless, as a highly popular textbook on obstetrics for the next 200 years.

Roesslin may never have assisted at an actual birth; he worked at his desk instead, compiling facts and fallacies alike from ancient writings. Yet his attitude was at least compassionate. He employed a talented artist, Erhardt Schoen, to illustrate his theories. Schoen drew thirteen figures on birth, one of which showed the foetus, as big as a child of ten — rambling within the spacious uterus. Such outlandish concepts were probably taken seriously by Dr. Roesslin. Just the same, his text was highly popular with mothers, midwives and doctors. In the *Rosegarden*, they found the first complete and outspoken codification of "facts" about childbirth.

In England, plagiarist Thomas Raynalde transformed the *Rosegarden* into the *Byrth of Mankynde*, (1545). The book became popular, perhaps because of Henry VIII's strenuous efforts to supply England with a future king. In 1537, his Majesty's third wife, Jane Seymour, bore him a son (Edward VI) but died in childbirth. The event galvanized the interest in obstetrics and with it in *The Byrth of Mankynde*. Though the book effected no immediate reforms, it contained some sensible suggestions and helped to stimulate a field bogged down by prejudice.

107

MEDICAL MEDDLERS

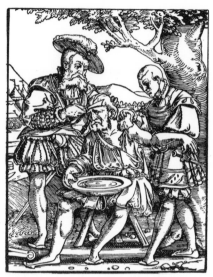

Doctor stood aloof at top of medical pyramid, looked down on lower forms of the healing art. His lofty bearing often drove ignorant public to quacks and empirics, who promised wondrous cures. Even minor crafts encroached on doctor's domain.

Surgeon dressed wounds, (above) healed fractures, and sometimes opened heads pretending to remove stones. Chyrurgeons frequently traveled with armies.

While the academically trained doctors served the sick, they kept one eye cocked on their competitors. The medical field had never before been so overcrowded with quacks and outsiders. In theory, the university-trained doctor stood at the head of the medical pyramid, with the minor crafts arrayed beneath him, each doing their appointed task as custom prescribed. Thus, the surgeon treated wounds and fractures, the barber pulled teeth and the bather cupped blood. But in practice, each craft offered to cure the sick. Even the apothecary dabbled in medicine, though pledged to obey the physician. This hopeless meddling confused the patient, and as in all medical bickering, he was the one who suffered most.

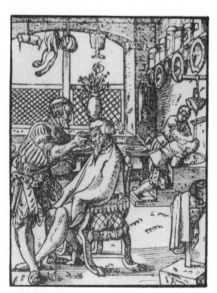

Barbers (above), pulled teeth, let blood and dabbled in surgery. This group eventually joined surgeons.

Bathers (right) cupped blood, did minor surgery, treated syphilitics.

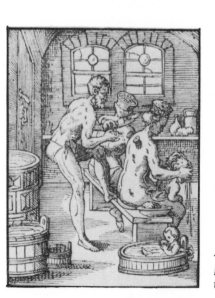

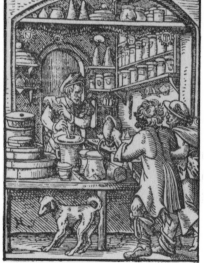

Apothecary, though pledged to obey physicians, could not resist the temptation to sell his own concoctions.

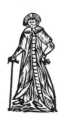

The Renaissance quack, like the great artists of the day, knew something about human nature. His miraculous cures were fashioned for an age intent on witnessing the seven wonders of the world. His assurances were as glowing as his imagination could make them. Hope was what his patients wanted and what they received, although they often lost their health or their lives in the bargain.

The age was ripe for quackery. The very word was coined at the time from "quacksalver," a name applied to itinerant doctors dealing in quicksilver, or mercury. Mercury was man's best hope against syphilis, and charlatans were quick to play it up as a panacea. Hence, the term quack, a man who deals in wondrous cures.

Legal traps were set to halt this flood of false physicians. Nuremberg promulgated a law which threatened to banish not only the quack but to punish the people who had consulted him. In England, in 1421, Henry V spoke out against practitioners who performed without the approval of recognized doctors and surgeons. But such laws could never be enforced fully, because the medical profession lacked the unity to fight impostors, and the public really wanted to be duped by the quack physicians. "We see the weakness and cedulity of man is such," said Francis Bacon, "that they will prefer the mountebank or

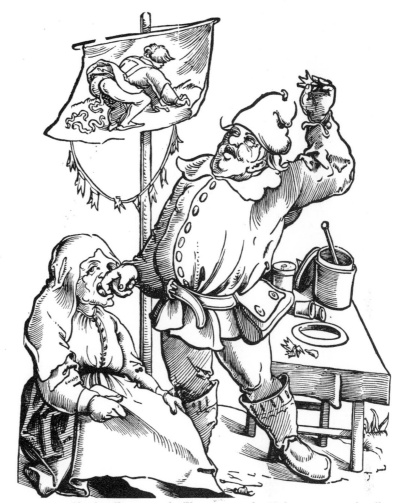

Toothpuller at work. Flag conveys forceful message to the illiterate.

witch before a learned physician."

Yet even here the doctor was partly to blame; his grave manners, his proud mien drove off the lower classes who needed the warmth and overt (though spurious) humanity offered by the quack. In contrast, the doctor-humanist dressed in long fur robes and recited Latin wisdom at the slightest provocation; he seldom touched a wound, but stood apart like an oracle, giving directions to his aides. Such conduct was too aloof, and perhaps too expensive, for the common patient.

Ultimately, the battle between quack and doctor was based upon human frailty. As Bass puts it: The quacks did not hesitate to promise the ignorant "an infallible remedy for every disorder," whereas "a man of real skill cannot venture a positive assurance that he can cure a cut finger." Indeed, the Renaissance physician could never hope to compete with the vulgar claims of the quacksalver in the above woodcut. His triumphant extraction of teeth was only one of his many specialties. As the shingle indicates, his chief stock in trade were laxatives of unquestioned power.

109

ENGLAND SETS UP
COLLEGE OF PHYSICIANS

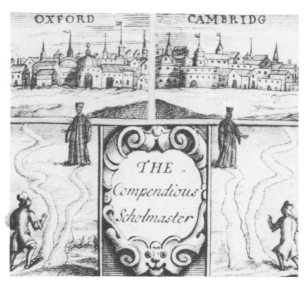

THOMAS LINACRE

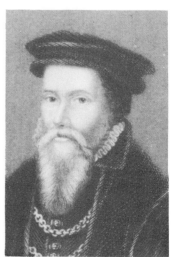

JOHN CAIUS

The great religious and intellectual storms of the 16th century struck England as well as the continent. But the sturdy island weathered the upheavals, as always, with a minimum of bloodshed and bombast. No angry Luther, not even a Paracelsus (that medical iconoclast) could thrive for long on English mutton. Nonetheless, the Renaissance was vigorously effective, especially in English medicine. Scholars of high calibre revived the healing arts through the careful study of ancient wisdom. If actual practice was neglected, philology and the humanities were pursued with quickened interest. Thomas Linacre, the humanist-doctor, gained fame with his flawless translations of Hippocrates, which included the first English version of the Hippocratic Oath.

This helped to provide the medical profession with sorely-needed prestige. As a court physician, Linacre moved to block the inroads of mountebanks in the medical ranks. In 1518, he had obtained a patent from Henry VIII to form a body of physicians to supervise the practice of medicine in London. To qualify, all doctors (except Oxford and Cambridge graduates) were required to prove their competence. From the supervisory group of 1518 was to emerge (in 1551) the Royal College of Physicians and with it, English medicine gained the basis for great professional stability. For Linacre had infused his followers with a deep sense of humanism, providing the leaven which raised the medical profession "above the dead level of a business" (Osler).

John Caius succeeded Linacre as president of the Royal College of Physicians. His travels through Europe had given him a first-hand view of Renaissance medicine. In Italy, he had lodged in the same house as Vesalius, who was then engaged in anatomical studies. When Caius returned, he revived the study of anatomy with his regular lectures on that subject. He had also hoped to make Cambridge the center of medical education, and he spent a fortune to establish Caius College. His labors, however, were not appreciated. A new generation of students had risen. They wanted a practical education; Caius' rigid classicism meant little to them. Yet it was on this ancient learning that the new science of medicine was grafted.

In Henry VIII the medical profession found a forceful, progressive patron. The Tudor monarch surrounded himself with doctors of the true humanist mold. He had been afflicted with an "ulcerous leg" (probably from syphilis) after his first campaign in France. This led to a frantic personal interest in "liniments," which he expressed by grinding up ointments from magic pearls, gums and aromatics. In typical fashion, he blamed the disease on Wolsey, who had "transmitted" it by whispering into the royal ear.

The monarch was in sympathy with the fight of the doctors against malpractice. He backed the establishment of the College of Physicians, the oldest purely medical institution in Europe. In addition, he sanctioned in 1540 the barber-surgeon pact. The surgeons had formed a small, exclusive guild, but were forced to compete with an increasing number of "tinkers, broom men, ratcatchers and rogues." To gain strength, they joined forces with the politically powerful barber's guild. Thomas Vicary represented the interests of the doctors at court, and with his aid the United Company of Barber-Surgeons was born.

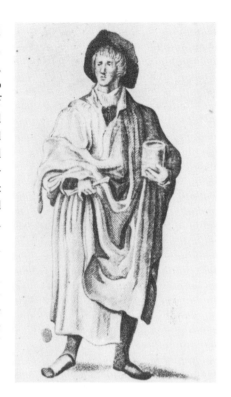

Andrew Boorde (right) said, "Myrth is one of the chefest thynges of physycke." A physician to Henry VIII, he ended in Fleetwood Prison. Some believe him to be the original "Merry Andrew."

The Barber-Surgeon Union (below) was an important landmark in surgical history. Holbein shows Henry VIII, haughty and majestic, handing the charter of union to Thomas Vicary, first master. The artist died before the work was finished, and guild members, intent on immortality, had themselves painted into the background. (Royal College of Surgeons.)

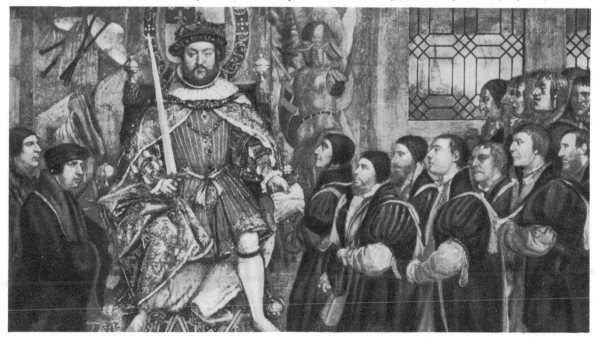

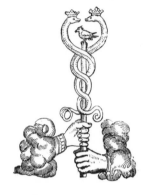

MEDICINE A DIVINE MISSION

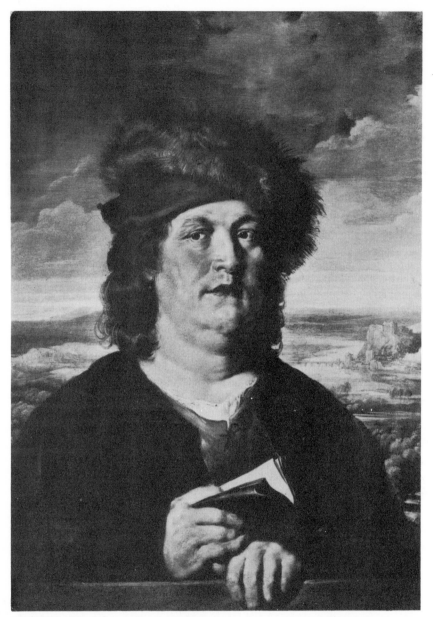

Paracelsus: Idealized portrait. (Rubens, copy of Jan van Scorel painting.)

To turn from English humanism to Paracelsus is like stepping from a quiet library into a three-ring circus. Aureolus Philippus Theophrastus Bombastus von Hohenheim, called Paracelsus, (1493-1541), modestly ranked himself as the savior of 16th century medicine. In his estimation all doctors who preceded him were consummate idiots — Galen, a liar and a faker; Avicenna, a mere kitchen master. "I am to be the monarch," shouted Paracelsus, "and the monarchy will belong to me."

Actually, behind all the smoke and bombast, there lurked a great iconoclast, a profound student of psychology and the acknowledged founder of medicinal chemistry. In truth, since Paracelsus, the entire field of medicine can scarcely claim to be the same. As Withington said, "He blew the trumpet, and he blew it loud, — and the Galenic walls came tumbling down." Past medicine had only succeeded "in the making of corpses." Physicians had traded common sense for empty knowledge. They needed experience, travel and humility. "The doctor must treat nature's book with his feet," said Paracelsus.

He practiced what he preached. As a young man, Paracelsus had trekked across Europe. Later, he visited England, Turkey, Greece, trying to uncover the very roots of medicine. All his life he remained a wanderer. Even the lectureship his printer-friend, Froben, secured for him at Basle (1527) did not last long. Here he labored past masters without mercy, and addressed his classes not in Latin but in lowly German, a language purportedly fit "only to address horses."

Needless to say, Paracelsus was shortly back at his private practice. He calmly compiled more facts about syphilis, cretinism and hospital gangrene. As for his former confrères at Basel, and all other orthodox physicians he said, "Even the flies would disdain to sit on them except to make their dirt."

All his life Paracelsus thundered against his colleagues. To expose their folly he set forth a tremendous corpus of ideas. In it can be found a composite of brilliant insight and abracadabra that defies unraveling. Most enlighted perhaps and pertinent to this day is what Paracelsus had to say on the comprehension and treatment of mental disorders. These teachings of the great magus have been elucidated in a profound study by Dr. Iago Galdston. It shows that Paracelsus was an astute psychiatrist and a forerunner of Freud.

Paracelsus felt that man was composed of antagonistic animal and godly spirits, and that the former had to be suppressed if man was to fulfill himself. This corresponds to the struggle between Id and Super-Ego in the system of psychoanalysis.

In distinguishing types of psycho-pathy, he compared the feeble-minded man to a healthy dog, and the psychopath to a mad one. He described the manic-depressive state, and held that all psychoses were "natural," as opposed to demonological, in origin.

Further, he knew that disease could result from mental problems, since the will, or spirit, had a powerful effect on the body. In such cases, he wrote, "You should treat the spirit, for it is the spirit that here lies sick." Faith could likewise create diseases and cure a good many as well.

More subtly, Paracelsus maintained that the "brute intelligence" is brought out by madness, while the "human intelligence" is unaffected and "not subject to sickness." Here was a clear discernment of primitive drives controlling the insane, while reasoning power remained lucid — witness the keen logic of the paranoid, based, always, on false premises. "It is a major achievement," wrote Paracelsus, "to understand the rantings of the lunatic."

Thus, the king of bombast showed

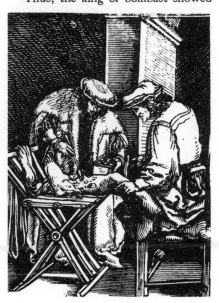

amazing profundity in his more quiet moments. He knew, for instance, that woman "is a different world" from man, and the physician must therefore treat her differently. He was even aware of the subconscious — "that which is without substance, and yet has effect."

This insight was based on an equally deep philosophy which seems especially pertinent today. In an age preoccupied with autopsy, Paracelsus considered the body "a living anatomy," a part of the universe. He was intensely concerned with the eternity, or soul, in man, and felt that a doctor was neither "pillmaker" nor businessman, but a legate of God, the supreme physician. Medicine was therefore a divine mission, and the doctor must raise his eyes from "excrements and salvepots to the stars." The perfect physician, he felt, was a philosopher, an astrologer, an alchemist and above all, a virtuous man. And the character of such a doctor Paracelsus proclaimed was far more effective than mere mechanical skill.

Surgeon treats ulcerated leg. (Woodcut from Paracelsus, Grosse Wundartzney.)

In 1526 Paracelsus saved the leg of Basle's famed publisher Johann Froben. When hearing about this, Erasmus of Rotterdam wrote a warm letter: "I cannot offer thee a reward equal to thy art and knowledge, but I surely offer thee a grateful soul. Thou hast called from the shades Frobenius, who is my other half: if thou restorest me also, thou restorest each through the other. May fortune favor that thou remain in Basel." But fortune and an angry faculty favored otherwise.

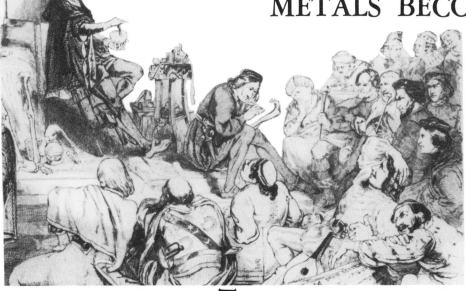

PARACELSEAN ALCHEMY: METALS BECOME DRUGS

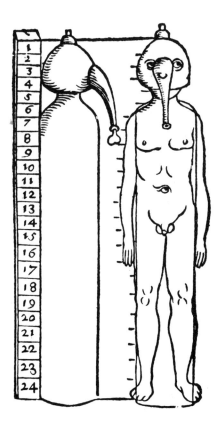

Paracelsian glass vessel (left), for the distillation of urine, was divided into 24 parts. Urine sediment was supposed to indicate locus of a disease on the miniature human body.

The most famous legend about Paracelsus deals with his brief, if highly pyrotechnic "lectureship" at Basel in 1527. (He never became a professor, for obvious reasons, though he called himself one in his famous manifesto to the students.) Paracelsus is said to have started his first course by dramatically lighting a brazier on the rostrum, then tossing the collected works of Galen and Avicenna into the fire. This was just his way of saying: "Gentlemen, let's begin once more at the beginning."

To change metaphors, the dynamic doctor was forever hacking out paths through scholastic underbrush, in search of new avenues leading to the basic sources of healing. Sometimes he succeeded, sometimes not. But he is generally acknowledged as the father of medicinal chemistry, and with it the godfather of modern chemotherapy.

Similarly, he preached on anatomy different from the one practised by the "Italian jugglers." The Paracelsian anatomist was to concern himself not with muscles, but with the chemical elements of the body.

Paracelsus applied alchemy with success to the field of therapy, which was then governed mostly by herbal remedies. He devised a kind of chemical view of life, in which the whole world was the physician's apothecary shop (an old biblical concept). On the one hand, God had created a plethora of diseases; on the other, He had provided the raw materials for a multitude of cures.

It was the alchemist's job to transform these raw materials by way of distillation into new remedies, or to isolate the health-giving quintessence of metals, called arcanum.

114

Paracelsus did in no way attempt to suppress the contemporary view that he himself carried a universal arcanum in the knob of his sword, a true philosopher's stone which could cure any and all disease.

The concept of the arcanum gave the alchemists something more tangible to work on than formulae to make gold. So, guided by Paracelsus, they invaded the mineral kingdom in search of new remedies. They selected simple substances — tin, silver or sulphur — to offset the complicated powders, plasters and potions mixed at the Galenic drugstore. As the master put it: "Which trousers are best, the whole or the patched? Bah! This miserable compounding business!"

But the conservative physicians soon hit back at Paracelsus. They warned the sick that metal remedies would poison them. The self-made super-doctor parried with an apt retort: "This poison, as you call it, has a far better effect than the wagon grease . . . with which you are so fond of smearing your patients." The point was well taken, and the trend toward the discovery of metallic remedies continued.

When Paracelsus died, on September 24, 1541, a few weeks after the Bishop of Salzburg had granted him a refuge in this hospitable city, the profession at large was unaware that one of medicine's greats had gone. The schools resisted his revolutionary teachings, put forth with the amiability of an intellectual bully. A band of faithful followers continued to praise him as the super-physician, which he believed himself to be. Unfortunately, they perpetuated his mysticism rather than his enlightened views.

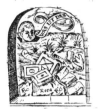

Laboratory of alchemist (below) shows preparation of quintessence. Snake-eating lion was symbol of melting process. Zodiac signs (lizard, snake, etc.) stood for various substances, important in creating curative "spirits."

Arcanum in knob of Paracelsus' sword could "cure all diseases" (below).

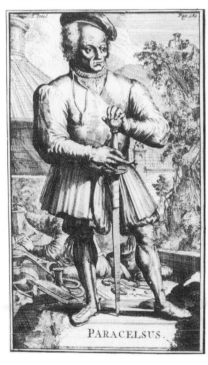

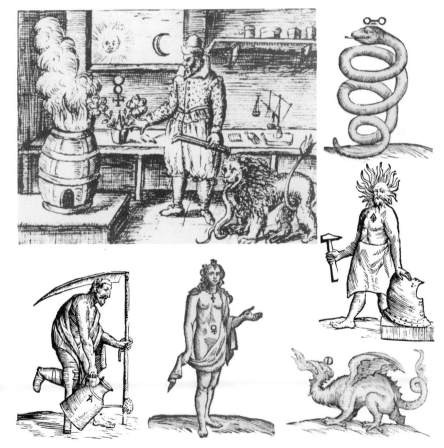

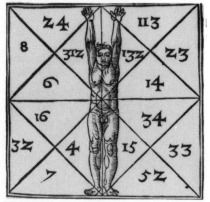

Thurneysser (1530-1596), mystic turned doctor, had his own printshop.

Horoscope shows regions of human body as related to transit of stars.

IN SEARCH OF DIAGNOSIS ..

To Paracelsus and his followers, the physician-alchemist seemed all-powerful. Since he "mastered the stars," he could cure the sick, — yes, he could even create a living being, because he obtained guidance from the secret laws of the universe. In practice, however, this doctrine was warped into outright mumbo-jumbo by men like Leonhard Thurneysser.

Thurneysser was seven years old when Paracelsus made his famous guest appearance at Basel. His father had decided to train him as a goldsmith, but the young man was so impressed with Paracelsus that he went to the Tyrolean mines to study metallurgy. A grant from Archduke Ferdinand of Austria enabled Thurneysser to travel across Europe in search of secrets for making gold.

Paracelsus had taken a similar jaunt, in search of new medicines, but the impressionable Thurneysser made no distinction between his own ends and those of his hero. Though never a student of medicine he pronounced himself endowed with the power to heal through "potable gold." He reasoned that knowledge of metals and their arcana made him a physician.

Apparently it did, in the eyes of high and mighty patrons. Thurneysser was soon given ample facilities to manufacture his secret remedies. Twelve secretaries were employed to handle his mail-order horoscopes and a press was set up to print his writings. But he was unable to produce gold from a stream in the neighbourhood of Berlin, as he had promised, and so fell out of favor.

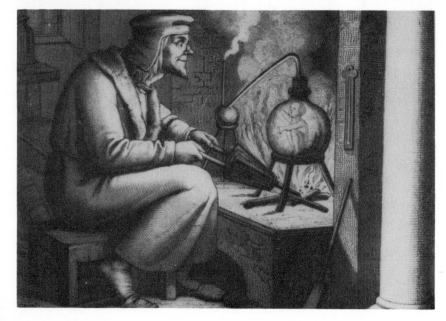

Birth of Homunculus. Paracelsus claimed small men (homunculi) could be made by placing human sperm, plus horse dung (which insured evenly-tempered "bed of heat") into retort, and baking it for 40 days. Such men, he said, had everything but a soul, which only God could implant.

DOCTORS CONSULT STARS

Jerome Cardan, mystic, mathematical genius and doctor firmly believed in astrological medicine and provided horoscopes with every diagnosis. At the same time, his healing methods were quite sound, and he served successfully as physician to dukes, cardinals, and kings.

When a black cat dragged his manuscript. *On Medicine*, off a shelf in his study, the superstitious Cardan resigned his post at the University of Pavia. Nonetheless, he continued his private practice.

In his most famous case, he traveled to Edinburgh (1552) to treat John Hamilton, Archbishop of St. Andrews. He remained there ten weeks, and reduced the "unhealthy temperature" in the cleric's brain by remarkably sound measures. The bishop, a prodigious worker, loved good food and certain carnal pleasures. So Cardan

placed him on a strict daily regimen: ten hours sleep, garden walks, head baths and light meals, predominantly of chicken broth and milk (he also prescribed "mastic," a forerunner of pepsin gum). The bishop recovered and Cardan left behind detailed instructions for his patient's conduct.

Later, Cardan lost public favor. His son was sentenced to death for poisoning his unfaithful wife. Cardan claims that a gradually reddening mark on his own hand exuded blood as the hour of execution approached.

The distraught physician spent his last years writing *De Vita Propria*, the story of his life. Morley, his biographer, says that Cardan's career was one of the most curious on record — full of extremes "the most wonderful sense and the wildest nonsense."

In spite of his signal success as a doctor, Cardan took a dim view of the profession: "that calling above all others (except the glory that attends it), is completely servile, full of toil, and (to confess the truth) unworthy of a high-spirited man, so that I do not at all marvel that the art used to be peculiar to slaves."

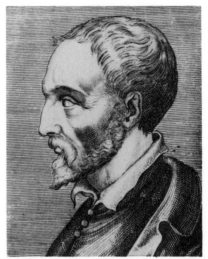

Cardan (1501-1576), doctor, mathematician wrote: The Book of My Life.

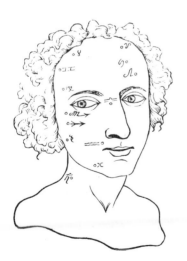

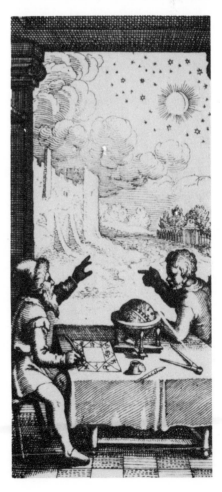

Astral influence shown by points on patient's head (left). Cardan made a system out of this divinatory technique, called it metocoscopy. Astro-physician (at right) draws diagnostic horoscope.

LAUGHTER AT THE BEDSIDE

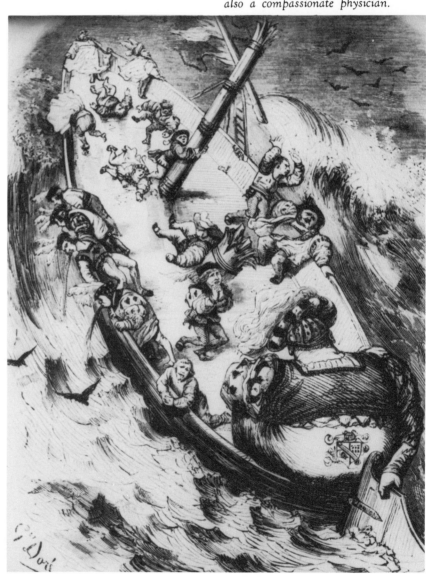

Francois Rabelais, French satirist, was also a compassionate physician.

In the medicine cabinet of Francois Rabelais there was hidden one magic remedy, the essence of laughter, which he had distilled after years of somewhat bibulous experiment. He administered this remedy with remarkable success through his books, *Gargantua and Pantagruel*. He had written them, originally, "for love of writing — and for lack of money." But upon his patients, especially those with gout, pox, itch or toothache, they exerted a decidedly therapeutic effect.

The great humanist was also aware of certain ailments peculiar to the medical profession. These too he tried to cure with his ribald pen by scuttling windy anatomists, herbalists, purgers, and astrological therapists like the prognostic Herr Trippa (Agrippa). He flayed the medical art because he loved it, and hoped to restore his profession to blessed sanity.

Feeding fish on voyage to the "Land of the Holy Bottle" (Pantagruel, Book IV). Rabelais scoffed at popular remedies for seasickness: "drinking salt water, covering the stomach with paper."

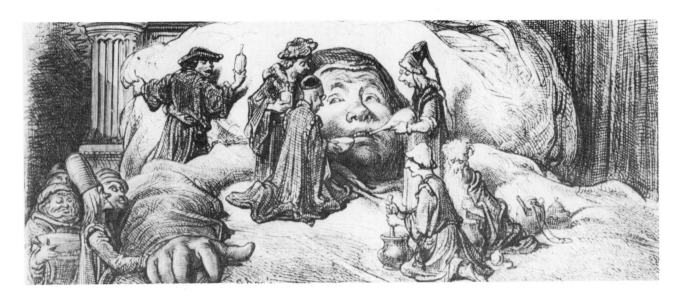

Francois Rabelais was a many sided man: monk, humanist, prodigious author, scholar, imbiber, and finally, "doctor of medicine by instinct and choice." His medical life began in 1530, when he discarded his monk's garb to study at Montpellier. He delivered bachelor lectures there on Galen and Hippocrates, whose work he later translated during his stay at Lyons. He refused, however, to submit to their authority. "Great as these masters are," he said, "they never knew all . . . the more we know, the more questions are presented to us for solution. Science like nature is infinite." At Lyons, he was appointed physician to the Hôtel-Dieu, and he delivered guest lectures on anatomy at the university. Here he described the human body with such contagious enthusiasm that one student expressed regrets, after the lecture, that he was not the corpse on the dissecting table, that enviable subject of "so divine a discourse."

Foolish physicians (above) mix "pharmaceutical hotchpots" to purge ailing Pantagruel (Book II). Servants later descended gullet in copper globes to dig out ordure. Woodcut by Doré.

Rabelais was later excused by papal bull for assuming secular garb. The same bull allowed him to reenter the Benedictine order and to practice medicine as well, provided he did not work for earthly gain. He was proud to be a physician, or, as he called it, a philanthropist.

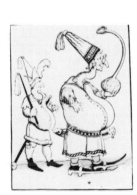

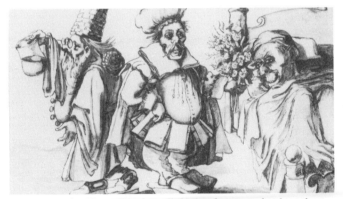

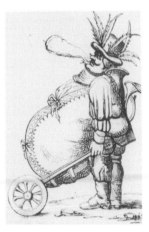

Caricature by Hans Weiditz, (left) lambasts medical profession as mercilessly as Rabelais' satires. Expansive patient (right) wheels surplus tonnage. Center: The Doctor's Visit by Mattioli.

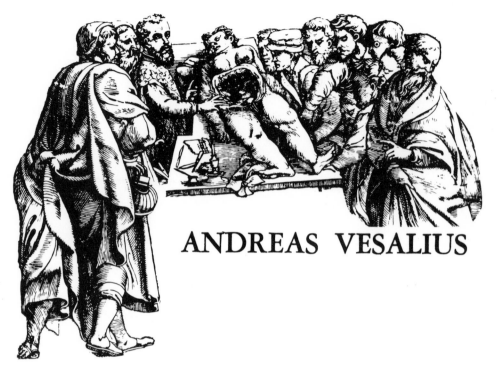

ANDREAS VESALIUS

Modern medicine began in 1543, with the publication of the first complete textbook of human anatomy, *De Humani Corporis Fabrica*, by Andreas Vesalius. Here was the most significant (and perhaps the most beautiful) text in all medical history; it served as a much-needed alphabet for future science, and just as important, the textbook provided an excellent example of objective research in action.

Vesalius, a truly great anatomist, can only be compared with Hippocrates in stature and importance. By limiting himself to actual evidence, he broke with many — if not all — of the obfuscations of the past. Further, he achieved the first significant fusion between science and art: his findings were presented through magnificent drawings probably by Stephen van Calcar, a pupil of Titian. Thus, at one stroke, Vesalius gave medicine an objective method, a visual medium and a firm foundation in anatomy.

André Vesal was born in Brussels; [his family had come from Wesel on the Rhine — therefore "Vesalius"]. He studied medicine at Louvain and Paris, but in the latter city became

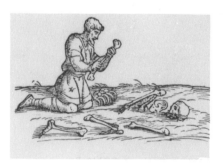

Anatomist at left gathers bones in cemetary. In similar fashion Vesalius and fellow students rifled skeleton heaps in outskirts of Paris. These young men prided themselves on being able to identify all bones of the human body blindfolded. At right, Vesalius and friend Gemma steal skeletons from gallows on outskirts of Louvain; they tore torso apart to smuggle it piecemeal through the town gates. Later, when Vesalius achieved fame, Padua readily furnished him with corpses.

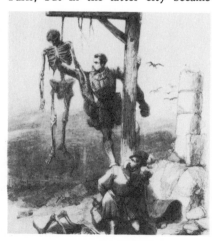

120

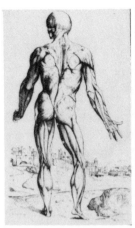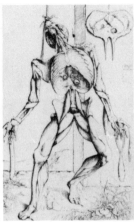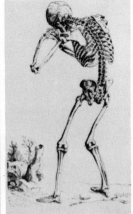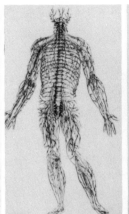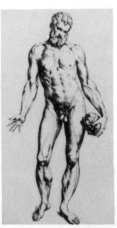

disgusted with the methods of anatomical instruction. His professors were
respectable Galenists who spoke from
the podium and used the corpse below to corroborate the master.

One day, when an instructor made
errors in dissection while the reading
from Galen went on, Vesalius was
asked to take over the demonstration.
He amazed the class with his skill.

Vesalius and his fellow students
also rifled skeleton heaps in cemeteries outside Paris. They placed bets
on their bone-identification prowess —
"within half an hour no bone could
be offered us which we could not
identify by touch." In 1536, Vesalius
returned to Louvain to lecture on
anatomy. A year later, he became
professor of anatomy at Padua, then

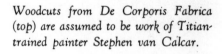

*Woodcuts from De Corporis Fabrica
(top) are assumed to be work of Titian-
trained painter Stephen van Calcar.*

the leading medical school in Europe.

His lectures at Padua attracted
record crowds of about 500 students
and doctors per session — all cran-
ing their necks to see him dissect.
He spoke with lucidity and enthusiasm, and supported his words with
charts of the portal, vascular, generative and skeletal system. It is quite
possible that these "visual aids" to
education were drawn by Vesalius
himself, assisted by his artist friend,
van Calcar. The charts were in great
demand among his colleagues, so in
1538 Vesalius had six of them printed.
These *Tabulae Sex* sold immediately
and have since been literally thumbed
out of existence. For the next five
years, Vesalius worked industriously
at his *Fabrica*. He was 29 when the
book was finally published.

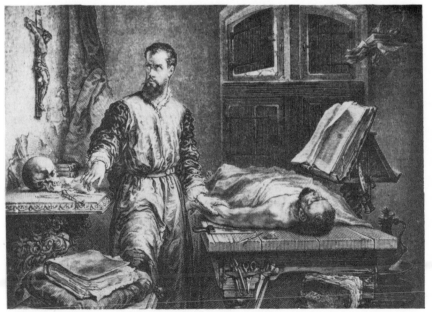

*Andreas Vesalius (1514-1564), at left,
performs clandestine dissection. (After
painting by E. J. C. Hamman.)*

VESALIUS Continued

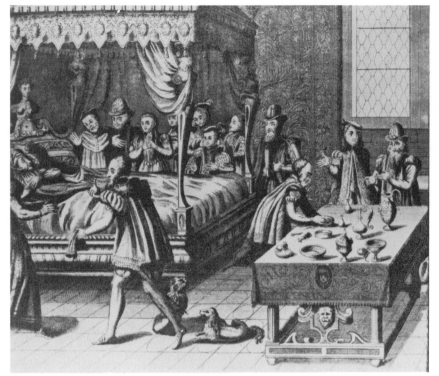

After the publication of *De Fabrica*, Vesalius left Padua to become court physician to Emperor Charles V. His teacher Sylvius had dubbed Vesalius "Vesanius," or madman. And perhaps he was mad to exchange his freedom for the duties of high office; more likely, he always had been pulled between pure research and the desire to heal — a familiar medical dilemma. So he abandoned anatomy, while his jealous associates moved on, along Vesalian paths.

But the indomitable Vesalius won fame as a physician as he had as an anatomist. Like Charles V, his successor Philip II often entrusted him with special missions. One day Philip's son Prince Don Carlos fell down a flight of palace-stairs in hot pursuit of a servant girl. The prince developed a fever and the court doctors despaired of his life. Vesalius, who was called to the rescue, made two incisions on the prince's forehead and removed a collection of trouble-making pus. The patient recovered shortly thereafter. It can be assumed that such cures made Vesalius' Spanish colleagues apprehensive, and that he became the victim of court intrigue.

It seems not improbable that this made Vesalius weary and disgusted with a country where "not even a skull could be had" for anatomical study. On a strange trip to the Holy Land in 1564 he stopped off at Venice, possibly to arrange for his return to teaching. But sailing back from Palestine his boat was shipwrecked and on the Island of Zante, he died from hunger and exposure, at the age of 50.

In 1559 Vesalius received a call to the death-bed of Henry II of France where Paré, too was in attendance. The king had been struck above the right eye by a broken shaft during a joust. Vesalius saw no hope, but used "guilty" lance-heads on four dead criminals to determine the nature of the injury.

SERVETUS, MEDICAL MARTYR

Bumptious Michael Servetus (1509?-1553) a friend and fellow student of Vesalius held that blood from the heart moved through the lungs, "where it is made red," then "after a long detour," returned to the left ventricle. He pronounced this theory of blood circulation on page 171 of a tract on Christianity (1533). Earlier he had sent a draft of this book to Calvin who was deeply offended by what he considered the book's heresies. In 1553 when Servetus was compelled to flee from his prosecutors in Catholic France, he turned South to "reformed" Switzerland. Here Calvin delivered him to the inquisition and had him burned in Geneva together with all traceable copies of his book.

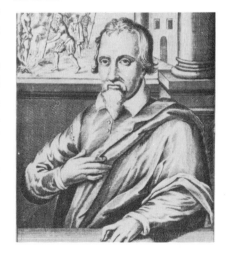

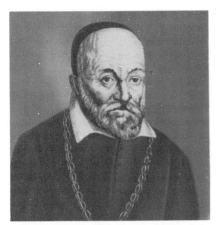

Fabricius of Aquapendente explored the vein valves used later by Harvey as proof for the theory of circulation

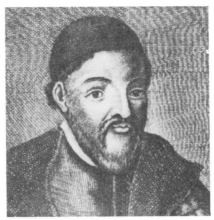

Fallopius succeeded Vesalius in Padua, discovered Fallopian tubes. He also named the vagina and the placenta.

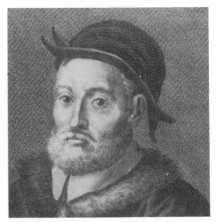

Cesalpino taught at Pisa, gave succinct picture of heart muscles, valves, pioneered in cardio-physiology.

Vesalius had seen man in his wholeness, as a "fabric" of interrelated parts. But his successors attempted a more piecemeal approach. They discovered new muscles, tissues or nerves and so won an entry in the anatomy text books. Fallopius went down in anatomical history by stamping his name on the female oviducts (Fallopian tubes), while Eustachius recorded an artery, a heart valve, and the auditory, or Eustachian tube. Sylvius, the friend, teacher, and finally the foe of Vesalius, lives on today through the various arteries and fissures he discovered.

These findings were important, but they lacked significant direction.

Meanwhile, other Vesalian converts had turned their attention to the heart. Galen (and Vesalius) had taught that the blood passed back from the right to the left ventricle through "invisible holes" in the septum. The anatomists who followed Vesalius found that these holes just weren't there; they discovered, instead, that the blood passed from the right ventricle through the lungs back to the left ventricle. Servetus had expressed this idea as part of his theological credo rather than as a medical fact. It is unlikely that his pronouncements became generally known. Among those who once more pursued this idea, Caesalpinus went furthest. He was actually the first to speak of "circulation" of the blood.

It was this group of Italian physiologists that changed the direction of anatomical research. They stressed the study of the function rather than the mere structure of the human body. Through these endeavors they paved the way for the research of Harvey.

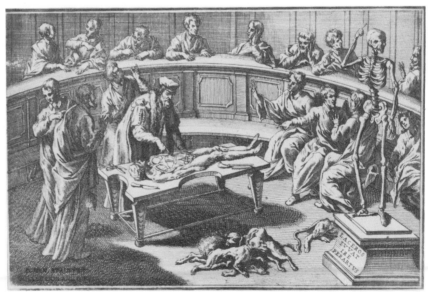

Eustachius teaching anatomy. He completed a few years after Vesalius, a superb anatomy atlas. This was lost for 138 years, until published by Lancisi, in 1714.

123

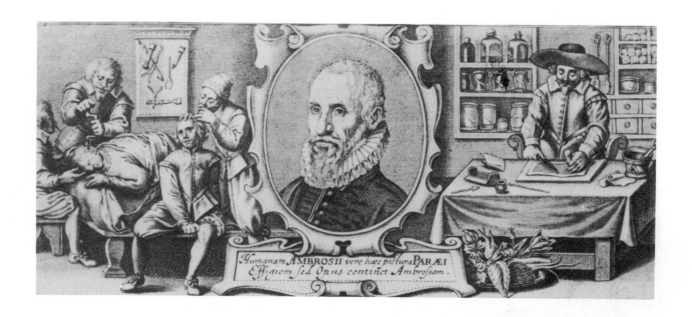

PARÉ: HIS KNIFE SAVES THOUSANDS

Ambroise Paré, a humble barber's apprentice, worked his way from the bottom up to become the greatest surgeon of the 16th century. He took up the knife where Guy de Chauliac had dropped it some 200 years before.

Paré salvaged his chosen profession from quacks on the one hand, and academicians on the other. The lowly army surgeon saved thousands of lives on the battlefield. He served four French kings, won recognition from the Collège of St. Côme, and discovered important new methods for treating wounds. No wonder, then, that the wounded cheered him at Metz, and the soldiers at besieged Hesdin (1553) carried him through the streets on their shoulders

Paré had no formal education. His university was the battlefield. In his 30-odd years as a field surgeon, he helped to place war surgery on a sane and democratic basis. Before his time, the common soldiers were often forced to rely on camp followers for treatment. But Paré was touched by the wholesale misery of the rank and file. He describes his feelings during the siege of Turin (1537), his first battle: "We entered pell mell into the city and passed over the dead bodies, and some not yet dead, hearing them cry under our horses' feet, and they made my heart ache to hear them." Once inside the city, Paré was asked by an old soldier if three of his severely wounded comrades perched against the wall had a chance to live. Paré said no, and the warrior promptly "cut their throats, gently and benevolently." The young surgeon was shocked, but the old man replied that he himself, if he were mortally wounded, would pray for such a merciful end.

From then on, the compassionate Paré did his best to cure the wounded and comfort the dying of every rank. One typical case occurred in the same campaign. A severely wounded man had been given up by his comrades. "Moved by pity," Paré asked the company leader for permission to serve the man as physician, apothecary, surgeon and cook. Permission was granted, and the man recovered under Paré's kindly care. Meanwhile, the common soldiers were so impressed by this charitable act that they collected a purse and presented it to Paré at the next review. "I dressed him and God healed him," wrote the humble surgeon. This was to be his life's credo.

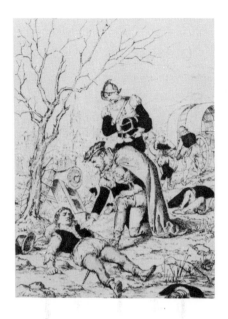

But if God was at hand, dressings were not always available. At the siege of Hesdin, for instance, Paré was forced to employ four fat prostitutes to wash bandages for the wounded. "Being kept at the job with the stick," wrote Paré in despair, "they only produced linen as hard as parchment, for there was not enough water, and less soap."

Paré considered each of his cases as a problem in rehabilitation, as well as surgery. His writings attest to the minute attention he paid to the convalescent's surroundings, food and bedding. In 1569, long after he had retired from the war and become a successful Paris practitioner, he was called to Flanders to attend the Duke

Ambroise Paré (1510-1590) treats soldier during siege of Metz. He used clear springwater and clean bandages.

d'Auret, who had suffered for seven months from a gunshot wound near the knee. Paré's description of the case is a classic in 16th century medical literature. Pacing through the ducal garden, he mapped out a complete campaign for the patient's recovery. First, he provided for clean bedding and requested that flowers be placed in the sickroom to counteract the smell of the wound. Then, to quiet the duke's nerves, he supervised the construction of a device which simulated rain. "By making water run from some high place into a cauldron," wrote the wise surgeon, "sleep will be promoted in him." For a final psychosomatic touch, he called for violins at the bedside, "to lift the patient's spirit," and for comedians "to make him merry."

Paré's important writings include the revolutionary treatise on gunshot wounds of 1545, which upset the whole brutal concept of cauterization. Later, he borrowed freely from Vesalius's *De Fabrica* to augment his own works, and thereby linked the teachings of the

great anatomist to the mainstream of practical surgery.

By joining the College of St. Côme, in 1554, Paré bettered both his own position and that of the surgical profession. The surgeons there were engaged in a battle for prestige with the physicians of the University of Paris, and with the lowly barber-surgeons who were slyly sponsored by the faculty. With the king's backing, the untutored Paré fought many verbal battles for his fellow-surgeons. And most of them he won.

During the slaughter of the Huguenots in 1572, Charles IX took Paré, an admitted Huguenot, into his own quarters to protect him from the mob. When the massacre ceased, he asked if Paré was ready to change his faith. The loyal surgeon is said to have replied:

"You have promised never to ask me for four things: to return to my mother's womb . . . to fight in a battle . . . to leave your services . . . to go to mass."

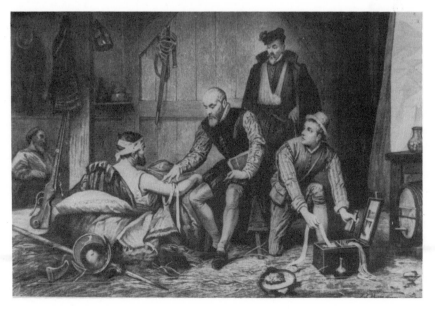

HORRORS OF CAUTERY CURBED

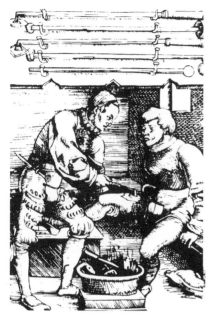

Old Method: Cautery to remove "poison" actually caused inflammation.

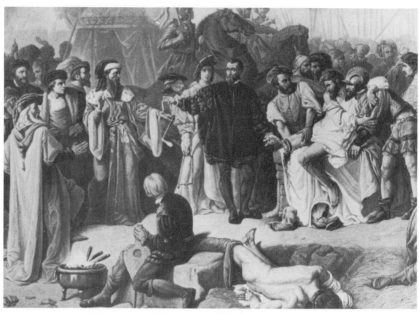

New Method: Paré ties up blood vessels (ligature) after amputation. He refused to use cautery, which was painful and dangerous. Paré washed wounds with water.

In Paré's time many prejudices blocked the advance of sound war surgery. None created more suffering than the belief that gunshot wounds were poisoned by the powder burns, and should be cauterized. Usually a boiling mixture of oil and treacle was poured into the wounds or they were cleansed by scalding irons. By accident, Paré was led to abandon this brutal practice.

In his first campaign, the inexperienced Paré did as he was told. He applied the red hot cautery or ladled boiling oil into the gashed flesh. Then one day in 1536 during the invasion of Italy, the oil supply ran out, and the young surgeon was forced to extemporize. He fashioned a cool, simple paste of egg yolks, oil of roses and turpentine, and applied it, apprehensively, to the wounds of new patients. Next morning, the surprised Paré discovered that the men treated with his makeshift "digestive" were resting comfortably, while their cauterized comrades were "feverish — with great pain and swelling about the edges of their wounds." Dramatically, Paré resolved "never more to burn thus cruelly men with gunshot wounds." Such wounds, he said, "are not poisonous, and the torturous use of the hot cautery is unnecessary."

In amputation cases, Paré continued to use the cautery, but only to staunch blood. Just the same he felt uneasy about smothering a battered stump. According to his own statistics, only about one-third of such cases recovered. Because of ghastly after-effects — fever, convulsions, renewed bleeding — most surgeons avoided amputation entirely. But Paré was now determined to make the process safe, and to this end, he experimented with the ligature. This technique, not unknown in antiquity, had been abandoned in favor of the cautery, but with boiling oil out of the way, it became feasible once more. Thus, when Paré amputated a damaged limb, he would simply tie up the blood vessels and apply his "digestives" to the wound, in place of the more popular dressings — ground rabbit's fur and mummy powder. His patients made an amazing recovery, and so did surgery.

126

Light *leather truss (right) replaced iron bandages in hernia cases.*

Artificial iron hand below was derived by Paré from knight's gauntlet.

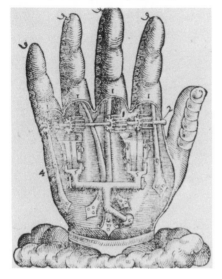

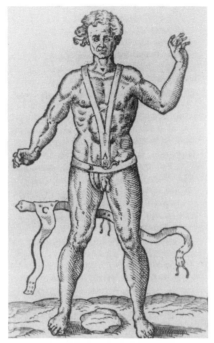

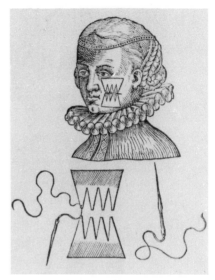

To avoid scars, Paré stitched adhesive, fastened on the outside of the wound lips.

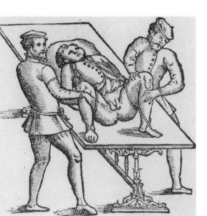

To cut her bladder-stone safely, Pare invented probe with outside slit. This left urinal passage unharmed.

Dislocated shoulder (right) was reset, according to Paré, by attaching pulley to elbow, then guiding dislocated arm into joint with the aid of a towel.

Paré's insight was not limited to surgery alone. He described sound methods for setting fractures and draining wounds; he constructed artificial limbs, surgical instruments and lightweight trusses to support ruptures. Further, he traced aneurysms to syphilis, and linked up pain in passing water to enlarged prostate glands. To avoid Caesarian childbirth, he revived the old podalic version of turning the fetus *in utero* and drawing it out feet first. He even devised a self-administrable syringe for women.

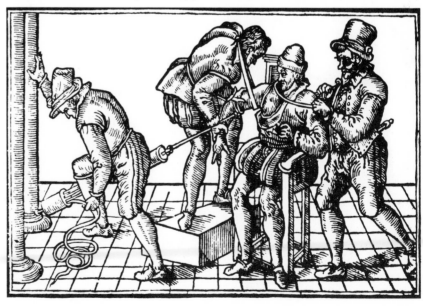

NEW FOUND REMEDIES ...
PHARMACY PROSPERS

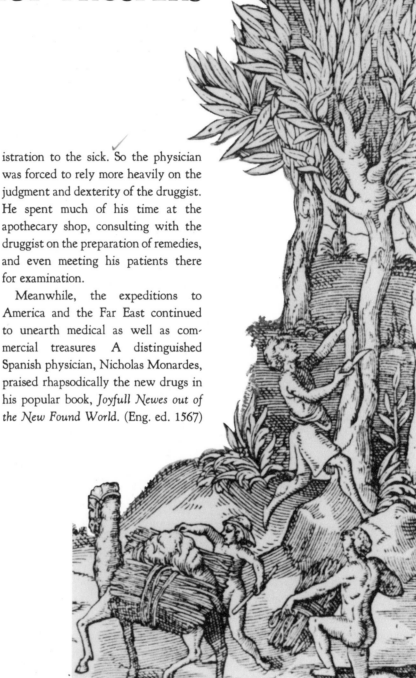

In the second part of the 16th century, the pharmacist was often ahead of the physician in equipment and scientific knowledge. On the one hand, Paracelsian alchemists were exploring the medicinal virtues of metals; on the other, new drugs were arriving from the Far East and West. Such drugs were costly; they had to be distilled, ground down or mixed with other substances for effective administration to the sick. So the physician was forced to rely more heavily on the judgment and dexterity of the druggist. He spent much of his time at the apothecary shop, consulting with the druggist on the preparation of remedies, and even meeting his patients there for examination.

Meanwhile, the expeditions to America and the Far East continued to unearth medical as well as commercial treasures A distinguished Spanish physician, Nicholas Monardes, praised rhapsodically the new drugs in his popular book, *Joyfull Newes out of the New Found World.* (Eng. ed. 1567)

Native lady hands medicinal tobacco leaves to Indian in search of cure.

Cinnamon bark, cut from trees in India, carried to European drugstores via camel caravan and ships. (right)

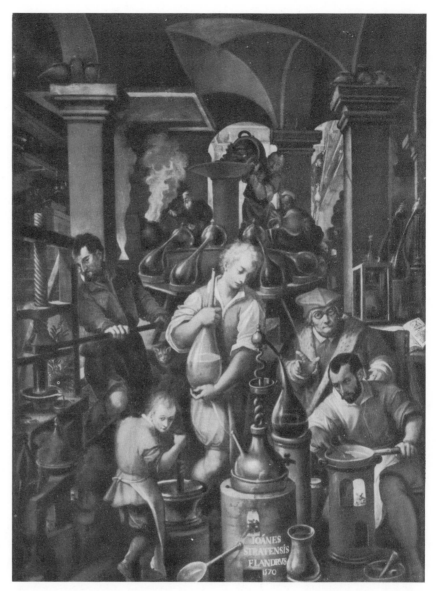

The doctors responded to the "joyful news" in Monardes' book, which ran to twenty editions in five languages.

Though Monardes stayed safely at home, other pioneers in medical botany set out for the Indies, East and West. Francisco Hernandez, court physician to Ferdinand II, spent seven years in Mexico experimenting with the local medicinal plants. He filled 26 volumes with drawings and observations, then labored for nine more years to shape his findings for publication. But he died before the work was finished. Forty years later, a tireless colleague completed a popular abridgement of the whole project. Unfortunately, the original Hernandez manuscripts were lost in a library fire.

Through wealthy Italian importers, the new drugs reached Europe: cinnamon bark from India, resinous balsam from the "weeping tree" of Peru, and most exciting of all — tobacco from America. According to popular belief, the tobacco plant had cured the Indians of many diseases; they used it, specifically, against syphilis, as an analgesic which took "the afflicted out of their minds so that they did not feel pain." Jean Nicot first saw the miraculous herb in Portugal. He brought some seeds to France, called them "nicotiana," and reported that the plant was infallible in whatever way it was applied: in leaf form for cancerous ulcer; as dried powder to snuff headaches away; or as smoking tobacco to alleviate asthma.

The flourishing trade in such cure-alls (balsam was as handy then as mercurochrome today) brought great prosperity to the druggists. They were quick to adapt their knowledge of chemical procedures to the new medicaments. By the end of the century the first crude gropings toward an exact science had begun in their laboratories.

129

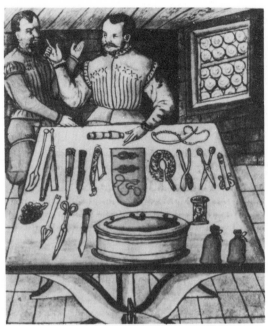

1 *Surgeon briefs aid on instru-*
ments; front box holds compresses.

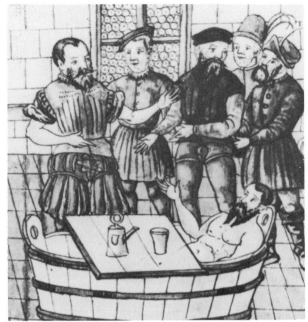

2 *Patient with hernia receives*
hot bath, meets doctor's aids.

SURGEON'S DIARY

Wound-surgeon Caspar Stromayr of Lindau (Lake Leman), completed his magnificent text on herniotomy in 1559.

It presented graphically the day by day activities of a surgeon.

Stromayr used 186 telling water-

3 *Doctor, patient and assistants*
pray for successful outcome.

4 *Patient is tied with heavy*
towels to operating board.

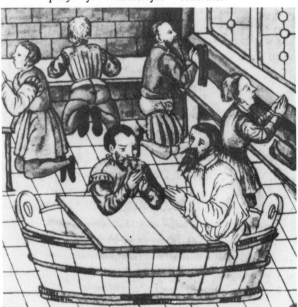

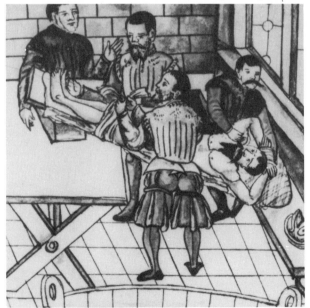

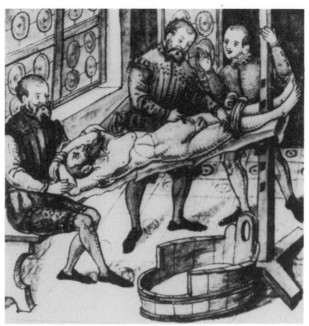

5 *Inclined position makes vis-*
cera sink back into abdomen.

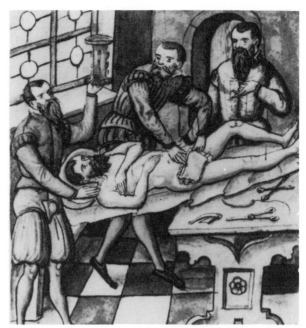

6 *Compress applied to wound;*
hour-glass shows speed of operation.

colors, probably by his own hand, to illustrate operations for the cure of hernias. He described each known form of rupture in great detail, and gave directions for post-operative treatment. The book was written out of compassion for patients who were then prey to the wiles of the wandering herniotomists.

7 *After operation, surgeon*
leads patient to nearby bed.

8 *Patient convalesces; doctor*
pleased — drinks his health.

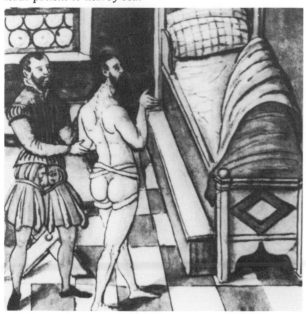

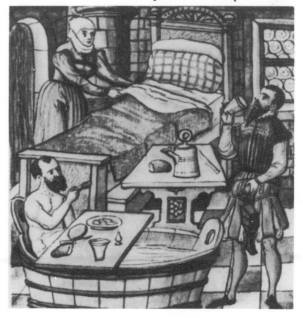

OCULIST TO THE RESCUE

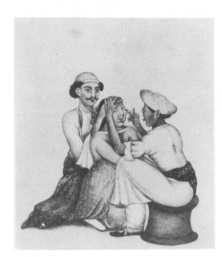

Indian doctor performs cataract operation perfected by Susruta, called the "Hippocrates of India."

In 600 B.C., a Hindu with cataract was better off than a European of 1500 A.D. with the same affliction. The Indian doctor (above) is performing a cataract operation perfected in the 6th century B.C. by Susruta, the "Hippocrates of India." Before operating, the great Susruta would wash his hands, cut his beard and fumigate the room with vapors. Then he would press down the afflicted lens ("couch the cataract") with minute precision. He was familiar, too, with the various forms of glaucoma, and passed on a host of ophthalmological lore to his successors. A Persian physician brought this knowledge to the Middle East around 600 A.D. and the Arabs adapted it a century later when they overran Persia. But ophthalmology remained degenerate in medieval Europe, where it fell into the hands of itinerant mountebanks.

A kind of one-man renaissance in ophthalmology occurred when Georg Bartisch, an empiric surgeon, published the first comprehensive text on the care and cure of eye troubles. Oddly enough, his *Augendienst*, 1583, had a serious blindspot: Bartisch dismissed spectacles — the current rage — as completely useless. "Man," he declared categorically, "has two eyes — he needs not four."

Bartisch's book was published at a time when ophthalmology was still largely in the hands of wandering peddlers and toothdrawers. For as little as seven cents, these "wanton fellows" would operate on cataract in the public market place. The gullible crowds which flocked to such performances were always impressed, since the "miraculous" operation was bloodless and almost painless; further, the procedure lifted the veil of blindness in a matter of minutes. As the theory ran, it was supposed to couch the humour causing the cloudiness; actually, it depressed the lens. Post-operative complications always ensued, and after the quack had made his getaway, it was highly probable that the patient became totally blind. Bartisch was enraged by these wandering "blindmasters" and "eye-destroyers." As court oculist to the Elector August of Saxony, he gained wide experience in eye-care. From Vesalius and his followers, Bartisch derived a working knowledge of ocular anatomy. Then, he wrote out his practical guidebook for oculists, and embellished it with detailed anatomical views of the

eye and brain. He also furnished an elaborate classification of cataracts — gray, blue, yellow and green. To correct such visual defects as convergent

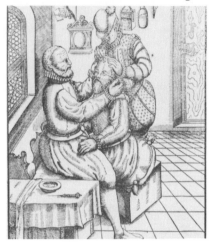

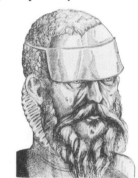

Surgeon operates for cataract

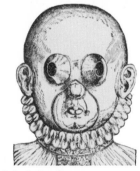

Shade for prevention of eyestrain

Mask for divergent squinting

strabism (eyes turned toward nose), Bartisch constructed special masks. For couching the cataract, he recommended a hard, sharp, silver needle and cautioned, moreover, that the surgeon stay continent for two days before the operation to insure a steady hand and high mental pitch. (As Bass says: the doctor might gain patients this way but also lose his wife.)

In spite of his many sound precepts Bartisch remained enslaved to superstition. He believed that amulets could prevent the devil from hampering the doctor; he believed, further, that eye-surgery was applicable to men only, since female humours made operations on women too precarious. Nonetheless, his book was the first step toward rational ophthalmology.

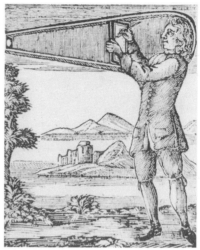

Camera obscura, for tracing landscapes, was modeled after human eye. Della Porta, Naples doctor, invented it.

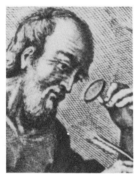 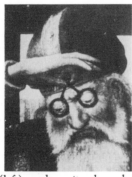 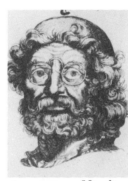

St. Jerome (left) reads script through transparent stone. Virgilius, Roman poet (center), holding up heavy iron-rimmed glasses (15th century painting). Scholar (right) wears improved spectacles.

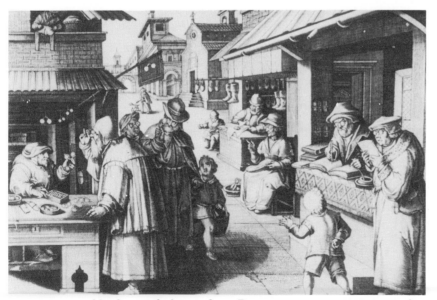

Nearly everybody in above Renaissance street wears spectacles. Wide usage resulted from spread of printed books. Customer at spectacle shop on left is fitted by trial and error method.

A BLESSING FOR THE OLD

If Pliny is to be believed, Nero watched the Roman circus through an eye glass. But the optical aid virtually dropped out of sight until the 13th century, when Roger Bacon recommended reading lenses for the old. A century later, spectacles were invented. They were used extensively during the Renaissance, when printed books began to circulate in great numbers. The practice of reading brought out unsuspected visual defects, especially in the aged. Bulky iron or brass glasses from Venice and Southern Germany were suspended above the nose by hand, and hardly improved a man's looks, and less a lady's.

Nevertheless, the spectacle shop did a thriving business. Though methods of selecting glasses were still primitive, the Renaissance made an earnest effort to alleviate defective eyesight.

133

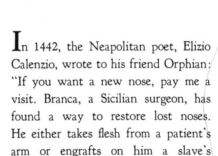

TAGLIACOZZI MASTERMAKER OF NEW NOSES

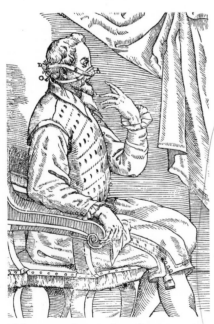

Tagliacozzi (1546-1599) grafted skin flap from arm to nasal tissue with aid of armor-like bandage (G).

After 20 days, rhinoplastic patient could point to rough new nose; further shaping was always necessary.

In 1442, the Neapolitan poet, Elizio Calenzio, wrote to his friend Orphian: "If you want a new nose, pay me a visit. Branca, a Sicilian surgeon, has found a way to restore lost noses. He either takes flesh from a patient's arm or engrafts on him a slave's nose . . . If you come hither, you can go away with as many new noses as you like."

But Branca and his family apparently kept this marvelous knowledge to themselves, for plastic surgery remained dormant for all practical purposes until in the 1580's, Tagliacozzi of Bologna took up the lost art. He revived and perfected it at a time when syphilis raged throughout Europe, disfiguring the human face and offending the newborn sensibilities of Renaissance man. At the same time, criminals and unfaithful women were being punished by having their noses clipped off, so Tagliacozzi arrived on the scene at the right historical moment.

Bologna was the new mecca of the noseless. Tagliacozzi taught anatomy there, and issued the first systematic work on plastic surgery in the form of a comprehensive treatise (1597).

To restore noses, a skin flap from the patient's arm was grafted onto his face, then artfully shaped by the surgeon. A few months later, the patient had a fine new nose. In fact, the noses were so fine that patients often preferred the new designs to God's original creation.

For two to three weeks, Tagliacozzi's patients were forced to sit upright, kept immobile by an armor-like body and arm bandage. The process was far from painless. This prompted the jurist, Paul Zacharius, to rule that a criminal who paid for a crime with his nose might have it legally restored. The plastic operation was twice as painful, he argued, as having the nose clipped off in the first place, so the culprit was thrice punished.

These new noses were also quite fragile, and had to be treated gingerly. It was recommended that metal caps be fitted over them for winter wear. The delicate nature of the new procedure is graphically illustrated by the tale of the "sympathetic nose" told in many variations after Tagliacozzi's untimely death at 54.

One story tells of a man who lost his nose in a duel. To avoid the usual arm incision he asked the surgeon to shape him a nose from the biceps of a porter called "Nock". Thirteen months after the operation, the new nose grew cold and lifeless. Then it dropped off. It was later learned that "the porter expired near about the punctilious time wherein the nose grew frigid." Or as Butler retells it in *Hudibras:*

But when the date of Nock was out Off dropt the sympathetick snout.

While much honoured during his life and praised as a pillar of the Church, many surgeons considered Tagliacozzi's work as sacrilegious. The face, they held, was God's creation, and no human being had the right to meddle with it. Some such trend of thought might also account for the story that the devil hounded Tagliacozzi after death. The surgeon had been buried at the Convent of St. Giovanni Battista, in Bologna. But his cries of everlasting torment are said to have disturbed the nuns' peace. An ecclesiastic court investigated the matter but found no evidence.

Bigotry and open opposition retarded the effective practice of rhinoplasty until the 19th century, when Tagliacozzi's art was revived once more. Today his treatise remains unchallenged as a classic.

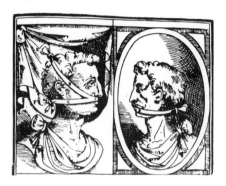

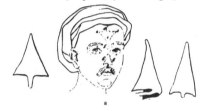

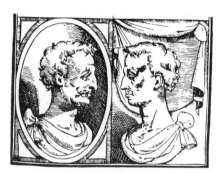

Indian surgeons transplanted skin flap from forehead (below). — Tagliacozzi's restoration of lips. (left and right)

MERCURIO, WRITER ON MIDWIFERY

While Tagliacozzi modeled new noses, his compatriot and friend of student days, Scipione Mercurio improved the hitherto feminine art of midwifery. Strangely enough, Mercurio started his career as a Dominican monk. After traveling through Europe he practiced with success in Venice and Padua. Mercurio's midwifery handbook, published in 1595, was filled with innovations. He gave the first lucid report of a Caesarian operation performed on a living mother. Further, he reintroduced the hanging-leg position (right) which Walcher revived in 1889.

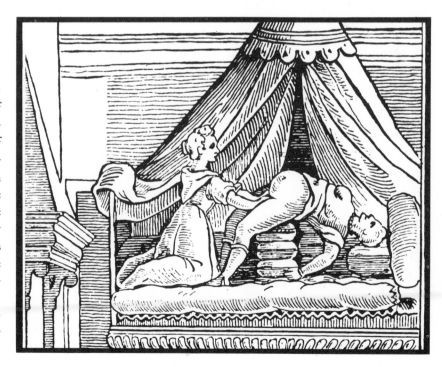

135

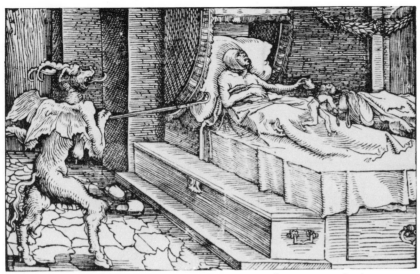

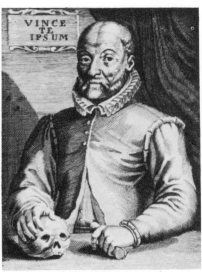

Bewitched woman shown during imaginary tryst with miniature devil.

Johann Weyer called "witches" insane.

THE INSANE .... PATIENTS, NOT WITCHES

Up to this time, mental disease was considered an outgrowth of witchcraft. This harsh doctrine had been proclaimed with religious fervor in the "bible of demonology," Spenger's famous *Malleus Maleficarum* (c. 1485) and many people believed it blindly. The devil had created madness, the credo ran; therefore, the mad were bedevilled and should be burned as witches.

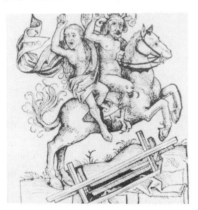

Since this belief excluded insanity from the medical domain, the prudent doctor left the deranged in the hands of law courts and witchburners.

Demented women who repeated their dreams in public were given short shrift in those days. The poor souls who believed in their midnight rides or erotic acts with Lucifer, were quickly trapped in court, and condemned to death. Witch-hunting was considered good form, and the more zealous citizens made it a point to flush the weird sisters out into the open. Fathers did not hesitate to denounce their daughters — if they behaved strangely, and sane and insane women died by the thousands. In such times, a bad dream was a good thing to keep to yourself.

But Johann Weyer (1515-1588), a courageous Belgian physician, defied

the times by declaring that witch-hunters were madder by far than many witches. In his *De Praestigiis Daemonum*, he defined the latter as deranged or perplexed old women who believed in their own fantasies. They were sick and not bedevilled, he added; they needed kindly medical care. "Our expenses would diminish considerably," he wrote, "if we would put to better use the logs and bundles used to burn innocent people."

To prove his point, he took some demented women into his own home. He observed their actions, and with the help of his good wife, he tried to alleviate their fears. Their affliction, he found, was comparable to physical disease. Like Paracelsus, he believed they should be released from dungeons, spared from the pyre, and placed in the hands of doctors. Weyer did in no way deny that demons existed. He contended, however, that insanity had no connection whatsoever with deviltry.

This revolutionary idea might have cost him his life, but his master, Duke William of Juehlich, shared his point of view and afforded him protection. It was heresy, in those days, to deny as Weyer did that the devil could enter the chambers of virtuous nuns via the keyhole. Weyer was therefore fortunate in having such a protector; nonetheless, to cut the

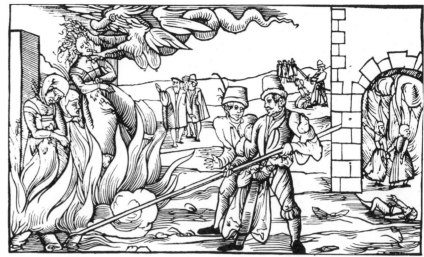

Demented women are burned as witches who consort with the devil.

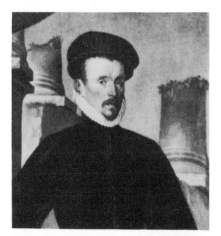

Felix Platter listed forms of insanity.

Gordian knot between witchcraft and insanity took a great deal of courage.

While Weyer's book passed through various editions his influence was not permanent. In Basel, Felix Platter visited the dungeons to classify insanity, but the general attitude toward mental disease remained appalling. When the insane dodged the stake, they were chained in cells or chased from village to village. There were a few "hospitals" which admitted mental cases, but such institutions simply "kept" the insane, and often exposed them to the ridicule of tourists. Until the 19th century, a trip through Europe's first lunatic asylum, Bedlam hospital in London, was popularly considered a hilarious experience that no tourist would want to miss.

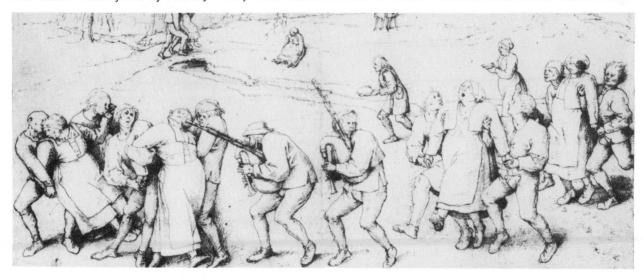

Peter Breughel's merrymaking males equipped with bagpipes poke fun at female victims of St. Vitus' dance.   137

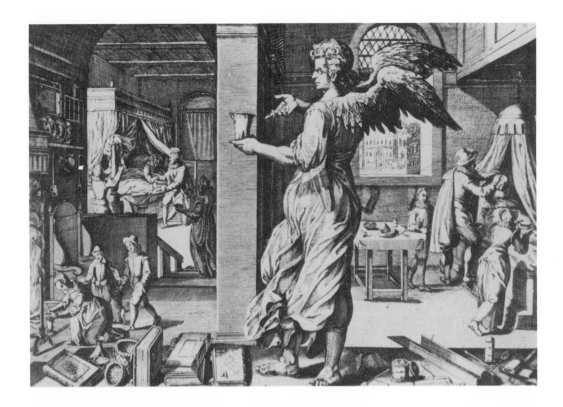

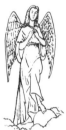

In Sickness:
An Angel.

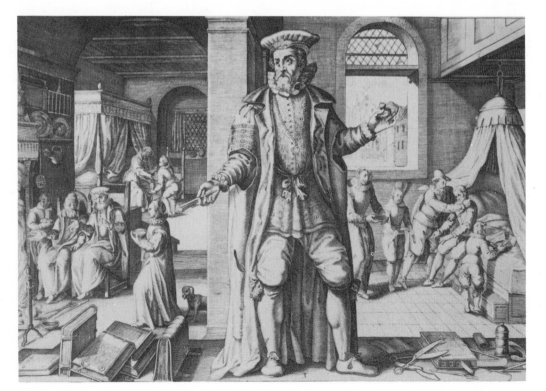

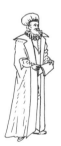

In Health:
A Man

THE DOCTOR'S THREE FACES

It was a paradox that the "enlightened" populace of the Renaissance regarded their doctors with an emotional rather than a rational attitude. This attitude was sharply satirized by the Dutch engraver Hendrik Goltzius. His allegorical drawings of 16th century sick chambers were based on the couplets of Euricius Cordus. These express, in turn, an all-too eternal truth: Whether the doctor is loved, liked or hated depends on the patient's condition.

God and the Doctor we alike adore
When on the brink of danger, not before.
The danger past, both are alike requited
God is forgotten and the doctor slighted.
— EURICIUS CORDUS
transl. by Chauncey Leake

Thus, the drawings show that people found the doctor godlike and angelic when sickness struck, only human when health returned, but diabolical whenever the bill was due. On the left, the kindly angel-physician attends to his patient's needs. But once cured, the patients ignore the devil-doctor's plea for a fee (below). Eventually, thanks to the mating of science and medicine, the doctor was seen from a less emotional viewpoint.

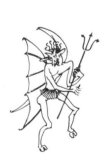

Asking Fee:
A Devil

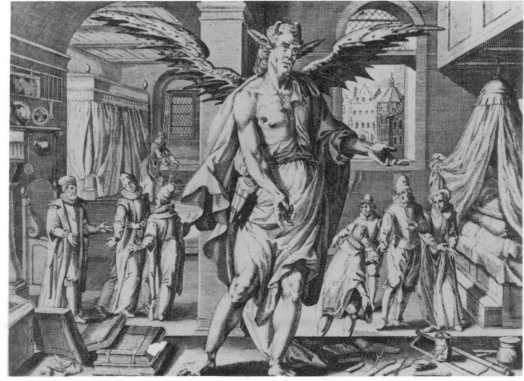

AGE OF MEASUREMENT

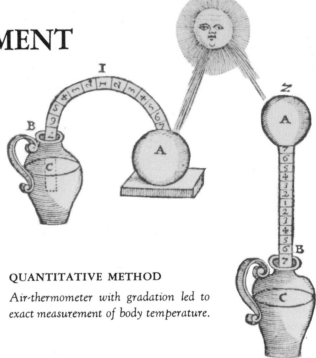

QUANTITATIVE METHOD

*Air-thermometer with gradation led to
exact measurement of body temperature.*

The "scientists" before the age of science were largely concerned with the quality of the elements which make up the world. They speculated on the nature of earth, air, fire and water, and related these elements to the human body. Their interest was "qualitative" predominantly. Then, with the Renaissance, the wonders of the world were examined more closely. By the time Galileo came to Padua, in 1592, the age of measurement was at hand.

At Padua, Galileo lectured on mathematics to an overflow audience with medical students much in prominence. He expounded his famous theories, and invented such instruments as the telescopic lens, the thermoscope and the pendulum. One of his students, Santorio Santorio, called Sanctorius, borrowed these devices to make comparative studies of the human temperature and pulse. Another graduate of Padua, William Harvey, later applied Galileo's laws of motion and mechanics to the problem of blood circulation. (It was a question of measurement — how much blood moves through the arteries — which finally

solved the riddle of the function of the heart.) And still other scientists took up the lens, the time-piece and the balances to examine minute or massive phenomena and to record their findings in quantitative terms.

Galileo had imbued his listeners from every land with an appreciation of experiment and exact measurement as scientific tools. Such tools provided them with an effective check against reckless speculation. From then on, even the plausible theory had to jibe with irrefutable experiments before it became acceptable.

Medical science eventually learned to utilize these new methods of research. The degree of fever, the pulse-count, could now be related to other symptoms, and at the same time, the whole panorama of disease could be mapped out in the laboratory. The new science of optics amplified man's vision downward as well as up, and an unknown, miniature world came into focus under the microscope. Dials, watches, rules, scales and lens: these were the tools which science and medicine now held in common.

These new tools and principles were often brought to the public's attention in a dramatic way. In 1654, Otto von Guericke, the mayor of Magdeburg, decided to startle the town's burghers with one of the wonders of the age (see below). After arduous study in the field of pneumatics, he had perfected an air pump.

With his pump, Guericke created a vacuum in a two-part metal sphere.

After this, two teams of ten horses each, struggled in vain to pull the sphere apart. Then air was admitted, and the sphere flopped apart with no external pressure. Guericke had successfully dramatized the type of experiment and research which made the 17th century a great age for science — paired with showmanship.

Unfortunately, the impact of these new scientific discoveries on the average physician was slight.

The four humours thrived in the examining room long after Harvey had killed them off in the laboratory. The pharmacies continued to dispense noxious ointments which had first been employed by Arabian herbalists. And blood was let in copious quantities, a true farce in an age that had discovered the principle of blood transfusion. Since the universities remained governed by dogma, the new savants were forced to band together in scientific societies all over Europe. Such groups were uniformly devoted to experimental research, and to this end, they pooled their instruments and their illustrious talents.

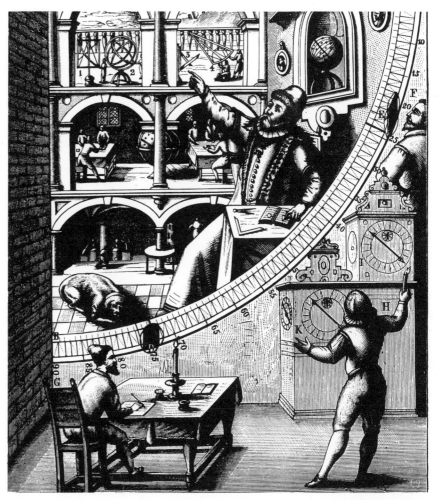

OBSERVATION

Astronomers make dial readings, compute findings. Doctors banded together in similar fashion to observe cooperatively the laws of the living body.

EXPERIMENT

Otto von Guericke demonstrated in 1654 workings of vacuum airpump. Doctor-scientists also began to experiment.

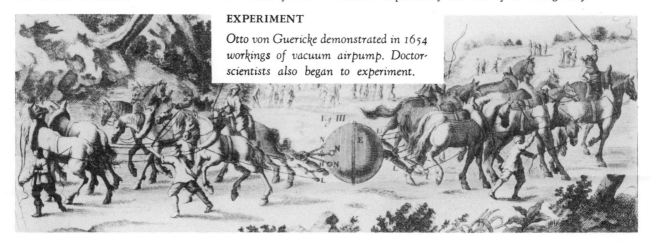

141

GILBERT EXPLORES MAGNETISM

"Gilbert shall live till loadstones cease to draw."

— *Dryden*

The word "electron" (Greek for amber) was introduced into the lexicon by William Gilbert, the president of the Royal College of Physicians who attended Queen Elizabeth in the last years of her life. According to Hakluyt, the great chronicler, Gilbert was "a gentleman no lesse excellent in the chiefest secrets of mathematicks than in his own profession of physicke." As a doctor, he had gained a large practice among London's aristocracy. But his experiments with magnets were to bring him even greater fame.

At that time, the loadstone was considered medicinal, and somewhat miraculous. It could "realign" a broken marriage, cure headaches, or, in mountainous form, pull the nails from passing ships, and thereby sink them. Gilbert exploded such nonsense with his classic treatise, *De Magnete*, which laid the foundation of the modern science of electricity.

Handily for the historian, the book was published in 1600. Gilbert had worked for years on the problem of magnetic properties. His home was filled with scientific apparatus and he had spent about £5000 (according to Harvey) on his highly objective experiments. He ruled out medicinal loadstones, but found that filed powder of iron was an excellent treatment for anemia. Most of the book was concerned, however, with physics, and only the methods of investigation proved valuable to medicine.

In the painting below, Gilbert entertains the court of Queen Elizabeth with some of his findings. He was considered her favorite physician.

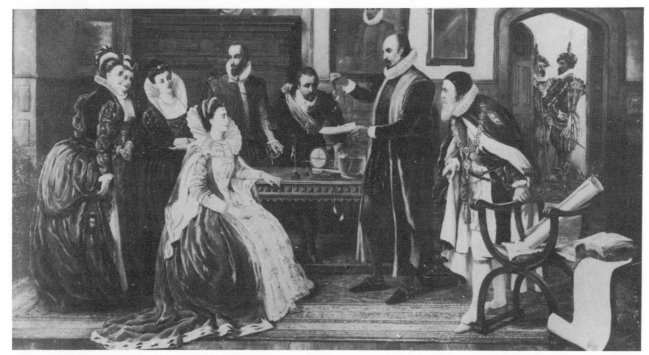

Dr. William Gilbert (1540-1603) President of the College of Physicians experimenting before Queen Elizabeth.

SANCTORIUS MEASURES METABOLISM

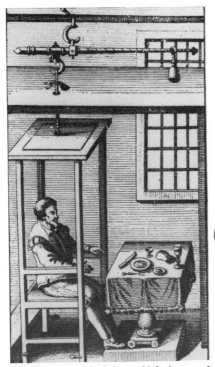

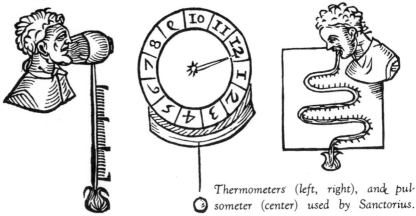

Thermometers (left, right), and pulsometer (center) used by Sanctorius.

Sanctorius weighed himself before and after meals in special chair (above). He was first doctor to conduct systematic quantitative research on metabolism.

Unlike Gilbert, Sanctorius used physics strictly as an aid to medicine. From his friend Galileo, he borrowed the pendulum and the thermometer for clinical research. He constructed the first pulse-watch (based on the pendulum), in order to gather data on the relation between pulse-beat and disease. When the length of the pendulum was adjusted until the swing matched the beat, the pulse was accurately measured on a dial (see above illustration). Sanctorius proudly claimed that his "pulsilogium" could "measure the pulsebeat with mathematical certainty . . . (it was) not feigned by conjecture."

The thermometer, too, could be used in diagnosis, said Sanctorius, "to learn daily with accuracy how much the patient's heat deviates from the normal."

In his most ambitious attempt to measure body behavior, Sanctorius utilized a "weighing chair." If a man was weighed before and after

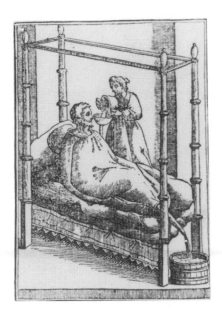

Leatherbag bath used by Sanctorius to counteract fever of bedridden patient.

meals and after digestion, part of the food registered in the form of added body-weight and part in excretion. But there would still be a difference between foodweight on the one side of the ledger and the sum of excretion plus added body-weight on the other. This difference was ascribed at that time to "invisible perspiration." Today we call these processes faintly fathomed by Sanctorius metabolism.

This indefatigable experimenter spent countless hours in his suspended chair, weighing himself after meals, naps and even sexual intercourse.

Sanctorius actually lived "in the balance." He placed his work table, bed and other necessities needed for existence, on suitable balances of his own devising. It was the first time in the history of medicine that a physician attempted to investigate physiological processes by exact measurement.

Unfortunately, he was too far ahead of his age, and most of his information proved useless. Pulse, temperature and body metabolism remained uncorrelated until modern physiology filled in the details.

WILLIAM HARVEY

"TRUTH IS MY TRUST"

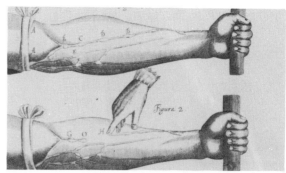

Experiment proving that valves let blood flow in but one direction was link in Harvey's chain of evidence.

At the Frankfort book fair of 1628, a slender volume called *De Motu Cordis et Sanguinis* was on display. Written by William Harvey, a London professor, its 72 badly printed pages dealt with a revolutionary theory: that the blood circulates throughout the body, and the heart functions as its pump. Today, this theory is a basic concept of medical science. Modern physiology, cardiology and hematology date from the publica-

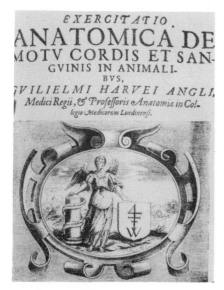

Title page of Harvey's epochal book on the circulation of the blood, 1628.

tion of Harvey's book. Transfusions, intravenous injections and shunting operations — all stem from the pioneer work of William Harvey.

As a young student at Padua, Harvey had learned from his teacher, Fabricius of Aquapendente, that the vein valves keep the flow of blood uni-directional. From Galileo, he had borrowed the quantitative approach of physics, and applied it to his later experiments with circulation. Thus, he was able to estimate that two ounces of blood were squeezed through the heart with every beat. At 72 beats per minute, 8640 ounces of blood (three times the normal body-weight and far more pressure than the tissues could stand) would pass through the body each hour. This proved that Galenic beliefs (that new blood wells up in an incessant ebb and flow from the liver) were ridiculous. Harvey concluded, instead, that a fixed quantity of blood flowed from the heart through the body via the arteries, and returned to the heart through the veins. Then a smaller cycle ensued, with the blood moving from the right chamber of the heart into the lungs, and from the lungs back to the left heart chamber and out into the

body again.

Harvey first expressed this theory in 1616, in a Lumleian lecture at the Royal College in London, but he took twelve years to publish his findings. He worked incessantly and methodically, setting down his experiments and conclusions briefly, and without rhetoric. In time, his findings changed the entire direction of medicine. Now that the mechanics of the blood-movement was known, disease could be tackled from within the body as well as from without.

Science was merely Harvey's avocation, a fact that makes his discoveries

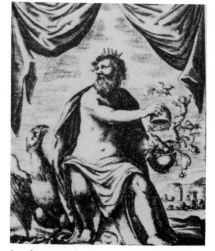

At the age of 73 Harvey published his second masterwork: De Generatione.

all the more impressive. For most of his life, he concentrated upon the practice of medicine, with Francis Bacon, the Earl of Arundel, James and Charles I as his most notable patients. Charles I took such an interest in Harvey's scientific pursuits that he placed the deer herds in the Royal Gardens at his disposal. When Harvey came upon some special find, he would demonstrate it before the king. Charles, in turn, would call strange cases to the doctor's attention. Once Harvey and the King peeked into the side of a courtier wounded in a fall. The beating heart was clearly visible, so they both touched it, and concluded that it was insensible.

During the Civil War, Harvey accompanied Charles as a physician. Later, he continued his embryological studies under the king's aegis at Oxford. He retired from the royal service at the age of 68, shortly after Charles defeat. He "retired" even further after the publication of his second great work, *De Generatione Animalium*, in 1651.

While this treatise on embryology influenced medical science profoundly, it was in his first book that Harvey set the classic example of medical research. His verdicts were proven by experiments and appraised by sound inductive reasoning.

Having mapped out the cycle of man's lifestream Harvey did not undertake to fill in the details. The scientists that followed him subjected individual regions to closer scrutiny with the aid of auxiliary instruments, Harvey had to rely mostly on what he saw with the naked eye. In spite of this, his verdicts have stood the tests of time.

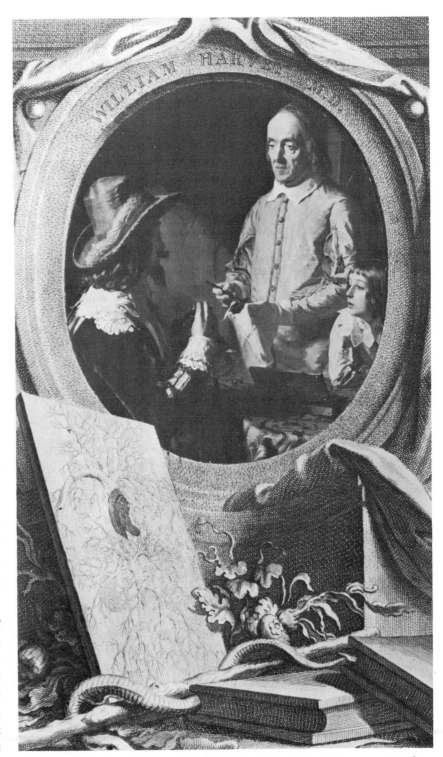

Harvey explains his theory to Charles I, his patron, whom he accompanied as physician during king's war with Parliament. (Painting by Robert Hannah.)

145

HARVEY: Continued

The giant of medicine was a lean, swarthy, undersized fellow who was forever playing with the knob of a dagger that he wore on his belt. If his works were restrained and objective, his pronouncements seemed overly bold to the stuffy Galenic academicians. Jean Riolan, his foremost opponent, called him "a circulator" — an itinerant quack. This French anatomist attacked Harvey's theories in a vicious pamphlet, but Harvey countered, in 1649, with a reasoned scholarly reply which disarmed his opponent. Yet the stark dogmatists continued to follow the slogan: "I prefer to err with Galen than to accept Harvey's truth."

Harvey possessed what Thomas Huxley has called "the fanaticism of veracity." "My trust is my love of truth," he wrote, "and the candour that inheres in cultivated minds." He sought out truth "through experiment," and through contemplation.

In the gardens of his country home, Combe, in Surrey, he is said to have had caves built so he might retire to a cool place to meditate. It was his lonely pursuit of truth that made him appear to the outside world as somewhat of an eccentric.

There is no doubt that he displayed many traits of the beloved physician, and one of his classic shortcomings —an illegible handwriting.

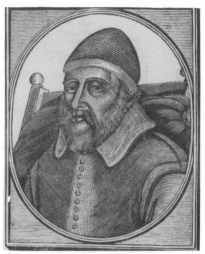

OLD PARR

At royal command Harvey performed an autopsy on the body of Old Parr. This rather remarkable individual was to become a symbol of longevity. He gave his age as 152 when the Earl of Arundel brought him to London. Parr was said to have married at 88 and committed adultery at 102. He was seen threshing corn for a living at 130. London's foul air and rich food soon struck him down. Harvey's famed report named peri-pneumonia as the cause of his death.

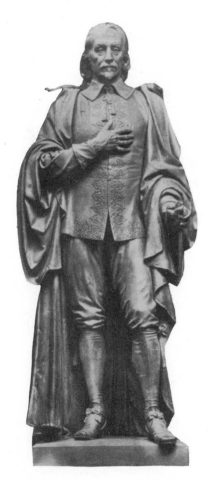

Memorial statue of Harvey, at Folkestone, where he was born in 1578.

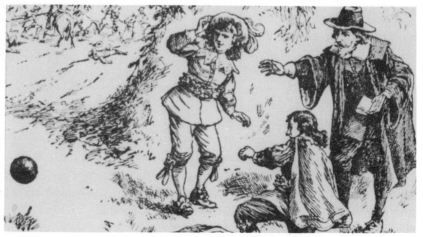

During Battle of Edgehille, 1642, Harvey took care of sons of Charles I. "He set to reading" but a cannon ball compelled him to "remove his station."

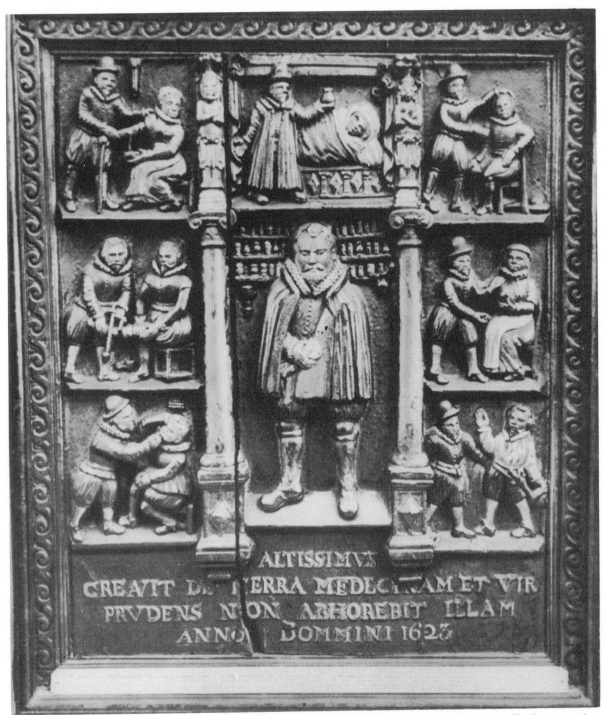

ALTISSIMVS
CREAVIT DE TERRA MEDECINAM ET VIR
PRVDENS NON ABHOREBIT ILLAM
ANNO DOMMINI 1623

A DOCTOR'S SHINGLE

The advertising sign of a Dorsetshire doctor (above) shows the state of practical medicine during Harvey's lifetime. From left to right, the "carved cartoons" illustrate the doctor's skill at dentistry, amputation, phlebotomy, urine-analysis, pulse-reading and the cure of backaches.

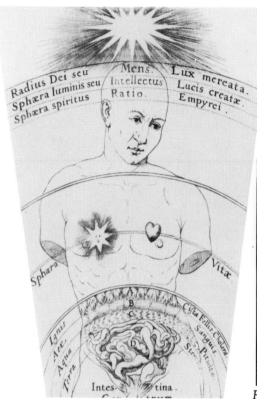

THE MYSTERY AND ..

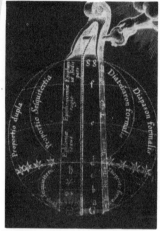

Robert Fludd (1574-1637) thought body was attuned to spheres, which were arranged in "musical" harmony. (left).

Mysticism was left pretty much intact — in spite of the advance of exact science. On the one hand, the minds of great scientists still had their dark corners: on the other, the minds of great mystics had their bright ones. It was an age of transition, and in some ways, a more tolerant age than our own. In 1609, for instance, Dr. Robert Fludd, an avowed mystic, was admitted to the Royal College of Physicians of London. Like Paracelsus, Fludd believed that astral bodies had an influence on health. He also believed in the harmony of the spheres. It was the doctor's job, he felt, to bring the sick body — the microcosm — back in tune with itself and the universe. In a mechanistic age, he reserved a safe place for metaphysical forces.

But Fludd distinguished himself also as a scientist. He was one of the first to applaud Harvey's discovery. Lengthy experiments were conducted in his house, which he had transformed into a laboratory. He designed ingenious machines along Galilean lines (among them, a wooden bull that bellowed and a self-playing lyre). Further, he compounded his own drugs and believed that consumptives might be cured by the use of sputum from cured patients.

ASTRO-HERBALIST

In 1649, Nicholas Culpeper, defied the Royal College by publishing an English edition of its famous *Pharmacopoeia*. This helped to popularize new knowledge, but it also incurred the wrath of organized medicine. Culpeper was labeled as "a frowsy-headed coxcomb who gallimawfried the *Apothecaries' Book* into nonsense." Actually, he had incorporated it verbatim into his own works. In 1708, Culpeper's *The English Physician* became the first medical book published in America.

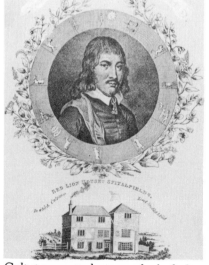

Culpeper, astrologer and herbalist, fought "filthy pretentions" of London physicians, plagiarized their books.

148

.. THE CHEMISTRY OF LIFE

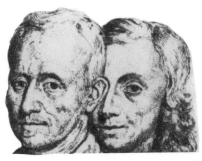

Another typical representative of this age of transition was Jean Baptiste van Helmont (1577-1644), the doctor-chemist of Brussels. Van Helmont was strongly attracted to the mystic gospel of Paracelsus. Like the master, he believed that life-secrets might be found in the chemical reactions of the human body. His research into the digestive processes led him to some valuable deductions. He was the first to observe weight changes in urine, for instance, and to point up the chemical functions of vital glands and their secretions: bile, chyle and gastric juice. His insight into body functions also led him to a virulent attack against bloodletting.

"A bloody moloch sits president in the chairs of medicine," proclaimed van Helmont.

He found his own medical chair by contracting scabies while shaking hands with an afflicted lady. When his Galenic physicians called it a liver ailment, van Helmont decided to cure himself, and did so with a sulphur ointment. Then he struggled through Galen and Avicenna, but discarded them in favor of Paracelsus. Like the latter, he believed medicine was the *ars suprema*. He conducted many experiments, then bundled his mystical and rational conclusions together in his ambitious *Opera Omnia*. In this book, he expounded the doctrine of immunity: "For he who has once recovered from that disease hath not only obtained a pure balsaamical blood, whereby for the future he is rendered free from any recidivation of the same evil, but the blood also infallibly cures

Jean Baptiste van Helmont (1577-1644) and his son, editor of father's writings.

the same affection in his neighbour."

Van Helmont turned down a doctor's degree at the University of Louvain, saying he felt disqualified to be a student, let alone a master of the Seven Arts. But his ideas on the chemical nature of life deeply impressed his contemporaries, especially when pruned and systematized by his pupil Sylvius. In addition to this, van Helmont easily ranks as one of the noblest practicing physicians who ever lived. He never forgot the Paracelsian concept of medical dedication, and refused to take money from his patients.

Title page of van Helmont's Opera.

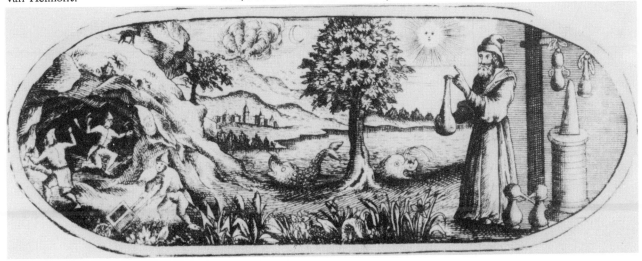

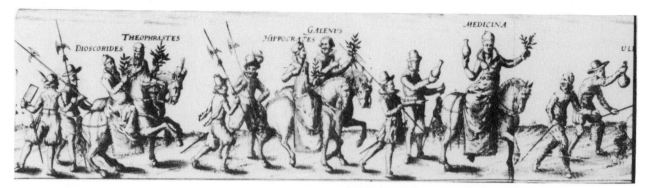

Medicine making its triumphant entry into Leyden, 1557.

HOLLAND'S RISE TO MEDICAL FAME

The Anatomy Lesson painted by Rembrandt at the age of 26.

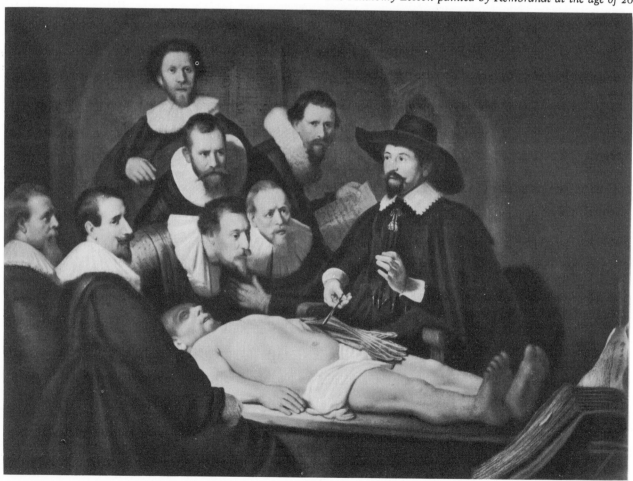

People today would consider a chance to escape legally from all taxes for ten years as a piece of good fortune. When the citizens of Leyden were offered such a chance in 1574 they didn't hesitate to say no. The city had just heroically withstood the onslaught by its Spanish besiegers. To reward the burghers for their gallant stand, William the Silent asked them to choose between two gifts: freedom from taxes for ten years, or the establishment of a university. Intellectual interests prevailed.

Leyden University opened the next year and its fame spread around the world. In the 16th century medical students seeking a higher education had gone to Padua and other Italian schools. Now the Dutch academies took up the bright torch of learning. Medically and politically, the Netherlands were making rapid advances. Trade with the New World gave the towns along the Atlantic coasts of Europe added importance. As the Dutch grew rich they showed increasing interest in science.

Leyden's rising fame as a medical school rested on two pillars, anatomical research and clinical instruction. Francis de la Boe Sylvius introduced bedside demonstration in Leyden in 1658.

This was a most important innovation. Sylvius himself described it. "I have led my students . . . daily to visit the sick at the public hospital. There I have put the symptoms of disease before their eyes; have let them hear the complaints of the patients . . . and have asked them their opinion in each case . . . Then I have given my own judgment on every point."

It was from the modest clinic that Leyden's fame as a medical center spread all over Europe.

Rembrandt entertained close ties with the medical fraternities of Delft and Amsterdam.

Among their members, none became better known through the master's brush than Dr. Tulp. He was both Rembrandt's friend and doctor. The artist once consulted him about a harassing idea. Rembrandt thought that "his bones were like jelly." Dr. Tulp, using psychotherapy, freed the artist from his obsession.

In the annals of research and scientific medicine, Dr. Tulp is well remembered through his classical description of Beri Beri. But Dr. Tulp did not like to share his knowledge with the laity. The trend of the time to popularize medicine found in him a vociferous foe. He felt that physicians who wrote in the vernacular actually hurt the public. As a case in point, he tells of a man who, dislocating his fibula, tried to cure himself by consulting a book by Paré. Shying away from the doctor's counsel, "he became sleepless and insane."

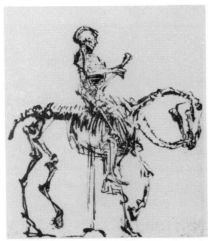

Horseman sketched by Rembrandt (above) in Leyden Anatomical Theatre. Equestrian skeleton served as basis for his Polish Rider, famed painting in New York's Frick Art Collection.

Anatomical theatre, pride of Leyden's citizenry had no seats, but fence rails, decorated with specimens (below)

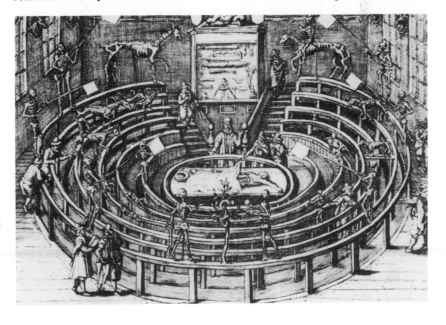

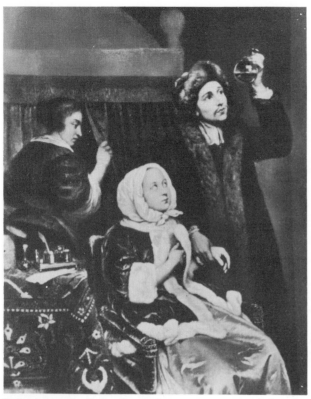 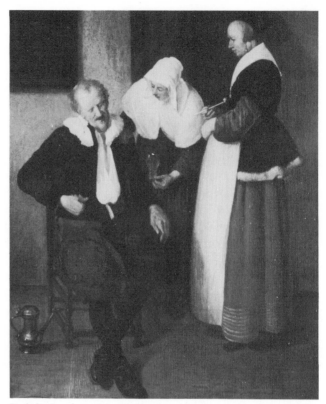

Caspar Netscher's handsome doctor scans urine, feels pulse of pining lady; maid disapproves.

Brekelenkam's tired old burgher clutches side after fainting spell; wine aids in recovery.

DUTCH DOCTORS ON CANVAS

As pouch and purse expanded, the benevolent Dutch burgher had his daily life depicted by the contemporary school of genre painters. His sensual, prosperous ways often led to body disorders, so medical scenes appeared quite frequently. Jan Steen alone painted twenty-odd pictures of the doctor at the bedside, and other artists followed suit. Their canvasses were peopled by two kinds of medical men: some showed the suave, fashionable practitioner; others the pretentious quack.

Though the thermometer and pulsometer had been invented, the Dutch physician still relied on the old standbys — the mysterious inspection of urine, and the rough guess at the patient's pulse. The more prosperous doctors seemed to be favorites with the ladies. Time and again, handsome young physicians are shown attending to female cases of melancholia and *febris amatoria* (love fever).

The itinerant surgeons were more colorful, since oafish victims inevitably came their way. Jan Steen's peasant, for instance (opposite page), was cured by an old medical hoax — "the removal of stones from the head." The stones were actually passed along a surreptitious assembly line from apprentice to surgeon to surgeon's wife, who caught them in a barber's bowl. Such itinerants lacked official recognition, but they tried to inspire confidence by printing medical bills-of-fare with prices for the cure or every ill from cancer to cataract. The charlatan wears his diploma right on the hat.

LOCKSMITH FREES HIMSELF OF BLADDER-STONE

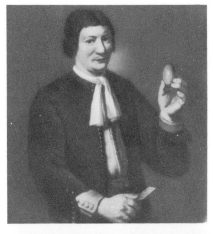

Locksmith Jan Doot, afflicted with calculus, was afraid to entrust his life to a wandering lithotomist, so he cut out his bladder-stone himself. (1651). The incision was made through the belly with a kitchen knife (right). A public notary covered the operation in the newspapers, an artist placed it on canvas (left). The stone (which weighed four ounces) and the knife (with wooden handle) are still preserved in the Pathology Laboratory of Leyden University.

Dr. Tulp, Rembrandt's famed friend called the operation "one of the most valliant acts in history."

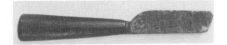

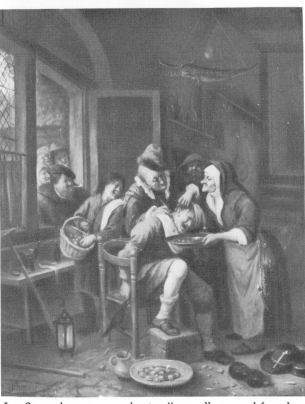

Jan Steen shows peasant having "stones" removed from head. Boy hands them to surgeon surreptitiously (above).

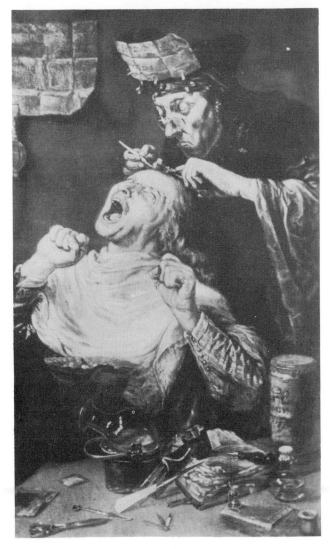

Diploma on quack's hat, document on wall, fail to quiet howling patient in Jan de Bray's painting (right).

FREDERICK RUYSCH, ANATOMIST EXHIBITS STRANGE SPECIMENS

The happy alliance between anatomy and art was revived in 17th century Holland. Great Dutch painters were attracted to anatomy, and anatomists, conversely, to art. Specimens were now prepared with an eye toward esthetics, and dissector Frederick Ruysch excelled at the new practice. His surrealistic sculpture groups were composed of skeletons, bladder-stones and veins, arteries and organs, the latter made solid with the aid of colored injections. In one of Ruysch's groups, a bony figure holds a fiddle formed from a sequestrum and a bow made out of an injected artery. In another, a uterus, complete with illegitimate foetus, is wryly labeled: "Fish may be found in pools where one least suspects them."

Peter the Great during his stay in Holland was touched by the charm of Ruysch's collection and especially by the body of a child embalmed with great artistry. He bent down, kissed its forehead, and promptly bought the whole specimen collection for 30,000 florins (about $100,000). Then he hired sailors to take it to St. Petersburg. Along the way the sailors drank much of the preserving alcohol. Part of the collection survived, however till recent times.

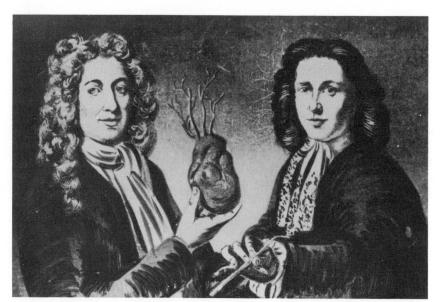

Heart is studied by de Boekelman and Six. These Amsterdam anatomists demonstrated in 1699 a method to solidify heart vessels by injections. (Painting by Pool.)

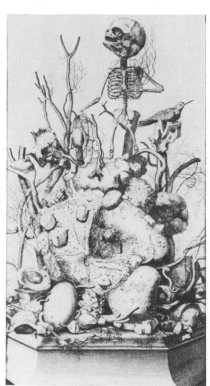

Ruysch combined organs, skeleton, calculi into grotesque specimen-groups.

In this period, the structure of the heart received closer scrutiny. Harvey already had indicated its function by explaining the interaction between heart, lungs and blood. Now the Dutch anatomists probed deeper by injecting the organ with solidifying liquids to reveal its finer vessels. Such work enabled the English physiologists at the Royal Society to move along still further. With the mechanics of circulation known they recognized that blood transfusion was a distinct possibility. It was this group which paved the way toward the practical application of Harvey's discovery.

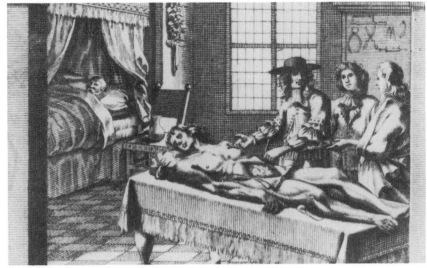

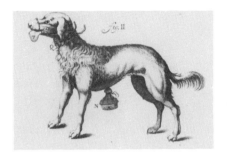

Dog (below) carries receptacle under pancreatic fistula created by de Graaf to observe the working of secretion.

Title picture of de Graaf's Of the Pancreatic Juice, 1671 edition.

DE GRAAF, PHYSIOLOGIST TAPS PANCREATIC JUICE

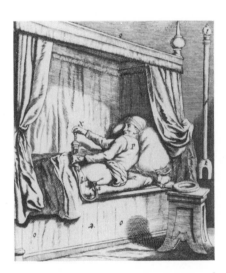

Enema for self-administration, invented by de Graaf. Long hose and exchangeable cannula enabled women to use this syringe for both anal injections and vaginal irrigation. This saved the embarrassment of calling in the apothecary, who usually gave clysters.

At the age of 23, while still a student under the great Sylvius, Regnier de Graaf wrote the treatise which established his fame as a pioneer biochemist. He had developed a method of collecting the pancreatic secretions of dogs through a fistula, with a receptacle attached. The salivary glands were tapped in similar fashion.

De Graaf was so intent on such studies that he once performed an impromptu autopsy on a French sailor who had just been killed by a falling mast. While the body was still warm, he drained the pancreatic juice and drank a sampling of it. Unfortunately, his treatise of 1664 was marred by absurd interpretations common among early iatrochemists. Though de Graaf had some inkling that glandular functions might offer the key to treatment of

disease, this idea had not yet fully ripened. Two hundred years later, Claude Bernard was to demonstrate the true function of the pancreatic juice in digestion.

Unlike Frederick Ruysch who lived to the ripe old age of 93, de Graaf was only 32 years old when he died. His accomplishments as a physiologist, embryologist, anatomist and practitioner are therefore all the more remarkable. As the picture at the top of the page indicates, he was fully aware of the important relation between disease and pathological study. Moreover, with insulin such a common and highly important factor in modern medicine, he deserves to be remembered today as the first investigator to focus attention on pancreatic research.

155

AS SCIENTIFIC FACTIONS FIGHT ...

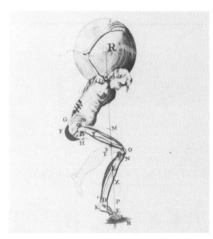

MECHANICAL DOCTORS

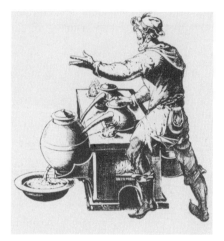

CHEMICAL DOCTORS

To the school of iatrochemistry then prevalent, the body was like a test tube, or a laboratory, in which chemical juices did all the work. To the opposing iatrophysicists, the body appeared as a machine. 17th century medicine was divided between these two schools, with Galileo and Sanctorius as the pioneer-mechanists, and Helmont-de Graaf as the proponents of iatrochemistry.

Italy was the stronghold of the mechanical school. Here Borelli decided that muscle movements were "rapid explosions" of blood mixed with muscle fluid, while Baglivi called the stomach a stove. Meanwhile, van Helmont at Brussels was intent on discovering "fermentation" as the cause of all vital action. But an apt statement from John Hunter resolved the argument a century later:

"Some physiologists will have it that the stomach is a mill, others that it is a fermenting vat, but a stomach, gentlemen, is a stomach."

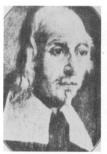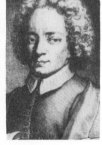

BORELLI (above left)
founder of bio-mechanics, studied workings of skeletal and muscular systems.

BAGLIVI (above right)
compared heart to bellows, teeth to scissors, stomach to stove.

PITCAIRNE (right)
thought stomach was pressure-cooker, with digestion due to muscle pressure.

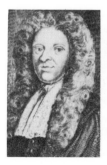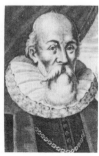

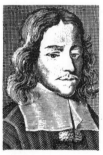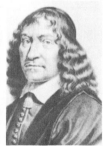

WILLIS (above left)
doctor was "vintner" who watched living processes activated by "ferments."

SYLVIUS (above right)
believed body actuated by changing mixture of saliva, pancreatic juice, bile.

SENNERT (left)
ascribed life to corpuscles, chemically propelled. He still believed in witches.

A DOCTOR GOES BACK TO THE BEDSIDE

When Hans Sloane came to London as a young physician, he presented himself to the illustrious Dr. Sydenham. Sloane who later founded the British Museum, handed Sydenham a letter of introduction which emphasized the bearer's skill as a botanist, anatomist and all-around scholar. But Sydenham was unimpressed. "Anatomy, botany — nonsense!" he exploded, "You must go to the bedside, it is there alone you can learn disease."

Sydenham was a practical clinician, with little use for laboratory knowledge or the subtle refinements of mechanical and chemical speculation. He did not deny the advances of science, he simply ignored them, since they proved useless to the practitioner. Thus, when Dr. Richard Blackmore asked him what books to read to improve his knowledge, Sydenham curtly suggested *Don Quixote*.

Actually, his patients were his books. Like his good friends Robert

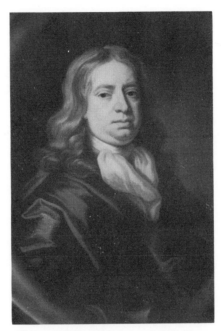

Thomas Sydenham (1624-1689) "I assist nature as Hippocrates bid me."

Boyle and John Locke, he believed in direct observation and the power of reason. Like Hippocrates, he charted the course of diseases. He believed

their course was orderly, and that nature had set up legible signposts along the way. Knowing these posts, the doctor could help to reestablish the body's balance by a sensible regimen: diet, rest and comparatively simple remedies.

This philosophy established him as the great outsider of his day. His practice was considerable, though he held no professorship and wrote no weighty treatises. At 52, he finally took his doctor's degree. Yet his character and teachings have impressed themselves upon succeeding generations. In the 18th century, another great clinician, Boerhaave of Leyden, was to remove his hat whenever he mentioned the name of Sydenham.

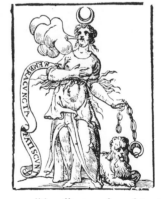

The term "fever" covered at this time a multitude of afflictions. Sydenham evolved differentiation enabling physicians to make concise diagnosis.

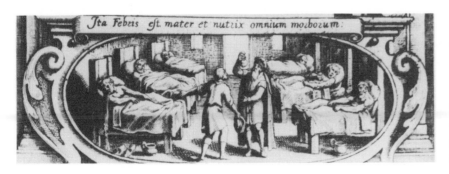

157

SYDENHAM TREATS GOUT

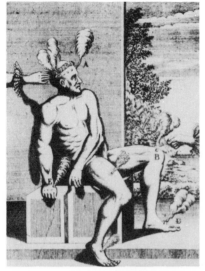

"The physician should bear in mind," wrote Sydenham, "that he is subject to the same laws of mortality and disease as others . . . he will care for the sick with more tenderness if he remembers that he himself is their fellow-sufferer." Sydenham spoke from

In China, cones of moxa leaves were lit on gouty parts (left). Moxa was used recently to treat atomic wounds.

experience. He suffered from gout for over thirty years, and in later life arthritic pain forced him to abandon his practice. Thus, the deep compassion in his treatise on gout is quite understandable. His description of the sudden onset and unrelenting progress of the disease has never been surpassed.

In treating gout, Sydenham refrained from strong-arm therapy. He was never wholly averse to bleeding and purging, but he recommended diet and rest instead. One of his own favorite remedies was "a draught of small beer," which he drank before dinner, after dinner, and before going to bed. As for wine: In one of the best known medical aphorisms he stated: "If you drink wine you have the gout. If you do not drink wine, the gout has you." He was strongly opposed to the sweat-cures prevalent at the time. Fresh air and plenty of horseback riding were far better for healing gout, said Sydenham. With regard to this latter concept, gouty and tubercular patients were commonly advised to get jobs as post-riders.

Sydenham comforted his readers by saying that gout attacked the rich more frequently than the poor, and that it rarely attacked fools. "Those who choose," he added dryly, "may except the present writer."

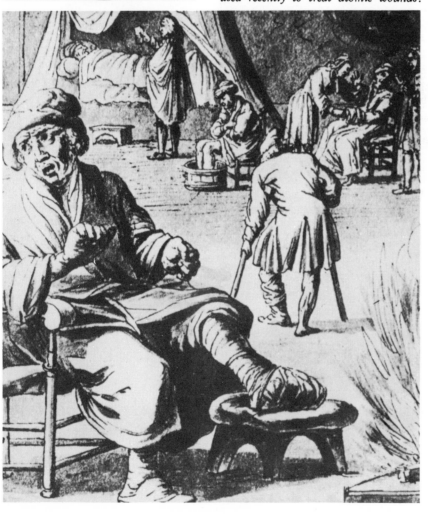

Sweat-cure for gout (left) was opposed by Sydenham. He prescribed fresh air, urged patients to "keep the mind quiet."

... CONCEDES: CINCHONA CURES FEVER

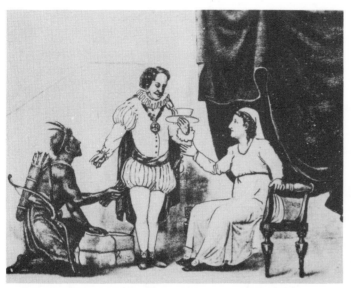

Countess of Chinchon receiving mythical dose of fever-bark tree.

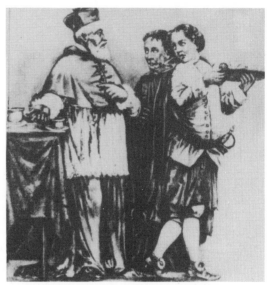

Cardinal de Lugo expanded cinchona market.

In the 1640's, a new wonder drug from Peru appeared on the European market. This powder ground from the bark of a tree cured the ague with truly amazing speed. The simplicity with which "fever-bark" could be applied left humoral physicians like Sydenham nonplussed. Malaria had baffled the profession for ages. It was a medical tenet that this disease could be cured only by the removal of peccant humours. To eliminate the morbific substances, it was thought necessary that the patient vomit, urinate, or sweat. Now the heathens of Peru had found an amazingly simple remedy: a few doses of "feverbark-powder" and malaria disappeared as if by magic. The physicians were sceptical.

There was a second objection to the Peruvian bark. The Jesuits, under Cardinal de Lugo, were trying to distribute it on a worldwide scale. In countries where malaria prevailed, they succeeded. In Protestant countries, they stirred up religious antagonism. When Cromwell contracted malaria, he refused to take any "Jesuits' bark," and died with his prejudice intact.

First Sydenham shrugged off the new cure, but eventually he changed his mind. When he saw that fever-bark was effective, he became one of the first physicians to work out rules for its use. Its efficacy even led him to the belief that "radical cures" — specifics — could be found for other afflictions like gout, plague and smallpox. This idea coincided with the theory of his friend Boyle who had emphasized that there were "intelligible causes" for each disease, and "specifick medicines" to cure them.

The feverbark tree was baptized Cinchona by Linné, after the Countess of Chinchon, who was supposedly stricken with malaria during her stay in Lima in 1630. According to the legend, an Indian arrived in the nick of time with some "fever tree bark" and the countess was saved. She then introduced the drug to Europe. Actually, the Countess did not go to Peru. It is doubtful whether she ever had malaria. Also, the curative properties of the drug were unknown in 1630, the date of her purported trip.

159

A MEDICAL FIASCO

THE LONDON PLAGUE 1665

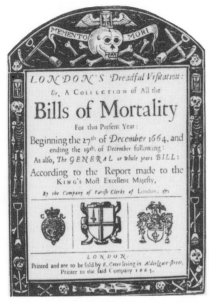

Bills of Mortality listed causes of death in each parish. Assembled by illiterats these statistics were unreliable. During plague, cause of death was often falsified. Families with victims feared long "lock up" in quarantine section.

When the Great Plague struck England in 1665, the new science of medicine proved helpless before the slaughter. A medical emergency service was desperately needed. But when the London aldermen asked the Royal College of Physicians for recommendations, it could offer nothing more than a weak rehash of 14th century measures. Four city physicians were hired to look after the plague stricken poor, where hundreds would have proved inadequate. A special anti-plague liquid was speedily concocted. But

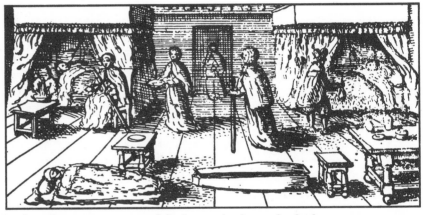

London: One vast mortuary of the living, the dying, the dead.

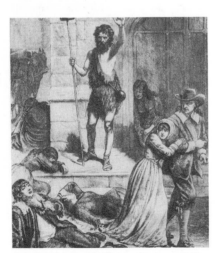

Mad Solomon Eagle strode through London with burning charcoal torch, pronouncing doom upon all inhabitants.

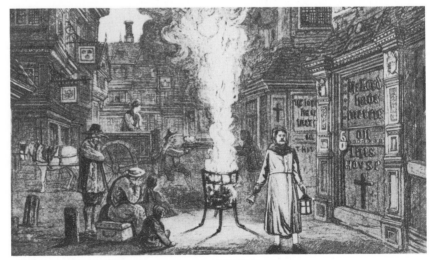

Watchman cries "Bring out your dead." Red cross, inscriptions mark homes of victims; fires dispell "miasmic air."

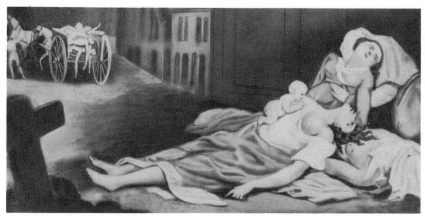

Dead victims were dumped in streets for pick-up by carts.

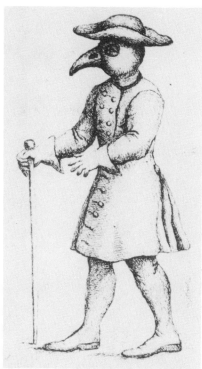

Physician's prophylactic garb made of leather. Beak held antiseptics. (above)

William Johnson, apothecary, who was assigned to distribute it to the poor, was himself struck down by the plague. As Defoe put it: "The plague defied all medicines. The very physicians were seized with it, with the preservatives in their hands."

Only a small group of heroic practitioners stuck by their patients. Dr. Nathaniel Hodges attended throngs of plague victims in his office or at their homes. Fortified by heavy "draughts of sack," he survived to write *Loimologia*, the best medical account of the great holocaust. Boghurst, the apothecary, proved almost as valiant. He is said to have dressed about 40 patients a day. Often he had to tie hysterical victims to their beds to prevent them from suffocating in the sheets. He even ate in the sickroom to save time, and was famous for his spiritual encouragement.

Meanwhile, the city had become "one vast mortuary — a reeking prison house of the living, the dying and the dead." When one member of a family caught the disease, the whole household was quarantined for weeks, which made their infection a virtual certainty. The houses themselves were locked airtight and closely guarded. Keyholes were plugged to keep the "miasmic air" inside, since the ignorant aldermen thought it endangered passersby and could even strike down birds in flight. This quarantine was instrumental in wiping out whole city blocks.

At the same time, official dogcatchers killed dogs and cats as the supposed source of infection, while flea-bearing plague transmitting rats were left unharmed. Fires were burned in the streets to clear the air, and in sickrooms, to destroy the clothes of deceased victims. Sufferers were awakened every four hours, since sleep was considered fatal. Buboes were kept open by blisters, so the "peccant humours" might escape. But such measures proved foolish. By the year's end, 68,596 Londoners were dead, according to an official but not very accurate tabulation. The next year saw a rapid decline of fatalities, partly due, perhaps, to the London Fire, which destroyed some of the disease-breeding slums. London has been free from major epidemics ever since.

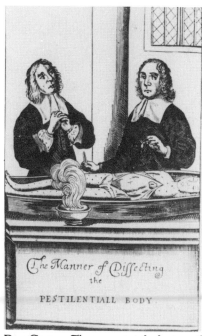

Dr. George Thomson tried daring if fruitless autopsies during plague.

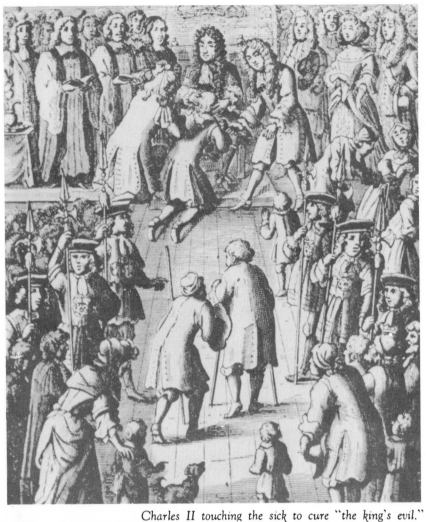

Charles II touching the sick to cure "the king's evil."

FAITH HEALERS

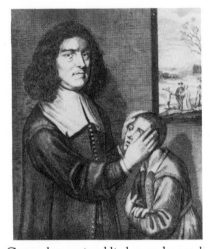

Greatrakes curing blind man by touch.

That the king's touch could cure the sick was an accepted belief since the days of Edward the Confessor. Now the practice was revived by popular demand. Charles II performed the "miracle" each year, and had given a grand total of 100,000 treatments by the end of his reign. Those afflicted by the "king's evil" (scrofula) or mere boils, thronged to London on the day of the ceremony. As they knelt before the king, he said, "I touch you and God heals you," then handed them a silver coin, called a touchpiece. Royal surgeons examined the patients beforehand to weed out the goldseekers from the truly sick. In March, 1684, Pepys the famed diarist wrote that "six or seven people were crushed to death by pressing at the chirgeon's door for tickets." William III often dismissed the sick with the sly remark: "God grant you better health and more sense." He knew that it was all a matter of mental suggestion or natural recovery. Those who remained sick were told they had lacked faith. The king couldn't lose.

Valentine Greatrakes, an Irish country gentleman, performed many miraculous cures "by the stroaking of the hands." He usurped royal prerogative in the apparently honest belief that he possessed a subtly "effulgent aura" which restored sick parts. Robert Boyle, the eminent chemist, supported him in this belief. Actually, Greatrakes brought a powerful psychological impact to bear on his patients, and succeeded with psychosomatic cases. He did unconsciously what Mesmer was to do by design a century later.

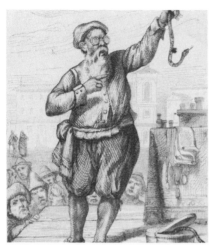

Medicinal snake-charmer, Bologna.

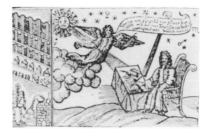

Handbill shows Dr. Case, notorious London quack receiving angelic instructions.

FAKE HEALERS

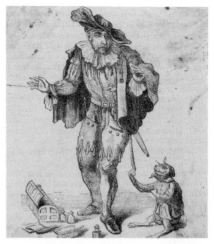

Monkey medicine-man, London.

During the plague, the doctor shortage gave the London quacks a field day. Though their cures proved either worthless or more deadly than the plague itself, their humbug was made to order for the panic-stricken populace. Thus, while medical service floundered, the charlatans moved in for a long and profitable stay.

The most successful quack of the day was a certain Dr. Case, a promoter *par excellence*. In 1660, when Case set up quarters in Blackfriars, he hung out his famous shingle: "Within this place lives Dr. Case." Then he sent forth pamphlets and leaflets studded with pleasant rhymes on his wonder drugs. "Good news for the sick!" ran a sample heading, and under this came such verses as the following gem on syphilis:

"All Ye that are of Venus' race
Apply yourself to Dr. Case —
Who with a box or two of pills
Will soon remove your painful ills."

Such tactics brought him wealth and hordes of patients. In the early 18th century, the *Tatler* was to remark that Case had made more money with his medical couplets than Dryden with his complete poetical works.

Though mountebanks thrived wonderfully well in the London of this period, quackery always has been a universal practice. Thus, the remarks on the quack by one contemporary observer seem valid for all times: "When people acquaint him with their griefs and their ills, though he knows not what ails them no more than a horse, he tells them it is a scorbutick humour caused by a defluxion from the osscarum . . . and the poor souls wonder that he should hit on their distemper so exactly."

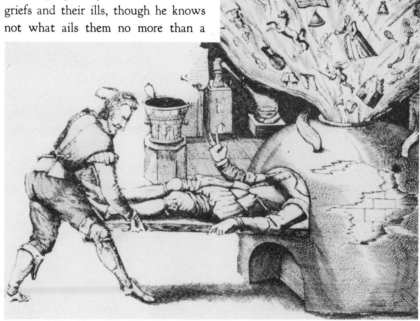

Inflated ideas "baked out" of patient's head by quack—fever-therapist.

MICROSCOPES REVEAL "LITTLE ANIMALS"

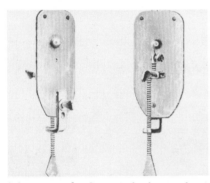

Anthony van Leeuwenhoek fathered bacteriology without knowing it.

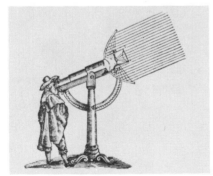

Microscope by Leeuwenhoek was lense mounted between two metal plates.

The plague ravaged many other places besides London during the 17th century. In France, almost half of the population of Lyons died; in Italy, Milan lost 86,000; Venice half a million. The doctors, though heroic, proved helpless. No wonder that the search for the cause of mass contagion was energetically pursued both by medical and non-medical men. In their quest they received unexpected help.

Since the early Renaissance, optometry had made impressive advances. It had developed the telescope to explore the universe and magnifying devices to peer into the strange world of little things. A long search for an instrument to overcome "the grossness of our unhelped senses" resulted in the microscope. Many scientists, including Galileo and Descartes, contributed to its gradual development. Once perfected, the instrument became "a miracle leading to countless other miracles." It enabled its early users to tackle the question of contagion from an entirely new angle.

Foremost among enthusiastic users of the microscope was Anthony van Leeuwenhoek. What bathtubs meant to Archimedes and pendula to Galileo, lenses meant to Leeuwenhoek. A linen draper by profession, Leeuwenhoek examined the structure of minute animals with the rabid passion of an amateur. He experimented relentlessly with his home-made microscopes and was fascinated by the minute animals he saw when he put sediments from his teeth under the lens. There were more animals in his mouth, "moving in the most delightful manner," than there were citizens of the United Netherlands, he boasted. What Leeuwenhoek saw under the microscope ranked in his mind as "exciting novelties." He had no clear idea of their portent. In a letter to the Royal Society (1683) he even drew pictures of them. The "Father of Bacteriology" never did quite know what he had sired.

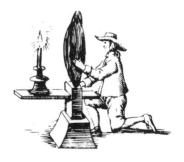

René Descartes' giant microscope had tubes filled with dear well-water.

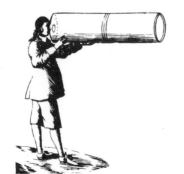

Kircher's "peep boxes" helped scientists explore "the hidden constitution of nature." Instruments were smaller than those shown in above engravings.

It was another inspired dilettante, Athanasius Kircher, priest, inventor, Egyptologist, who utilized the microscope to gain a deeper insight into the nature of epidemics. When the plague raged in Rome (1656-1657), he put a few drops of blood from a plague victim under the microscope. To his astonishment he saw "innumerable swarms of worms." From that observation he concluded that animate corpuscles caused and carried contagion.

Kircher probably did not see what today we know as bacteria. What he noted undoubtedly were blood corpuscles. Yet these supposed "worms" inspired him to present the world with the idea that a living parasite — a thin, elusive vermicle, invisible to the naked eye — was the culprit causing the plague.

The microscope, plus remarkable flashes of insight, helped him to formulate the basis of our modern germ theory. His idea proved wrong in only one point. The blood "got wormy," he believed, when worms developed from putrid matter by spontaneous generation. Aristotle's shadow still blocked the path of truth.

Nonetheless, Kircher proved — or at least thought he proved — by visual tests what Fracastorius had fathomed. In attributing contagion to living organisms, Kircher observed: "Flies feeding on the juices of the diseased and dying, hurry off and deposit their excretion on food, and persons eating it are infected."

Unfortunately, the medical profession did not pursue this trend of thought. Dust collected on the microscope and the doctors turned to the old furrow.

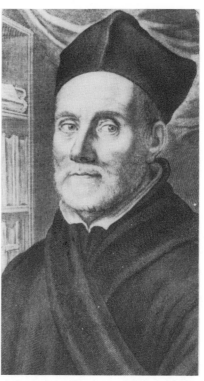

Athanasius Kircher, Jesuit scholar, pronounced "worms" plague carriers.

KIRCHERIANA

Kircher was active in many other fields. He founded an archaeological museum, tried to decipher hieroglyphics, drew up a device to project slides ("never saw anything more pleasant"), designed sound transmission apparatus. (see right). The appraisal of this Jesuit priest has varied widely. Some call him a mechanical genius, others a "dabbler in science."

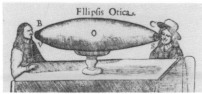

Cigar shaped otical elipse to help converse with the hard of hearing.

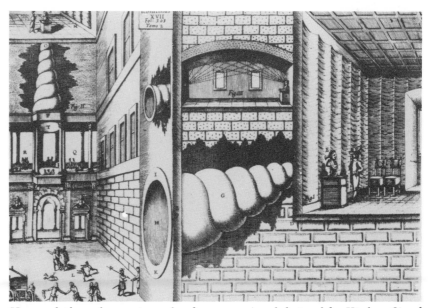

House telephone from private chambers to courtyard designed by Kircher. Sound channel was modeled after cochlea (snail-like cavity of ear).

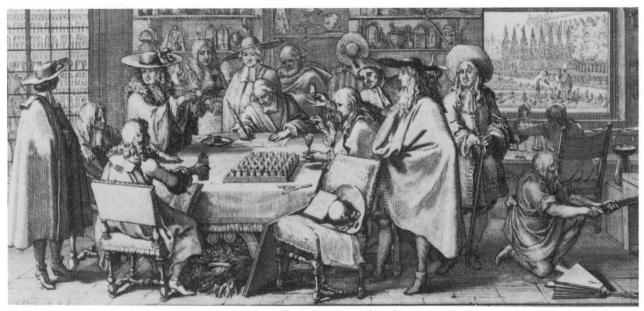

Members of learned society demonstrate new-found wonders of science and medicine.

BLOOD TRANSFUSION POSSIBLE

In this age of science, most universities remained hostile to the new discoveries. To promote more rapid progress scholars and amateur scientists banded together to form Learned Societies. These groups were bent on independent research into problems of "Magneticks, Chymicks and Mechanicks." Though they saw the world as a wonderful toy box, their experiments were rigidly objective, and the results were vigorously debated among the members.

The most effective of these groups, the Royal Society of London, exerted a marked influence on progressive medical thought. It was the first to champion Harvey's theory of circulation, and to use microscopes extensively for physiological research. Hooke, a live wire of the group, discovered that cells were the basic unit of all living tissues, while Malpighi,

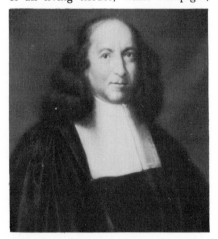

Marcello Malpighi (1628-1694) observed with aid of microscope, blood pass in frog's lungs from arteries to veins, through hair-fine tubules called capillaries. This provided final link for Harvey's theory of blood circulation.

a corresponding member, spotted the all-important capillaries. Then, in the 1660's, the Society embarked on a series of daring experiments.

An architect, a chemist and a doctor pooled their talents within the Society to perform the first successful blood transfusions. From Harvey's theory, Christopher Wren deduced that the blood stream might be used to carry liquid medicaments to the various parts of the body. Accordingly, the great architect fashioned a makeshift syringe from a quill and a dog's bladder, and used it to shoot medicinal substances into "divers creatures."

As the Society's historian puts it: "The animals were immediately purged, vomited, intoxicated, killed or revived, according to the quality of the liquor injected."

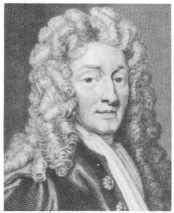
Christopher Wren, architect, introduced medicinal injections.

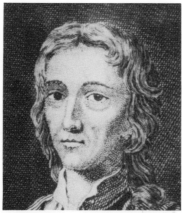
Robert Boyle, chemist, coordinated group experiments in transfusions.

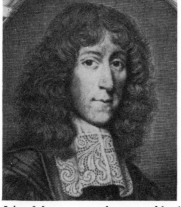
John Mayow proved venous blood absorbed air by way of lungs.

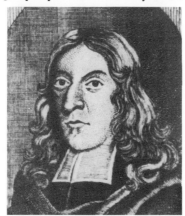
Richard Lower described first blood-transfusion in his De Corde, 1669.

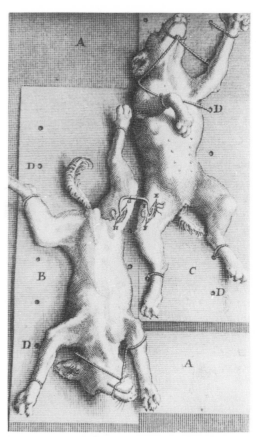
First animal transfusion was staged by Lower in 1665. This proved that blood could be passed through silver tube from artery of one dog to vein of another. Animal receiving blood survived.

EXPERIMENTS SUCCEED ON DOGS FIRST

Robert Boyle, the skeptical chemist, immediately sensed the significance of Wren's technique, and tried to co-ordinate the work of the various Oxford participants. He mapped out further experiments, and backed the project with his active interest. Meanwhile, the medical members saw their chance to treat disease internally by using the blood stream as a carrier for medication. One eminent physician, Richard Lower, went a step further: blood itself could be infused into the ailing body, he reasoned, in an attempt to control sickness. After many experiments, Lower and his associates performed a public transfusion, in February, 1665, before the Society. They used a silver tube to join the cervical artery of one dog to the jugular vein of another, then let the blood flow. The recipient animal survived. In successive experiments, Lower used various species, mixing the blood of lambs, oxen and dogs. This led to the final practical triumph of the Society's cooperative venture. Blood transfusion was to be performed on humans.

LAMB'S BLOOD INFUSED INTO AILING HUMANS

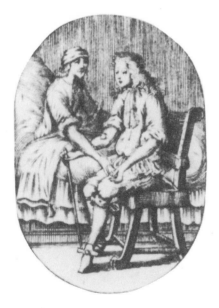

Early type of transfusion was practiced by Johann Elzholtz, who injected donor's blood into open vein.

On November 23, 1667, the Royal Society, "Section Bloodtransfusion" met for an epochal experiment. It set about to inject twelve ounces of sheep's blood into the bloodstream of one Arthur Coga, a poor clergyman. The program ran off smoothly and added up, it seems, to a complete success. Samuel Pepys jotted down his impressions of the "infused" patient: "He speaks well . . . saying that he finds himself much better since, and as a new man, but he is cracked a little in his head."

Here was a startling new process that promised to control sickness, to insure longevity or even immortality.

On the other hand, if blood could determine one's character and physiology, transfusions were opening interesting perspectives. Sheep's blood injected into a dog was believed to result in a healthy sprouting of wool on the canine's back. As Christine of Sweden observed in a letter to her counselor, Dr. Bourdelot: transfusions were fine, but she wanted no part of an injection of sheep's blood. If lion's blood were available, she jested, she could be much interested: "for turning into a female lion, — nobody can devour me."

In France, Jean Denis tried to vindicate the therapeutical aspects of blood transfusion. Early in 1667, he repeated Lower's tests with animal transfusions. Then, on June 15 — four months before Lower treated Coga — a feverish young man was brought to Dr. Denis. He had been bled endlessly by his physicians, so Denis immediately infused eight ounces of lamb's blood into his body. The boy

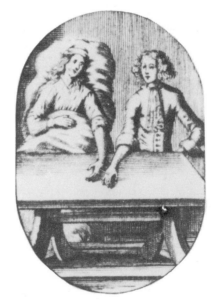

George Mercklinus discussed various forms of transfusion but they probably were not performed.

Later, Erasmus Darwin was to revive the practice of transfusion to sustain sufferers from cancer of the throat.

felt much better, and Denis thought himself established as the discoverer of therapeutic transfusions.

On July 29, 1667, Denis performed a similar experiment on a healthy carrier of sedan chairs. Ten ounces of blood were drawn from one of the man's arms, while twenty ounces of lamb's blood were infused into the other. The patient bounced up after the operation, helped to bandage the lamb, and confessed to a "feeling of warmth." He spent his reward in a nearby tavern, rested up for a day, then returned for a repeat.

The experiment was next tried on a man who would have died in any case, and promptly did. Then came monsieur Saint Amant, the valet de chambre of Madame de Sévigné. He suffered from frenzies, during which he was inclined to beat his wife. But after two transfusions, the man was converted into a loving husband. Unfortunately, his madness returned by the end of January, 1668, so a third transfusion was confidently undertaken. This time, Saint Amant died under the knife, and a great commotion started.

The patient's wife accused Denis of murder. Denis replied that she had either poisoned her husband or led him to certain death by encouraging his natural bent for debauchery. After several months of charge and countercharge, the courts exonerated Denis. Then the medical faculty of Paris stepped in, and forbade any further transfusions without its permission. Although textbooks continued to discuss the procedure, nobody dared to apply it, at least not openly. The 19th century was to revive it as a life saving therapy.

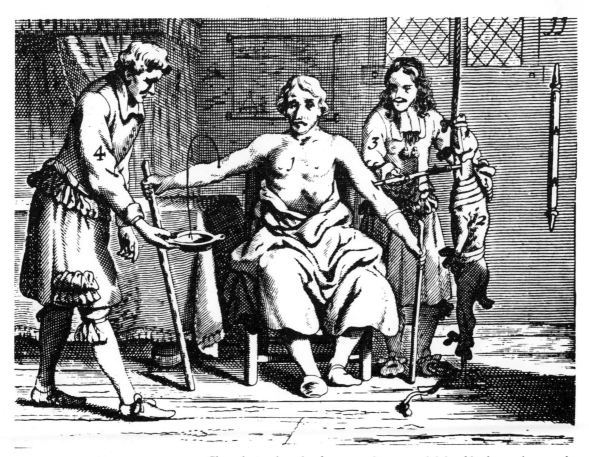

Transfusion from lamb to man. Surgeon at left lets blood to make room for incoming flow from lamb. Actually vessels adjust to increased supply. 169

PARIS SHUNS "NEW MEDICINE"

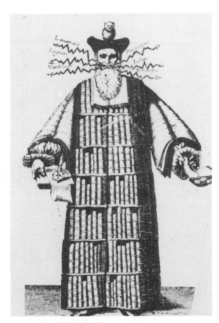

Doctor bound by books.

Though the Royal Society had spread the news of its amazing discoveries, only faint echoes reached the coast of France. From Paris, the fog of academism spread out across the countryside, and cushioned the medical ear against all heretic sounds. True, Jean Denis had been able to profit from Harvey's theory, but his experiments in blood transfusion were effectively scuttled by 1670. The Paris medical faculty was bound by tradition, and tradition was found in books, not laboratories.

To this end, a doctor's competence was judged by his ability to quote from the classics. When arch-conservative Guy Patin wanted to make doctors out of his two sons, he locked them in his study and forced them to learn the classics by heart. "This is the way I taught my two sons," he said with parental pride, "and it succeeded very well." In such an atmosphere, there was no place for Harvey's *De Motu Cordis*. Hippocrates, Galen and Avicenna had said nothing about circulation of the blood; therefore, the blood did not circulate. As for Paracelsus, the name was blasphemous.

"The physicians of this school," wrote Garrison, "had become sterile pedants, red-heeled, long-robed, big-wigged, pompous and disdainful in manner." In lieu of medical treatment, they attempted to overawe their patients with an adroit barrage of technical drivel. The important thing, to the Paris faculty, was to guard its rights and privileges against all comers. "Foreigners" from Montpellier were shunned. Apothecaries and barber-surgeons were classed as vile conspirators against the medical profession. And within the faculty's own august ranks, intrigue and petty jealousy flourished.

Their therapies included all the old standbys: bleeding, purging and cleansing the bowels. Guy Patin, the faculty spokesman at mid-century, described the typical medical approach in his letters. When he took over a case, blood flowed like the River Seine and the poor patient was stuffed with purgatives. He subjected his own family to such treatment, which at least proved his sincerity. Patin bled his wife twelve times to cure a fluxion in her chest, and bled his son twenty times to cure him of a cold. Such bleedings, he held, could only help if prior attempts had been made "to repress the impetuosity of the vagabond humour, and to chastise the intemperance of the liver." Though Harvey and his successors had disproved such nonsense long before, the dogma remained untouchable.

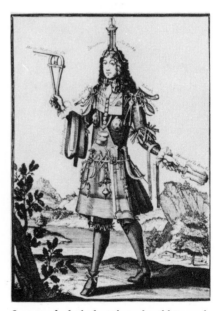

Surgeon bedecked with tools of his craft.

170

Patin was particularly upset by the encroachments of new-fangled medicines. He conducted a violent crusade against antimony which the faculty at Montpellier had praised as a panacea. Patin said it was poison. He claimed it had killed more people than the Thirty Years' War. Such outcries touched off the famous "antimony war" between Paris and Montpellier. Appropriately enough, Patin's party received a severe setback in the opening rounds. Young Louis XIV fell ill with a strange disease in 1658. The court physicians called it typhoid fever, but no one seemed able to cure it. Then Villot, "the charlatan," who had treated the king previously for venereal disease, was called in. Now he gave the monarch a dose of antimony, and the patient recovered (either because of it or in spite of it). Though Patin's angry attack had been decisively blunted, the war between

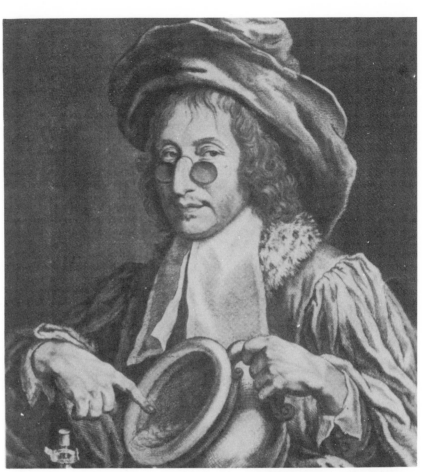

Patin, Paris faculty whip points at result of his purgatives.

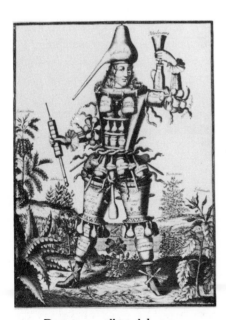

Doctor, a walking laboratory.

the two schools dragged on.

With all his subservience to the past, Patin ultimately proved to be a man of some stature. When he hated, he hated well and venomously. All through his life, for instance, he had nothing but vicious words for "his good, dear enemies, the apothecaries." But this time, unwittingly, his attacks were on the side of progress (though he was mainly grieved about their use of antimony). The druggists were then engaged in polypharmacy, strictly for business reasons. The more ingredients a prescription contained, the more sweetly rang the cash register. Patin found this fraudulent, and preached a return to simple remedies. He had no use for mixtures with 60-odd ingredients, or for such pharmaceutical staples as crab's eyes, and bezoar stones.

Patin also opposed the barber-surgeons, since they, too, were trying to usurp the province of the academicians. With Mencken-like vigor, he called them "booted lackeys who flourish razors." But here, too, Patin was foiled by the ailments of Louis XIV. Thanks to a fistula in the royal anus, the surgeons soon moved up in their professional status.

171

THE SUN KING -
A PICTURE OF MISERY

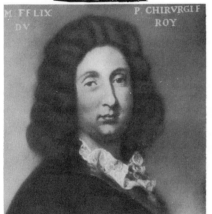

Félix: his operation on king's anus helped raise status of surgery.

Fagon (right): hunchbacked medical advisor to Louis XIV was universally admired for his scrupulous honesty.

Maréchal (far right): successor to Félix, chief surgeon at Sun-King's court was knighted, became fabulously wealthy.

The medical profession prospered by its close association with sun king Louis XIV. A staff of trusted physicians supervised his every move, and recorded his progress in the invaluable *Journal de la Santé du Roi.* This book gives an intimate picture of an outwardly radiant monarch who suffered, physically, almost every day of his life.

Ever since early youth, Louis had suffered from a plethora of ills: smallpox (he was pockmarked), gangrene, venereal disease. At one time a long tapeworm gnawed on the royal intestines. Such ailments occasioned daily visits by the court doctors, who quickly appropriated a few bright rays of royal infallibility.

The Paris faculty was inevitably jealous. It considered the royal doctors quacks and politicians bent on unseating the acknowledged leaders of medicine. Nevertheless, an appoint-

ment to the royal staff was highly coveted. The chief physician was actually a member of the royal cabinet, and the undisputed leader of his profession. The position was a rich political plum, but it had certain drawbacks.

Louis was an abominable patient. In later years, he ate too much, chewed too little, and therefore suffered from indigestion. The doctors were blamed if his pains were not speedily alleviated. They were forced to purge him, then stand by in the bathroom to see that all went well.

In 1685, Louis developed a small lump in the rectum. The court doctors and apothecaries failed to remove it, so a surgeon, Charles François Félix, was summoned. First, he explained to Louis how surgery would bring relief. Then he set the date of operation six months ahead. This gave him time to practice on more lowly

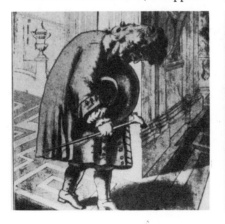

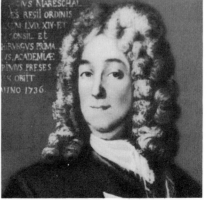

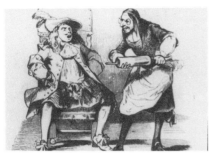

patients, the greater part of whom died under his knife. They were buried at night, to keep the news from reaching the public ear. Finally, on November 18, 1686, Felix performed his operation at Versailles, in the presence of Madame de Maintenon and the court medical staff. It proved a complete success. As Louis recovered, his sycophants walked around the court with their bottoms bandaged, to show their sympathy with the king's posterior discomfort.

Félix received 300,000 livres for the job, three times the annual salary of the chief physician. He was made a nobleman, and the year 1686 became known as "l'anée de la fistule."

Louis had rendered the same service 16 years earlier to obstetrics. He endorsed Dr. Jules Clément as midwife to his mistress, Madame de La Vallière. After watching the birth from behind a curtain, Louis made Clément the official *accoucheur;* and so godfathered the male midwife.

The Paris pedants were further stung by the sharp needle of Molière's wit. He exposed their vacuous bedside chatter in four comedies, each a vivid picture of medical life at the time of Louis XIV. Molière hated pomp and pretense. He struck several blows for reform by presenting the members of the Paris faculty as living mummies. Through his studies with Gassendie, the naturalist, he had become familiar with the new scientific spirit. Further, he had suffered himself at the hands of the Galenists. Molière had pulmonary tuberculosis, but he found his doctors such avowed enemies of progress that he turned from medicine in disgust. Only Dr. Mauvilain remained his friend. When Louis XIV asked how Molière got along with this physician, Molière replied: "Sir, we talk together; he prescribes remedies for me; I do not take them and I recover."

Appropriately enough, Molière died after playing the hypochondriac in his *Malade Imaginaire.* On February 17, 1673 when he appeared in this role, the public roared at his coughs, but this time they were deadly serious. He was carried home from the play, spitting blood. When he died the same night, there were no doctors at his bedside.

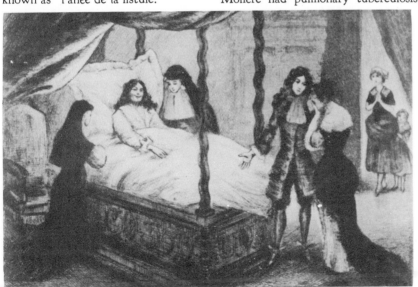

Death of Molière. After satirizing pompous Paris faculty, Molière died appropriately without doctors. His wife and friends were at his bedside.

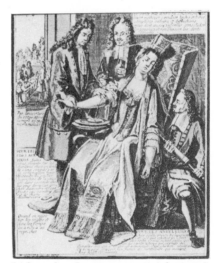

Lady reduced to prostration by triple threat of bloodletting, purgatives and enema-clyster. These remedies for all diseases were lampooned in Molière's comedies. Doctors always leaped up with simple motto: Clysterium donare, postea seignare, ensuita purgare.

173

17th CENTURY SURGEONS OPERATE FOR CANCER

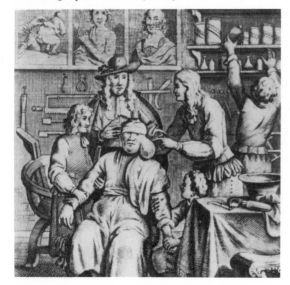

Tracheotomy after Casserius.

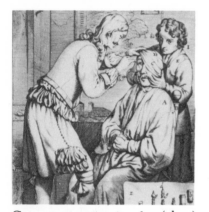

Cataract operation in 1653 (above).

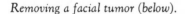

Removing a facial tumor (below).

There were no great surgeons in the 17th century, but there were a great many good ones. Central Europe was torn by 30 years of warfare, and as usual, the army surgeons gained knowledge and experience. They also attempted more daring operations, since the research of learned societies had penetrated down to the surgical craft. The textbooks of Purmann and Scultetus devoted ample space to blood transfusion, and to the tapping of the abdominal cavity, which required some insight into the workings of the stomach.

But if experience gave them more self-assurance, the surgeons were still labeled *feldschers* (fieldbarbers). The barber's apron kept them out of the ranks of legitimate medicine, though in France, the court recognized the surgeons at the Collège de St. Côme.

The wandering lithotomists ranked even lower, but some of them were very proficient operators. Frère Jacques de Beaulieu acquired renown for cutting stones by a new method: a lateral incision of the perineum. In 1698, he was called before the court to demonstrate his technique. The surgeons admired his dexterity, condescendingly. Soon Frère Jacques went back to "cutting charitably for the stone, as the poor implored him."

Frère Jacques, wandering lithotomist, cuts stone via perineum.

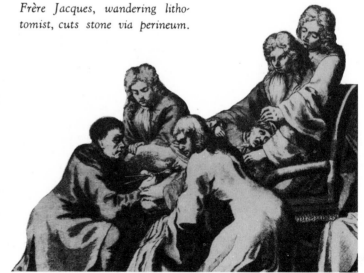

174

The panel at right shows what steps the 17th century surgeon took when a cancerous breast was to be removed. The Greeks had tried it long before, though their methods, according to Celsus, "never did any good to anybody," probably because they shrank from a radical extirpation. Lanfranc pointed out in the 13th century that total removal was the only possible cure.

Now Purmann took up Lafranc's idea, and expressed it forcefully in his *Lorbeer-Krantz*. First, he railed against his conservative colleagues, who treated cancer by corrosives, "which will only lead to added irritation." Then he called for radical extirpation, especially when the growth was easily discovered, as in cancer of the breast. Once the growth had been removed, Purmann suggested that the wound be thoroughly cauterized.

This "searing" process helped to keep edges sterile; it severed lymphatic vessels without undue bleeding, and prevented cancer cells from re-entering the circulatory system. Though the 17th century surgeon had only a hazy idea about such benefits, he knew that the cautery often achieved good results, and he used it empirically, as the modern surgeon handles the electric knife. As a result of this procedure, cancer was at last removed from the list of surgical untouchables.

Excerpt on cancer from Peter Lowe.
Whole Art of Chirurgerie, 1634.

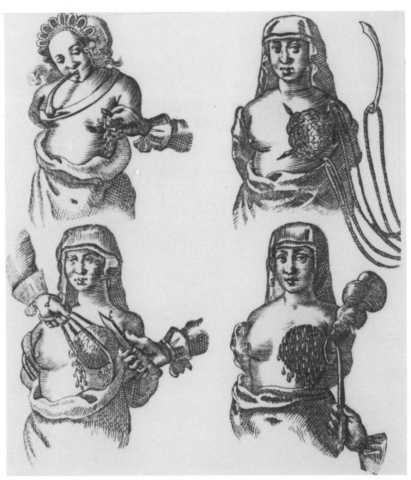

Four steps in extirpation of cancerous breast.

¶ Of *Cancer*, which the Greekes called *Carsinoma*.

Although that Cancer bee comprehended under the schirrous humors, yet there is great difference: for Cancer is a hard tumor, round, unequall, with dolour, punction and pulsation: it groweth sooner than Schir, and hath great vaines about it, tumified and swelled, full of melancholicke blood, and doth resist being prest upon. It is sometime taken for the sore of a beast, and is called Cancer, because it sticketh fast to the part as doth the Crabbe-fish to that which it taketh hold on; as also the vaines which are about are like unto Crabsfeet. It is of colour libide or blacke, hard, and rough, eating, gnawing, and going, like unto the Crabbe-fish

Pa.li.4. cap.24
Definition.

Celsi.5. ca.28

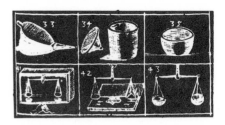

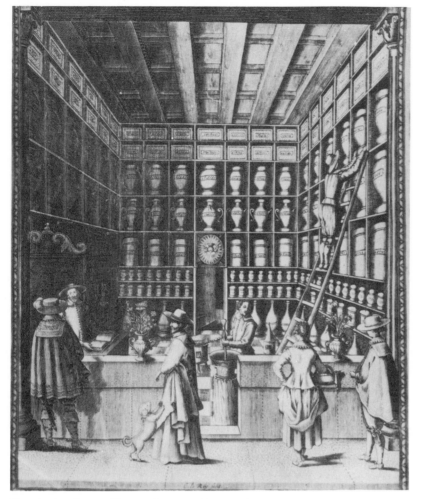

French Apothecary Shop at the time of Louis XIV.

sweep. The famous Dr. Baldwin Hamey, for instance, had nothing but praise for a colleague who treated his pharmacist as his serf.

In England, France and Germany the general idea was to keep the drug-sellers in their place, socially and professionally. But the scheme was doomed to failure, since the pharma-cists had also taken on added stature. During the plague, they had stayed at their posts, while many doctors fled. This naturally endeared them to the populace, or what was left of it. They had profited also from the fact that chemistry and experimental sci-ence often revolved about pharmacy. Consequently, they had few qualms about dispensing remedies to their customers, along with free medical advice. This practice reduced the doctors' fees, so the public liked the druggists all the more. As one ob-server put it, "the doctors of that day knew so little that the druggists found it easy to know as much."

"MAD POISON MIXERS"

Relations between doctors and drug-gists had never been too friendly. They reached the breaking point in 17th century England. On one hand, the "mad poison mixers" overstepped the bounds of their profession; on the other, the doctors behaved with abominable arrogance. The result was open warfare, with no prescriptions barred, and the patients caught in the midst of warring factions.

Though the average physician was far from scholarly, he often carried himself with the aplomb of a barn-yard rooster. He considered the apothe-cary of equal rank with the chimney

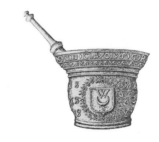

Mortar of Claude Cordier of Toules.

176

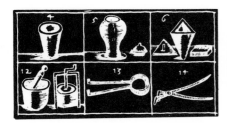

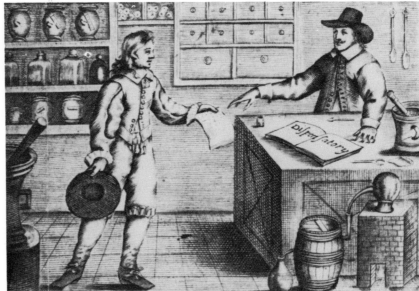

London druggist conforms to law of 1618; he holds ready dispensatory book for entry of doctor's prescription. Apothecaries resented supervision by College of Physicians.

In 1618, London apothecaries were placed under the guardianship of the Royal College of Physicians. Doctors could now inspect the drug shops and punish malpractice. But the prosperous druggists ignored the law almost entirely. They continued to charge exorbitant fees for pills (e.g., 30 shillings apiece) and to milk the rich by as much as 100 £ per case. The average patient found it impossible to buy medicine, and druggists were soon dubbed "thieves and swindlers."

They countered with an offer to dispense drugs to the poor at cost, but it was largely a public relations gesture. So the College decided to try its own hand at pharmacy. In 1696, it opened a dispensary for the poor.

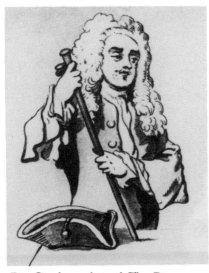

Dr. Garth, author of The Dispensary, cheered patients with his jests.

Some doctors disapproved of the step. They received good money from the apothecaries when one of their prescriptions caught the public fancy. But others had watched too many "mean medicine mixers dash by in their elegant carriages." So, as the century closed, the profession was split into dispensarians and anti-dispensarians.

As this dispute gathered momentum, Dr. Samuel Garth took pen in hand to write a goodnatured poem, *The Dispensary.* This rhymed dispatch from the front sided with the physicians, but at the same time, it poked fun at both armies. The poem was an instant success, since, in Johnson's words, it coincided "with passions and prevalent prejudices."

Dr. Garth was an eminently sociable man. His wit earned him entrance to the exclusive Kit Kat Club, which met in a London bakery. As the only medical member, Garth amused his fellow bon vivants with his rhymed account of the great drugstore debacle.

The doctor was careful, at all times, never to let his practice interfere with his pleasure. Once, while seated in a tavern with his friends, he was discreetly reminded that his patients were waiting for him. To which he gave the classic, if indiscreet, reply: "It's no great matter whether I see them tonight or not, for nine of them have such bad constitutions that all the physicians in the world can't save them; and the other six have such good constitutions that all the physicians can't kill them."

It is only fair to add that even Garth's patients cherished his bon mots more than his medicines. When his poem was published in 1699, it helped to dispell some of the seriousness of the dispensary war, and so provided a pleasant *finale* for 17th century medicine.

PRIEST-PHYSICIANS PRAY AND HEAL

For a century tales of fabulous wealth waiting to be tapped in America had floated back to Europe. Lured by the prospect of booty, or driven by religious intolerance, a small group of brave and restless spirits set out during the early 17th century to conquer the wilderness on the new continent. It was a new world indeed that these pioneers faced — but, medically, in no way a better one.

From the very first permanent English landing at Jamestown, Virginia, in 1607, epidemics ravaged the settlers. Beriberi, smallpox, malaria and yellow fever brought more havoc than all the arrows and tomahawks of the Red Man. In 1610, for example, 338 out of the total population of 398 in disease-ridden Jamestown died.

In New England the Puritans at first rejoiced that God had sent a "providential" plague to wipe out the Indians and make room for the white pilgrims. The onset of typhoid fever, tuberculosis, pneumonia, scurvy and other indigenous ills of great virulence soon dampened their righteous enthusiasm. During January and February of 1621 these diseases, aggravated by a lack of proper food, carried away about half of the colonists of Massachusetts.

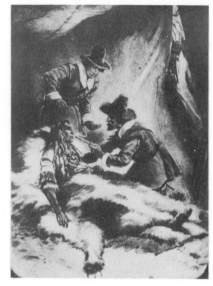

The need for doctors in America grew desperate. True, the mother companies that organized the expeditions across the Atlantic attached doctors to each group. But both in number and caliber they proved totally inadequate to cope with the emergency. America in those days had no more attraction for Europe's medical talent than the Matto Grosso jungles today have for the successful New York practitioner. The better doctors of Leyden and London had their own comfortable offices in the heart of civilization. Why give up a good life to venture into the far-off wilderness?

Most of the doctors arriving in the colonies were ships' surgeons, classed in the passenger lists on par with the bricklayers. These doctors opened shop with a scanty medicine chest, and their stock of remedies soon melted away. As early as 1608 Captain John Smith had to go all the way back to London for treatment of a wound, "for there was neither chirurgeon nor chirurgery at the fort" (Jamestown).

A Dr. John Pottes, sent to the colonies in 1621 from England, did have experience in "Chirurgerie and Physick" but proved more of a trouble-maker than a consoler of the sick. Colonists accused him of poisoning the Indians and keeping company with "inferiors who hung upon him while his good liquor lasted." In 1625 he became one of the first American physicians ever hailed into court by a patient. A woman accused him of causing her miscarriage by failing to satisfy her craving for hogmeat. The court absolved the doctor, however, and he continued his "porkless" practices till 1628 when he was appointed — of all things — temporary governor of Virginia.

Yet the colonists did have other medical assistance. Divines took over where physicians failed. Many priests assumed medical as well as spiritual duties. The old "angelic conjunction" of the priest-physician who ministered to both soul and body flourished once more along the Massachusetts coast.

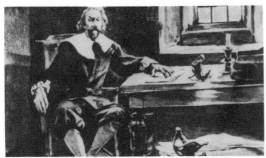

John Winthrop, Sr., first Governor of Massachu-setts, imported medicines from England to help sick.

Like the courageous members of the clergy, Governor John Winthrop, Jr., of Connecticut stood by the sick. He was a learned man, trained at Trinity College, Dublin, a member of the Royal Society. The state's citizens looked upon him as an oracle in cases of illness. Petitions for medical advice reached him from far and wide. While some of his prescriptions made sense, others showed him hopelessly entangled in the superstitions of the age. He prescribed "buttered musket balls" for stomach ache, to be taken on the full of the moon. Then he added "a bit of lion's mane hung under the left arm, he said, would also help!"

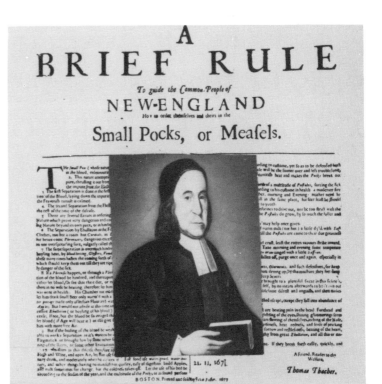

Smallpox Manifesto (1677) of Rev. Thomas Thacher, pastor of Old South Church, Boston. This is the only known medical publication printed in 17th century America. It was based on tract by Sydenham.

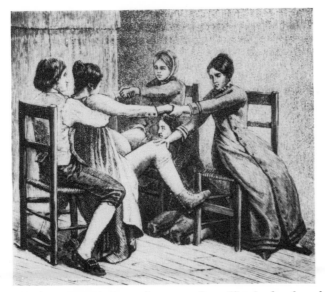

Obstetrics among Pennsylvania settlers. The husband and mother-to-be join hands with strong-armed neighbors.

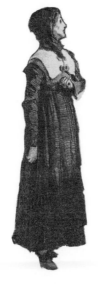

Anne Hutchinson, pioneer midwife.

PIONEER MIDWIFE

American obstetrics started in mid-ocean. In 1630 a woman passenger aboard the pilgrim ship "Arabella" fell in labor and was delivered by a midwife rowed over from the sister ship "Jewell." Among the early American midwives none achieved greater notoriety than Anne Hutchinson. First highly esteemed in Boston, she stirred up trouble by voicing enlightened views on the rights of women, and was banned from the colony. Later, the Indians killed her and her family near Pelham, N. Y. The Hutchinson River Parkway, near New York, perpetuates the memory of this pioneer in midwifery and woman's rights.

179

REASON REIGNS...
AND CHARITY IS REBORN

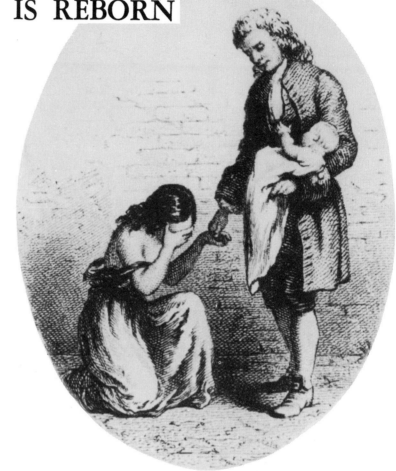

Science had taken tremendous strides during the 17th century, and for medicine, moving somewhat behind, the promised land seemed just over the next hill. Harvey and Boyle, with their experiments, had planted the flag on or near the summit; Leeuwenhoek had thoroughly explored the approach and Sydenham had patiently marked out the network of trails. But at the end of the century, when the excited corps of physicians caught up with the vanguard, there were only more hills to climb. The average doctor felt duped, and a reaction was inevitable.

In the first place, the use of quantitative methods had resulted in a baffling multiplicity of medical "facts." Physiology, microscopy and chemistry had left the physician unable to act. He could not generalize on his new knowledge, partly because there was not enough of it, and partly because the evidence was often conflicting. For instance, when Sydenham's careful classification of symptoms was methodically carried out, it resulted in the listing of some 1800 different diseases. The doctor had no "laws" of symptomatology to guide him.

In the second place, many of the new facts had no immediate bearing on medical practice. Of what use, for example, were Harvey's discoveries in the face of a yellow-fever epidemic? Pure research, after a seemingly long reign, had resulted in almost no practical benefits. The patients were unrelieved; they still suffered from the same old diseases. Obviously, it was time to take stock, to bring order out of chaos. If possible, the rich but perplexing heritage from the 1600's had to be assimilated.

This assimilation process took place in what is familiarly called "The Age of Reason." For the time being 18th-century rationalism replaced the old empiricism. The new medical leaders began to sort and pack the accumulated data into neat systems. Where the data proved inadequate, logical analysis was used to cover the gap. Thus, elaborate structures could be built up from a few simple, and usually valid principles. Order seemed once more in sight. But the net result, unfortunately, was confusion heaped upon confusion. Almost anyone could begin with a simple premise and work out an elaborate structure, and almost everyone did. John Brown, for instance, reduced disease to a process of over- and under-stimulation, then worked his way outward again. Benjamin Rush did the same with "hypertension." So many simple systems appeared on the scene that the befuddled practitioner was now unable to choose among them. Before he could say Hippocrates he was caught up once more in the age-old battle of medical ideologies.

But if medicine had bogged down, temporarily, as a science, it did serve to speed up social progress. Humanitarian and democratic movements were on the march in the 18th century. The conviction had grown that even the humblest man had a right to happiness. As urbanization took its toll, society began to recognize its obligations toward the welfare of *all* its members. All were imbued with reason, and therefore equal, if

Eighteenth century Medical Life: Doctor at sickbed (right); in his study (below left); doing surgery in polyclinic (below right).

only by virtue of being human to the same degree.

Such convictions broadened the field of medical care to include new groups: the poor, cripples, even political prisoners and criminals. Medical men led the fight for more humane treatment of these unfortunates, and helped to ease their suffering. Even the wealthier classes joined the crusade, for practical as well as charitable reasons: sick and impoverished workers meant economic waste; waste reduced the ability to produce goods, and undermined a nation's wealth.

But whatever the motives, everyone felt that Reason would solve all social problems and bring happiness to mankind. The physicians of the age were imbued with a belief in reason; consequently they pioneered in prison reform, in child care, and in the all-important hospital movement. As Garrison has pointed out, they were probably the most charitable members the profession has ever had.

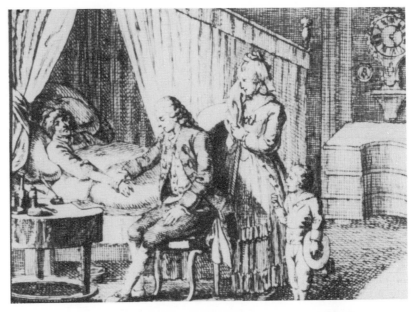

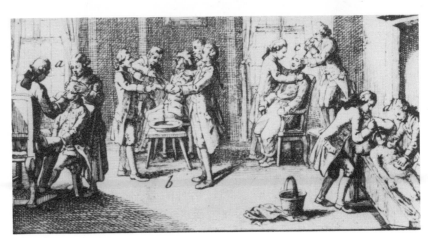

181

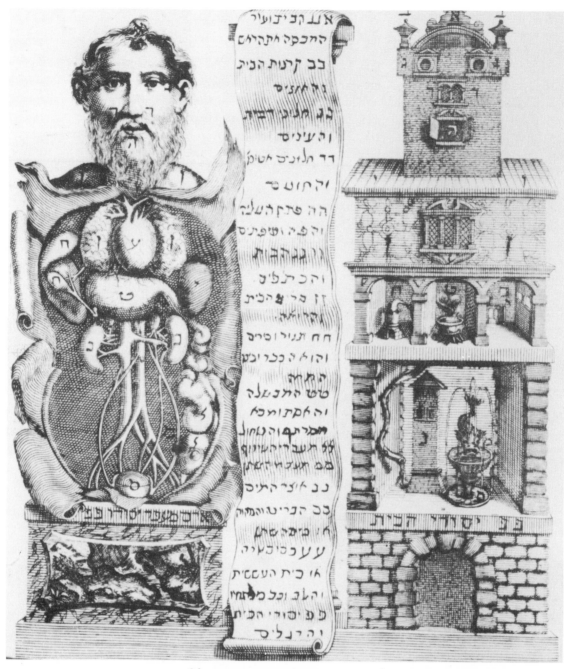

MAN IS A HOUSE

18th century iatromechanist compares human organs with parts of a house: eyes are lookout windows; stomach has function of kitchen; kidneys serve as water supply; intestinal tract invites comparison with cellar complete with trap door — anus.

Dr. Tobias Cohn from whose Maaseh Tuvish, (Venice 1707) the above illustration is taken, was born in Metz, studied in Cracow, took his degree in Padua, practiced in Poland, wrote in Adrianople, taught in Constantinople, died in Jerusalem.

"THE SOUL RUNS THE BODY"

GEORG ERNST STAHL

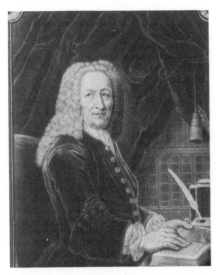

Friedrich Hoffmann, wrote medical system filling whole bookshelf (27 vols.). Compounded "Hoffmann Drops."

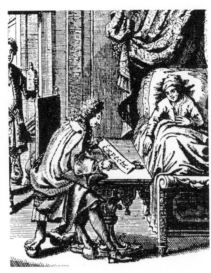

Dr. George Ernst Stahl — "the sourfaced metaphysician" at the bedside. He believed that the "invisible soul"

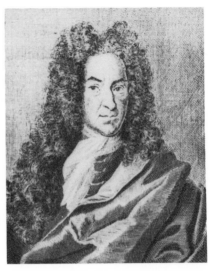

cured all ills. This doctor's recipes just showed: Expecto — Let's wait and see. Naturally, Stahl was not popular.

In the 18th century as in the preceding era doctors still were divided into two camps, iatrochemists and iatromechanists. In addition another system came to the fore.

To Georg E. Stahl of Halle University, life had qualities not expressible in terms of chemistry and physics. Stahl's doctrine of animism determined his course of action as a physician and had a decided influence on medical thinking in this age and succeeding generations.

Stahl, a man of considerable genius, clouded by an unfortunate temper, was called the "sour faced metaphysician." Of mechanics and chemistry he wanted no part. These sciences,

had, in his estimation, nothing to do with medicine. He declared emphatically that the physician's domain begins where that of the physicist's ends. The living processes, in Stahl's system, are directed by man's "sensitive soul" — a term closely akin to what today may be called the subconscious personality. The soul knows more about the body and how to rectify its malfunction than any physician. All the doctor can do is watch the soul's efforts to realign the body's imbalance. Since the blood is the mainstream of life — the blood has to be brought back to normalcy and water is best to "dilute the blood."

The name of Stahl is usually linked to that of Friedrich Hoffmann. The two were born in the same year, and had been friends during their student days. However, it was not long before their friendship cooled into open estrangement.

Stahl's animism appeared rather nonsensical to Hoffmann, a friend of Boyle and an avowed mechanist. To Hoffmann all life was explainable by contraction and dilation. Movement is the essence of vital action. All organs and muscles show a normal "tonus" when health prevails. On the other hand, the doctor must adjust the tonus if in a state of overtension.

183

BOERHAAVE
of EUROPE

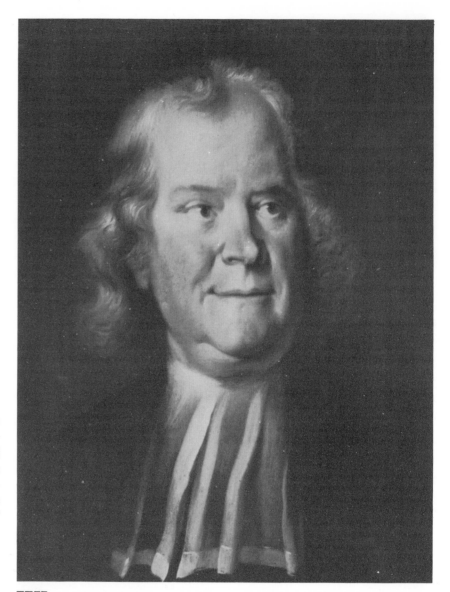

He was said to be so popular that the churchbells of Leyden once signaled his recovery from gout, and jubilant crowds welcomed him in the streets as he returned to the university. He said the poor were "his best patients, for God paid for them." (Portrait by Cornelius Troost.)

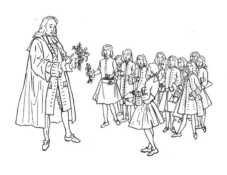

When the celebrated Dr. Hermann Boerhaave died in 1738, people said that he had left behind as a bequest an elegant volume which contained, according to the title-page, "all the secrets of physicks." Every page of the volume was said to be blank, save one. On that particular page the good doctor had summed up his medical knowledge: "keep the head cool, the feet warm, and the bowels open."

This was a fairly accurate estimate of actual medical practice in the 18th century. Though medical science had made some progress, the results were often lost in the preposterous war between the chemical and mechanical schools of medicine. The air bristled with these hostile theories, but the judicious Boerhaave, whose system it was to have no system, cut through all theories.

Like Hippocrates and Sydenham, he placed the patient in the center of medical attention. He was an eclectic, in the best sense of the word, borrowing from each system with one goal in mind: to find therapies of proven value at the bedside.

Although he was not a great innovator, nor a great writer, Boerhaave's success was preeminent because of his simplicity, clarity and eclectic wisdom. His personal warmth, and his acute discernment at the sickbed, made him a great and beloved physician. His radiant personality and uncommon good sense made him the natural medical leader of his day. Most important of all, his teaching methods were sound and often revolutionary.

Boerhaave himself was a voracious student. He was able to hold four professorships in medicine, chemistry, pharmacology and botany, and to lecture on these subjects four to five hours a day. He reorganized the botanical gardens at Leyden, and students visited there under his guidance. His most effective reform was to bring students directly into the hospital. There were only two wards of six beds each at his disposal, but every case was studied exhaustively. As a result, the hospital and postmortem room soon ranked in importance with the library, the lecture hall and the botanical garden. Finally, Boerhaave was a superb orator, clear in diction and thoroughly systematic. Students flocked to Leyden from both Europe and America to hear him. The city fathers were compelled to break down the town walls, according to a contemporary report, to make room for the overflow.

Boerhaave reached his calling by a somewhat circuitous road. As a young man, he studied for the priesthood at Harderwick. One day, while taking the packet boat home to Leyden, he overheard a group of people railing against the books of the "heretic" Spinoza, who had startled Europe with the belief that God was everywhere. Boerhaave interrupted to ask one violent speaker if he had read the works in question. A rumor spread from this chance remark that the young divinity student was a Spinozist, so he was promptly excluded as a candidate for the ministry.

When Boerhaave became a doctor instead, he quickly achieved a remarkable reputation. His enormous general practice brought him a fortune estimated at two million florins. Hundreds of patients clamored to see him daily. A Chinese mandarin is supposed to have addressed a letter to "Boerhaave of Europe," and it reached him promptly. Peter the Great reportedly spent the night in his bark near Boerhaave's country home, just to have two hours' conversation before the professor left for his lectures.

Boerhaave's success in training a medical elite was his greatest contribution to the healing arts. A Leyden graduate outranked a competitor from Oxford or Cambridge at this time, and the converts of Boerhaave spread his gospel throughout the western world. They established or revitalized schools in Edinburgh, Vienna and Goettingen. His teachings were to become the prevailing medical gospel in Europe as well as America.

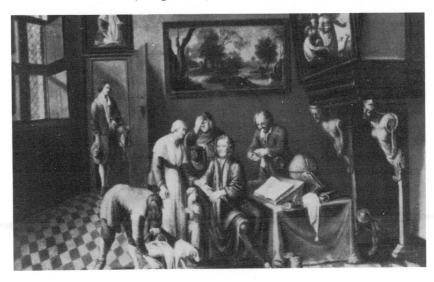

Office of Boerhaave at his palatial home outside Leyden. Patients filed in not individually but in groups — a procedure enabling him to see more than a hundred sufferers a day.

THE MONROS MOLD
A GREAT NEW SCHOOL

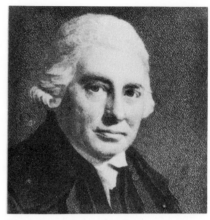

Monro Secundus, held chair of anatomy for 50 years. Though consulted in surgical cases, he did not operate.

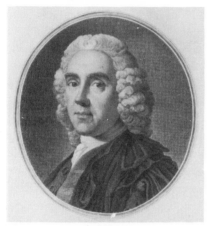

Monro Primus taught anatomy for 38 years, initiated Edinburgh's fame, organized Infirmary, Medical Society.

Three of Boerhaave's 400-odd pupils at Leyden in 1718 were destined to spread his gospel across Europe. Gerard van Swieten brought clinical medicine to Vienna; Albrecht von Haller, a young and poetic Swiss, established physiology through his inspiring work at the University of Goettingen and in 1719, Alexander Monro began the reign of the "Monro dynasty" in Scotland. For the next 126 years, his family was to occupy the chair of anatomy at Edinburgh.

As efficient and worthy instructors, the Monros helped to establish Edinburgh as a great training center.

Aside from some anatomical discoveries, they made no lasting contributions to science. Yet they provided a remarkable example of medical clan rule.

John Monro, an army surgeon under William of Orange, had settled in Edinburgh in 1700. He was determined to transform the town into a first-class medical center, and his only son, Alexander, was to do the transforming. He himself trained the boy in medicine, then sent him to study at London and Leyden. By a neat arrangement with the Town Council, young Alexander became professor of anatomy upon his return. He was then 22.

For the next 38 years, "Alexander Primus" reigned at Edinburgh. There had been a bad moment at the very beginning, when he left half of the manuscript for his first lecture at home; but he quickly shifted to extemporaneous speech, and this duly impressed the city fathers. As time went on they continued to be impressed. When Alexander retired, he had no trouble in securing his chair for his youngest son. Fortunately, Alexander "Secundus" proved a worthy successor. In his 50 years in office, he lectured to about 14,000 students — nearly 300 per class.

For 10 years, the second Alexander shared his chair with his son, "Alexander Tertius," who continued to hold it for 38 years thereafter. But the dynasty had obviously petered out, for Alexander III was a mere epigone. He rested on the family laurels, and, literally, on its notebooks, by faithfully repeating his grandfather's written lectures.

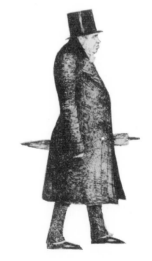

Monro Tertius, lectured for 38 years. His courses were but a weak recital of his grandfather's note-books.

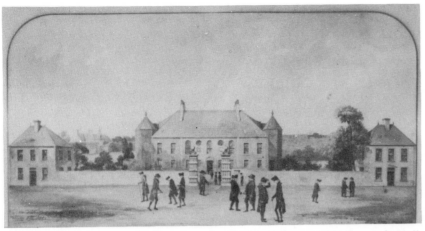

Edinburgh's practitioners during informal gathering in front of Old Surgeon's Hall.

SCOTTISH DOCTORS HAVE SENSE OF HUMOR

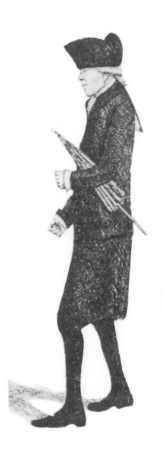

Old Surgeon's Hall was the acorn from which Edinburgh's Medical School sprouted after the appointment of Monro Primus in 1720. Four other Boerhaave students joined him here in 1726 to teach medical theory and practice.

At this time Edinburgh teemed with doctors — colorful, true originals, a bit queer in their habits but devoted to their patients' welfare.

A doctor could then afford an eccentric bedside manner. The Scots liked their doctors human and humorous.

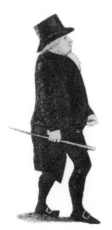

Benjamin Bell, the Edinburgh Infirmary's first surgeon, was bold with knife and lucky in his real estate speculations. At the end of his life he "owned" an Edinburgh suburb. Dr. Joseph Bell, the prototype of Sherlock Holmes, was his descendent.

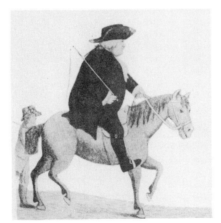

When Dr. John Shields, "becoming latterly very corpulent," could no longer make his rounds on foot, he hired a boy to help him into the saddle of a "sagacious and surefooted grey pony." Although he charged little for his visits, Dr. Shields became quite rich.

Alexander ("Lang Sandy") Wood was typical of the Scottish doctors of the day both in humor and humanity. He was the first person ever to carry an umbrella in Edinburgh. A pet raven and a sheep accompanied him on his rounds. His pleasant manner and amusing wit sweetened the social life of his fellow doctors. Lang Sandy had two enthusiastic hobbies — golfing and drinking good wine. Because of his talent for "working all day and laughing all night," his medical brethren honored him with a diploma as "Doctor of Mirth." In spite or perhaps on account of his peculiarities, the townspeople held him in great esteem.

187

FRAYED NERVES CAUSE SICKNESS (Cullen)

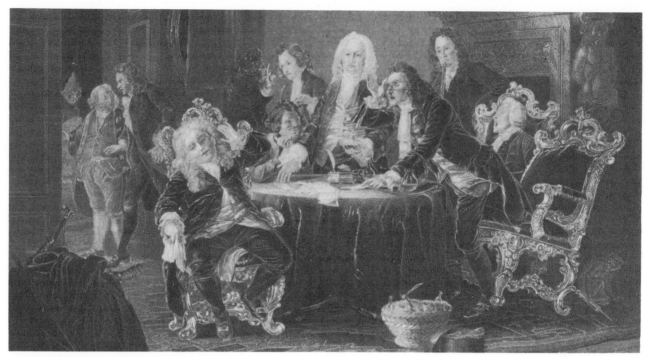

Consilium Medicum. Doctors noisily defend their respective systems while the patient silently passes away.

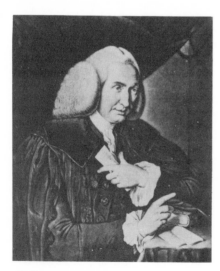

William Cullen (1710-1790) Edinburgh's outstanding clinician, teacher of a generation of students from the Old and the New World.

The Monros achieved distinction for their local patriotism, anatomical research and length of service. But Edinburgh's "Starlight of Physic," William Cullen, even outshone that reigning medical trio. As a clinical teacher Cullen ranked second only to Boerhaave. From all parts of the globe students journeyed to Edinburgh to hear his lectures, which were unsurpassed in vividness and logic. New York's Samuel Bard was among the young doctors inspired by the Scot's glowing personality.

You cannot teach medicine without a system, Cullen believed. "You cannot huddle facts together," he declared. Yet he wanted to hold theories in a light rein, as Sydenham did. Cullen's system stressed nervous irritability as the cause of disease. When a modern doctor ascribes a disease to frayed nerves, he is harking back to Cullen.

The system of nosology, which Cullen advocated, classified diseases in the way that Linné, the Swedish botanist, grouped the species of animals. It had the virtue of clarity but contained no original facts. Cullen ignored the advances in pathology and diagnostics that had been made by outstanding men like Morgagni, Lancisi or Auenbrugger. For science Cullen did little; for medical practice, a great deal.

"HEALTH DEPENDS ON EXCITABILITY" (Brown)

As a practising physician, Cullen was ideal. His manner was so open and so kind that he became the friend of every family he visited. Unlike the proverbial thrifty Scot, he always had a "noble carelessness about money." He kept all he made in an unlocked drawer where he could help himself freely. In spite of his great success — when he died in 1790 the desk drawer was empty.

Cullen divided all disease into four groups, but John Brown his erstwhile assistant, topped this by his claim that there was just one simple principle at work in all the ills of the human body — "excitability." A natural state of excitability meant health. An excess of stimuli, creating over-excitement,

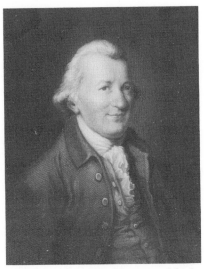

John Brown (1735-1788), praised by his adherents as the "Paracelsus of Scotland." His system reputedly caused more deaths than the Napoleonic wars.

or a lack of stimuli, resulting in sluggishness, caused disease. The doctor's job was easy — all he had to do was decide whether the patient had too much or too little stimulation.

In "sthenic" diseases (stenos: strong), such as fever, measles and smallpox, the body's over-excitement must be tuned down by purgatives, bleeding or debilitants. On the other hand, if the body was not sufficiently agitated to function normally, Dr. Brown prescribed stimulants: plenty of food, horseback riding and heroic doses of drugs. So appealingly simple was Brown's system that his disciples insisted upon his continuing to lecture even when he was locked up in Edinburgh's debtor's prison.

PATIENTS STUFFED AND STARVED

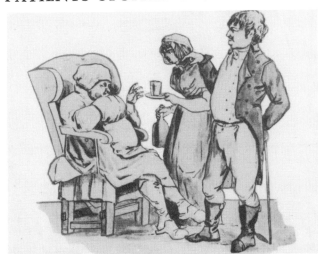

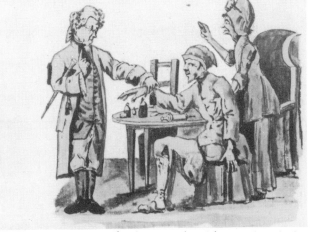

The Brunonian doctor (left), believing that most diseases are asthenic, stuffed his patient with powerful stimulants. Dr. Brown declared that gout was a "minus" disease and prescribed lots of food, strong wine and large doses of drugs. Later in the century, the pendulum swung in the other direction, when Hahnemann recommended infinitesimally small doses. He called it the "Theory of Potency."

The Boerhaavean doctor (right), afraid to tax the sick organism, insisted on a starvation diet for his patient and expelled the disease-causing matter by drastic purging. Boerhaave's system still clung to the tenets of the humoral theory.

189

ENGLAND

CANE-CARRYING PHYSICIANS
ARE WELL-HEELED · WELL-WHEELED

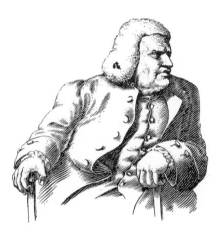

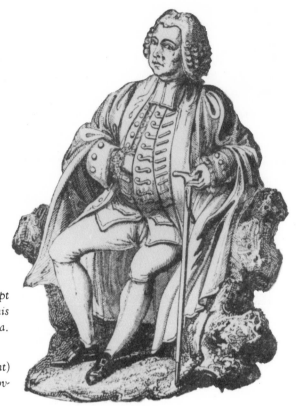

Dr. Samuel Johnson (left) kept London doctors busy with his chronic ills: dropsy and asthma.

Dr. Anthony Askew (right) shown holding the much coveted gold-headed cane.

In the first half of the 18th century London was rated below Leyden and Edinburgh as a medical center. Yet the great town did do something for the profession. Its literary Golden Age established a close link between the intellectual elite and the medical practitioner. England's great poets and wits, such as Swift, Pope and Johnson, counted doctors among their coffee-house brethren. Pope called the doctors "the most amiable companions, and the best friends, as well as the most learned men I know." Dean Swift encouraged Dr. Arbuthnot, physician in ordinary to Queen Anne, to publish his "John Bull," which created the prototype of the Englishman.

These doctors were raised in their status by the intellectual leaven of the time. They also benefited by the wave of prosperity that was a result of England's foreign trade and early excursions into manufacturing. There is an air of expansiveness about the doctors of this period. They are both prosperous and likable, full of good-fellowship and humor — outstanding as men and practitioners.

That loquacious genius and arbiter of English letters, Dr. Samuel Johnson, reflects in his writings the doctor's newly won distinction as a man of the world. Dr. Johnson's own frailties made reliance on medical art a daily necessity. As a scrofula-suffer-

ing youth, he had been sent in 1714 by Dr. John Floyer, of pulse-watch fame, to be touched by Queen Anne. (She died the same year.) Johnson kept all his life the touch-piece he had received on this occasion. He took to the grave with him his tubercular swellings, abiding testimony to Anne's inability to heal by the touch.

From his twentieth year on, Johnson rarely had a painless day. He suffered from general flatulence caused by all kinds of endocrine disturbances and was plagued throughout his life with attacks of aphasia, asthma and dropsy. All this made him a great dabbler in physic, and his writings an eloquent commentary on the doctors of his day.

Symbol of the physician's rise in social standing was the gold-headed cane. This badge of honor was bestowed on the city's outstanding doctor by the College of Physicians.

Dr. William MacMichael's enchanting, though not entirely authentic classic, "The Gold-Headed Cane" (1827), tells of the adventures of the medical stick with its six masters. John Radcliffe (1650-1729) was the first to carry the cane and Matthew Baillie (1761-1823), the last. "After his death,

it ceased to be considered an appendage of the profession," Dr. Mac Michael relates in his story.

The cane most doctors used during this period not only served as an outward sign that physicians had become gentlemen, but it also had a practical value. The stick's knob contained vinaigrette or other disinfectants. The doctor always held the cane up to his nose when he approached a sick person, "so that its fumes might protect him."

Five holders of the gold-headed cane, Doctors Askew, Mead, Radcliffe, Baillie and Pitcairne, are pictured on this page. One of the most elegant holders of the cane was Dr. Askew (left). His lavish house on Queen's Square in London became so crowded with fine books that he was advised to build shelves out on the street. Askew never allowed his friends to touch his bibliophilic treasures. He showed them under glass or, from afar, while atop a library ladder.

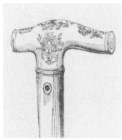 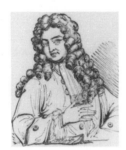 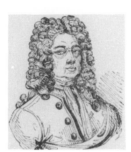 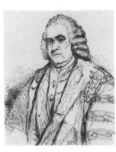 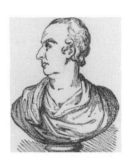

The **Goldheaded Cane**   **RADCLIFFE**   **MEAD**   **PITCAIRNE**   **BAILLIE**

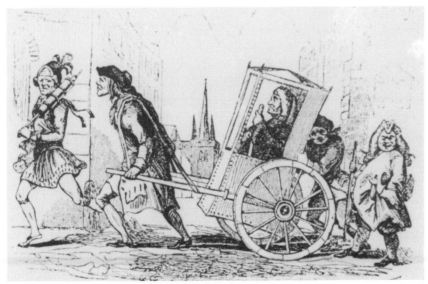

Man-drawn sedan chair takes doctor on his round. He is paced by apothecary shouldering enema. Less fortunate colleague follows on foot. Knob of stick held disinfectants.

As the doctors prospered in London's gay social life, the carriage joined the gold-headed cane as a sure index of professional prestige. The times had passed when a fashionable doctor could walk his rounds or go on horseback, without serious loss of prestige. To arrive in a sedan chair was the least one might expect from a prosperous doctor. The beginner was compelled to keep a flashy team of horses and maintain them in proper style or face medical ruin.

The size of a doctor's wig and the number of its curls — three or more — also had social significance. During the winter a successful London doctor equipped himself with a warm muff.

191

PEPPERY RADCLIFFE

PRINCELY MEAD

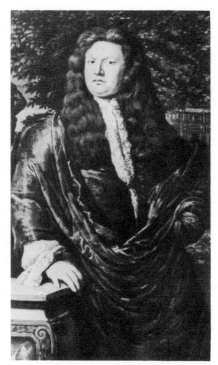

Dr. John Radcliffe, (1650-1729) feared as a man, trusted as a doctor.

"**I** would not exchange your majesty's legs for your three kingdoms!" Dr. John Radcliffe exclaimed when King William III of England uncovered his dropsical ankles. Although he was coarse, violent, hated by his colleagues and notoriously impolite to the ladies, Radcliffe was the first doctor to receive the gold-headed cane.

Never a learned man, his acute judgment commanded confidence. He brusquely diagnosed Queen Anne's complaint of distemper as something like "hysterical nonsense." This finished him as a court physician. Yet he was asked to appear at her death bed. "I have taken a physic and cannot come," Radcliffe replied to the royal summons. His answer set off an indignant uproar at court. Radcliffe was accused of willfully denying the queen his lifesaving presence. That, in the eyes of the world, made him a "negative murderer."

Dr. Radcliffe represented a new type of doctor, one who enjoyed the full power of the profession's rising prestige. Though born in the middle of the 17th century, he was decidedly a product of the Age of Enlightenment. He is credited (among others) with the remark that as a young practitioner he knew 10 remedies for each disease and that in his old age he knew 20 diseases — but not one remedy.

In spite of trouble, threats and animosities he became a great power.

That he treated his patients with merciless candor did not impair his popularity. While his bluntness hurt, it gave the patient confidence in his integrity and skill. The doctor openly admitted that his scientific training was defective. Asked for his office, he pointed to a few vials, a skeleton and a herbal: "This is Radcliffe's library."

Though his enemies accused him of being a miser, Radcliffe generously bequeathed most of his fortune to Oxford University. He endowed the Radcliffe Observatory, Hospital and Library. This prompted Dr. Garth to remark slyly: For Dr. Radcliffe to found a library was, "about as logical as if a eunuch should found a seraglio."

Dr. Richard Mead fell heir not only to Dr. Radcliffe's fabulous practice but also took over his house and became the second practitioner to carry the gold-headed cane. Mead and Radcliffe were a strange pair. Where Radcliffe was blunt, Mead was polite. The former was a frank despiser of all learning; the latter a gentleman with highly cultured tastes and a medical thinker of note. On the other hand, both came from humble families and attained success in their profession by their own initiative.

"Use all mankind ill" was the word that Radcliffe passed on to his younger colleague when Mead became his heir. Mead, however, climbed to success by a philosophy of singular humanity and goodness of heart. He lived in princely style, with his annual income of more than £7,000 putting him in an economic class with today's $100,000-a-year men.

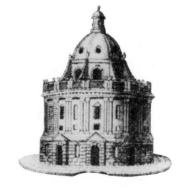

Radcliffe Library (Oxford) perpetuates name of generous Dr. John Radcliffe.

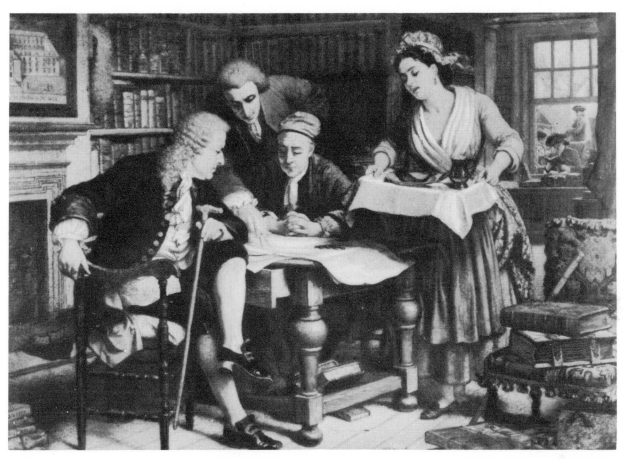

Dr. Richard Mead (left) discussing with his friend, Thomas Guy (right), the building and endowment of Guy's Hospital. Guy was probably the only University Press Printer who left a fortune. He had been successful with South Sea Bubble investments.

"Ever reknowned Richard Mead! Thy pharmacopoeial reputation is lost in the blaze of they bibliomanical glory!"

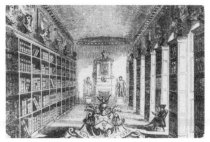

Dr. Mead's library was freely used by his scholar and artist friends.

Like many of his contemporaries, Mead earned his fees not only at bedsides but also in the coffee houses. Here, apothecaries presented verbal reports of cases to him, and he prescribed for the patients on that basis at ten shillings apiece, a fee smaller than his usual one pound for a personal visit. In his day, Mead was called "a physician who made the most and spent the most," but he never lost his humane approach. He strongly advocated a government agency similar in function to a national health council for the planning of sanitary reforms.

When the plague broke out at Marseilles in 1719, the alarmed British government asked Dr. Mead to outline measures to counteract mass infection. In a short but classical discourse on pestilential contagion published in 1720, he condemned the practice of locking up infected victims and suggested that they be isolated by removal to plague houses.

193

THE
NEGLECTED
LITTLE ONES

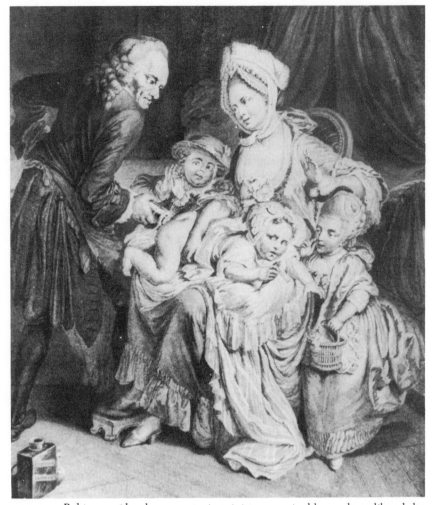

Babies considered grown ups in miniature received heavy doses like adults.

Before the coming of the humanitarian 18th century no group of beings was more abused than were "the little ones". The rich, busy with their worldly pleasures, usually turned their "brats" over to nurses. For the poor there were no nurses. Children were just a troublesome burden.

Lowly parents, hard-pressed for even a miserable livelihood, often wilfully crippled their poor children so that they would incite pity, and thus inspire more alms-giving when sent begging through the streets.

Queen Anne, who ruled England from 1702 to 1714, set a dismal example of improper child care for her subjects. Between 1684-1688 she had four miscarriages. Not a single one of the 18 children that the queen brought into the world survived to maturity.

Such wastage of child life was considered natural. Parents viewed the loss of 75 per cent of their infants before the age of two as a normal condition entirely in keeping with nature's plan.

Also there were ways to get rid of unwanted children: A mother always could claim that "overlaying" had killed her child. Since a mother slept with her baby in the belief that "maternal warmth does the little ones good," it was easy for an unmarried mother to toss about in her bed

and thus "accidentally" crush her baby to death without fear of apprehension.

Many unmarried mothers chose another way out. They dropped their offspring at the doorstep of a rich woman in the hope that she would provide a home for the foundling. Doctors were not alarmed by the heavy death toll of babies, since they believed children outside their orbit.

No wonder, then, that child care was in an abominable state. When the young received any treatment at all they were drugged and bled just like their elders. Children in general were considered grownups in miniature. They were believed able to eat like everyone else, only not as much. Diets that upset adults taxed young stomachs even more. Roast pork was recommended to free the little ones from their longings for mother. Nurses also gave them liquor "to harden their systems."

A weak trickle of pediatric literature had come down through the ages. There had been attempts to deal with diseases of early childhood. Thomas Sydenham had written about it, and treatises on the subject had appeared sporadically in Holland, France and Germany. Yet the medical profession at large had left the nurses and mothers to deal with the worrisome little nuisances. Since they were unable to speak and thus tell about their complaints, how could a learned doctor be expected to bother with them?

A growing humanitarian movement stirred society from its criminal neglect of the young and made the medical profession aware of its obligation to the underprivileged. The child in its innocent goodness now began to appeal strongly to the century's mood of romanticism.

Strangely enough, the man who crystallized this feeling against "the massacre of the innocents" into practical action was neither a doctor nor a father. Thomas Coram, a bachelor, established the first children's hospital and also roused physicians to extend their care to the suffering young.

Thomas Coram (1668-1751), a maritime trader who had spent some profitable years in America, pitied the many babies left on the highways

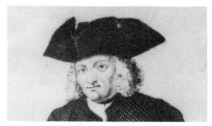

Bachelor Thomas Coram pitied foundlings, started child welfare movement.

leading to London. He spent his old age fighting to save such infants and in 1739 helped to found London's Foundling Hospital. Its opening took London by storm. The best minds of the day helped support the institution. Dr. Richard Mead, acted as one of the governors. Hogarth volunteered as its official artist, and Handel's Messiah was performed annually for its benefit.

Though not a hospital in the modern sense, this child shelter drew generous aid from the medical profession.

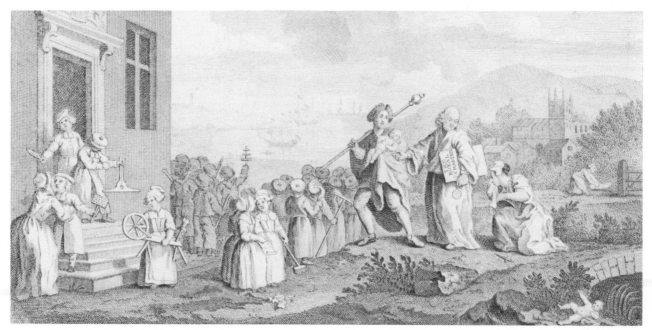

Foundlings Hospital focused attention on proper childcare. Engraving commemorating Hospital's opening (1741).

STOP TIGHT SWADDLING

CADOGAN TEACHES SENSIBLE CHILDCARE

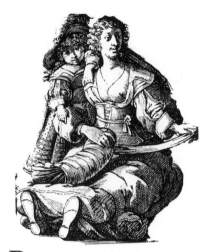

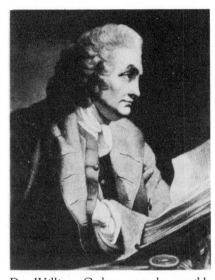

Dr. William Cadogan taught sensible child care, advocated frequent diaper changes — gave infant "right to kick."

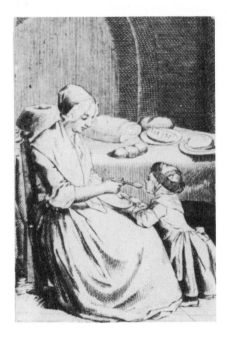

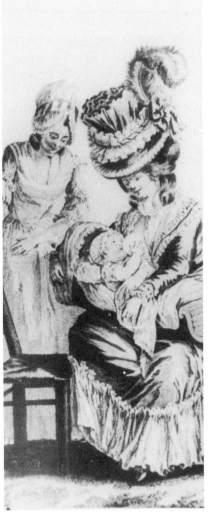

Doctors recommended breast feeding (above) to reduce infant mortality.

Mothers fed children food of grown-ups (left) injuring delicate stomachs.

Probably the worst of all hazards facing the young was tight swaddling. The baby looked like a mummy, and often ended up like one.

A heavy, airtight wrapping of bandages was meant to keep the bad air out and the "nourishing juices" in. It was considered dangerous to change diapers too often. Of course, these babies were apt to become ill.

During the 1740's a group of pioneer pediatricians appeared on the scene to liberate the babies from their life-strangling bundles and to offer sound advice to mothers. The most eloquent of these educators was Dr. William Cadogan of London. He told mothers it was dangerous to swaddle babies tightly, and his *Essay upon Nursing* (1748) thundered against feeding infants an "unwholesome mess." Many mothers, he observed, were not nursing their babies "for fear of getting fat."

In the first part of the 18th century England could boast of more books on the care and cure of horses than on the handling of babies. But pediatric interest increased at last after William Cadogan and others had sparked this vital branch of medicine.

CORRECT FAULTY POSTURE

ANDRE ASKS PREVENTIVE ORTHOPEDICS

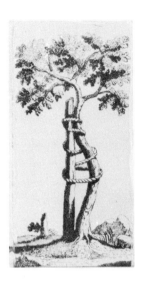

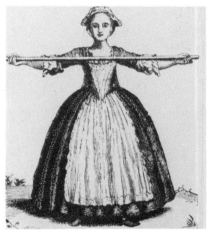

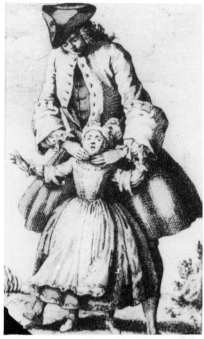

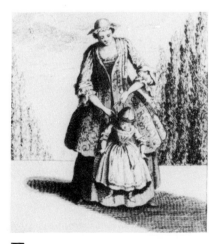

Illustrations from André, Orthopédie: nurse lifting baby into midair causes wry neck (left); correcting mal-posture through exercise (center); slanting neck straightened through doctor's "conservative adjustment" (right).

Free and straight as a tree — that was how Jean Jacques Rousseau thought children should grow up, unimpaired by civilization's hampering conventions. His idea found a medical counterpart in the science of orthopedics.

This very word had a programmatic ring. As its originator, Nicholas André says: "I have formed it of two words, namely orthos (straight) and paidios (child)."

In his famed treatise on the art of preventing and correcting corporal deformities in children (1741), André devotes much space to the proper posture, dress and exercise that will enable the child to develop into a sound and useful member of society.

Since surgeons before him had engaged in fracture treatment, it would be incorrect to say that André actually founded orthopedics. But influenced, no doubt, by current ideas on child welfare he did put this specialty on a safe footing and stressed its preventive aspects. He recognized the fact that man and society as a whole can be saved much suffering if abnormalities are adjusted at an early age.

Rousseau had postulated natural education. André, on the other hand, provided the medical instrumentalities and the necessary common-sense procedures to achieve this aim.

One of the hurdles that hampered children in the development of their normal physical powers was the rigid way in which they were dressed. Trussed up in stays and restrained in their movements, the children of the upper classes presented a pretty, but thoroughly unhappy picture. They were dressed for show — not for play. Toward the end of the 18th century their hour of liberation arrived, when enlightened doctors backed the demands for dress reform.

JOHN HOWARD
DEMANDS PRISON REFORM

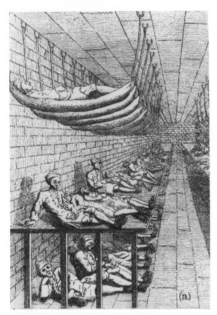

Gate of Debtor's Prison, London, from pamphlet, The Cry of the Oppressed.

England's men of good will had taken the lead in fighting the disgraceful neglect of helpless children. The same stirrings of conscience now roused interest in the miserable conditions in English prisons.

The debtor's cells harbored many innocents, whose health was jeopardized by the dark, narrow quarters, the poor food and the lack of sanitary facilities. The wretched prisoners fell prey to jail fever, suffocated or died of debility.

One of the great humanitarians of this age, John Howard, was moved to action by his shame and anger at prison conditions. He visited prisons and hospitals throughout Europe and had himself locked up at times to experience the ordeals of the inmates.

Through Howard's irrefutably documented exposés the reformers gained public support for broader social and hygienic improvements in other areas, such as London's slums.

The prison-reform movement thus provided a rallying point for one of the greatest forces of meliorative medicine.

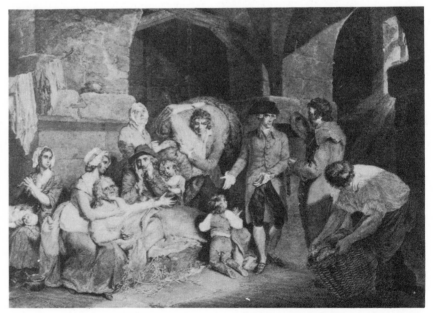

Cruelties in the Marshalsea Prison, London. Scene in sick men's ward.

John Howard (1726-1790) conducted a survey of international scope on prisons and hospitals. The English government was shamed into action by his courageous exposé.

STEPHEN HALES
GAUGES BLOOD PRESSURE

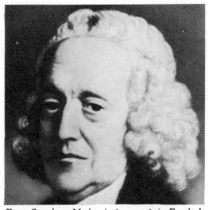

Rev. Stephen Hales (1677-1761), English clergyman, humanitarian, physiologist.

In 1681 Robert Hooke wrote a treatise entitled "A Supply of Fresh Air Necessary to Life." It took nearly a century for the social implications of this thesis to be recognized.

The 17th century had produced many scientific facts. The 18th century finally learned to use them in the interest of social welfare. Physiology joined forces with humanitarianism to alleviate, or at least mollify, the sufferings of the oppressed.

"A Supply of Fresh Air" was desperately needed — and the Reverend Stephen Hales set out to supply it. Recognizing that noxious air caused epidemics and great sufferings in prison, he constructed a "windmill ventilator" (right). This was no amateur gadget of a country tinkerer but a significant health invention. The Aldermen of London realized its value and had one installed in Newgate Prison. The ventilator reduced the death rate from eight to two a month and was enthusiastically received, even on the Continent.

But "air conditioning" in the interest of health was only one of Hales' many contributions to medical science. Probably his most remarkable foray into physiology was the one he made in December, 1711. After casting a white mare to the ground and tying her to a stable door, he laid open the cartoid artery. Into it he inserted a brass pipe which in turn was linked to a glass tube 12 feet 9 inches high. When the blood was admitted it spurted up in the glass tube to a height of 9 feet 6 inches. In a similar experiment, probably performed at the same time, Hales measured the pressure in the veins of a horse (see illustration below).

With his simple glass gauge the ingenious curate performed the first blood pressure measurement ever recorded. In the history of physiology Hales ranked in originality and experimental acumen with the immortal Harvey.

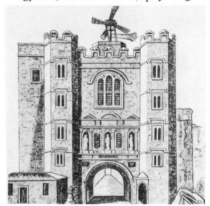

Newgate Prison ventilator invented by Rev. Stephen Hales (1751).

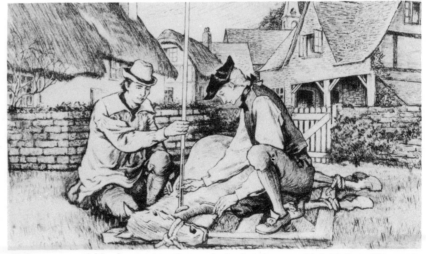

Hales measured blood pressure of mare he had tied to an old field door. Glass pipe inserted into jugular vein showed blood pressure column. It measured 12 inches when animal was quiet, 64 inches when animal stirred and became excited.

CURES FOR WORKERS...

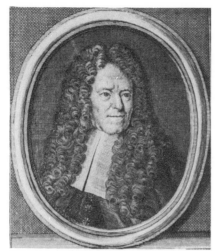

Bernardino Ramazzini recognized ills caused by dismal working conditions, asked doctors to consider patient's occupation in making diagnosis.

As the eyes of the humanitarians began to see the sufferings of the underprivileged, the doctors turned their attention to group diseases. As Dr. Richard Shryock observes, in this age medicine transferred its ministrations from a personal to a social plane.

In Bernadino Ramazzini the workers found a stanch champion. His *Treatise on the Diseases of Tradesmen* which appeared in 1700, was far in advance of its time, and remained for long a standard reference work.

In his *Treatise* Ramazzini admonishes the doctors to study occupational hygiene. On a guided tour through the city's working quarters, he shows them the misery of the scavengers "who clean out privies and sewers." He admonishes his colleagues not to shy away from unpleasant smells and sights for as Hippocrates said, "a doctor must inspect the unseemly and handle the horrible."

Ramazzini goes from shop to shop. There are the grinders whose lungs are going to waste and whose limbs are tortured by their unnatural posture as they bend over the stones. He describes their dizziness and tells how the monotony of their task results in mental uneasiness and sleepless nights with the grindstone still spinning in their heads. The millers, carrying their loads, suffer from hernia.

Looking beyond the mere cure of occupational diseases, Ramazzini suggests ways to prevent them by personal prophylaxis — bathing, frequent change of clothing, correct posture, physical exercise, and covering the mouth in the "dusty trades." His principal thesis has remained the credo of industrial hygiene to this day:

"'Tis a sordid profit that's accompany'd with the destruction of health."

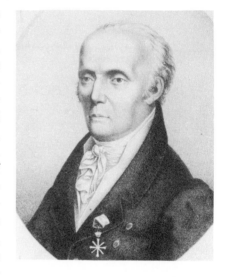

Johann Peter Frank pronounced state responsible for people's health, proposed strict legislation to enforce sensible living "from womb to tomb."

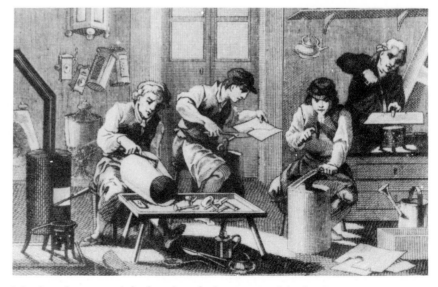

Metal workers get sick by breathing bad vapors, and by bending position.

SAILORS AND SOLDIERS

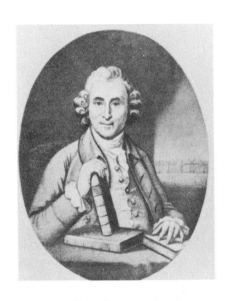

James Lind fought scurvy with citrus fruits, described dehydrated soup. Admiralty made lime juice part of navy diet in 1795—one year after Lind's death.

While the British Navy was sailing to greater glory in this age of colonial expansion, its sailors lived under murderous conditions. Their diet consisted of putrid beef, rancid pork and moldy biscuits. Scurvy was rampant.

James Lind, a Scottish naval surgeon who sailed aboard the H. M. S. Salisbury in 1747, found that 80 out of 350 sailors were laid low by scurvy. In other instances, fatalities rose to 75 per cent on a single cruise.

In his *Treatise of the Scurvy*, published in 1753, Lind showed that scurvy was both curable and preventable by an amazingly simple measure —

the addition of lemon juice to the sailors' diet. Not until more than 40 years afterward did the British Admiralty make lemon juice an official part of the diet on all British warships. This was in 1795 — one year after Lind's death. Scurvy disappeared practically overnight.

Lind's research on scurvy not only turned sickly British tars into healthy "limeys" but opened the way for today's nutritional science that has eliminated scorbutic suffering and brought many other deficiency diseases under control.

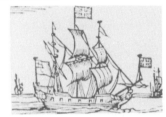

The hygienic conditions of the soldiers also presented a sordid picture. To the hazards of the battlefield were added the dangers of unsanitary camps rampant with wound fever and exposed to malarial swamps.

Dr. John Pringle, a thoroughly practical man as well as an outstanding scientist, recorded the sufferings of the soldiers in his treatise, *"On the Diseases of the Army"* (1752). Here he analyzed questions of diet, water supply, and personal cleanliness. This book helped in no small measure to raise the standard of preventive military medicine.

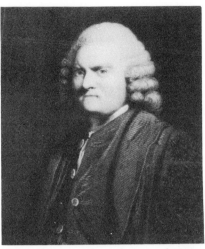

John Pringle reformed army hygiene, became president of Royal Society.

Pringle introduced the word "antiseptic" into our terminology. A pioneer of The Red Cross idea, he worked tirelessly to have hospitals recognized as sanctuaries.

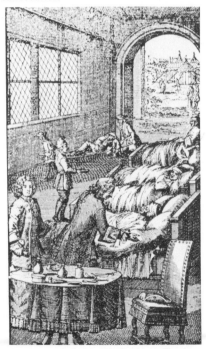

Army camp hospital shows well organized medical service, as outlined by 18th century "social physicians."

201

YEAR OF TWO GREAT BOOKS

1761

In the first half of the 18th century doctors tried to build valid systems and put medicine to work for man's social betterment. Despite great strides in bedside teaching, the scientific harvest remained poor. Then in one memorable year, 1761, two men, Morgagni and Auenbrugger, published two books that were to rejuvenate medicine with the spirit of observation.

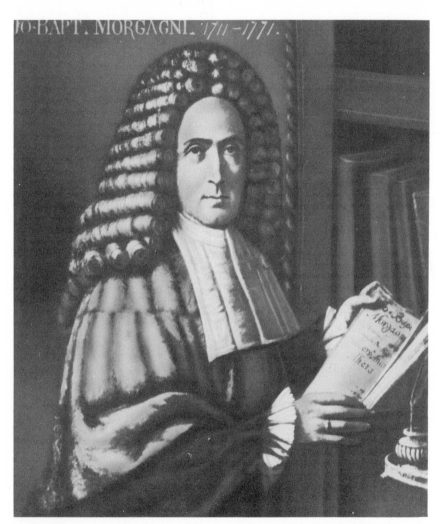

G. B. Morgagni correlated clinical disease pictures with organic lesions. He anticipated strategic importance of Pathology Department in today's hospital.

Not until Giovanni Battista Morgagni was nearly 80 did he publish his great two-volume book, *On the Seats and Causes of Diseases*. The title is significant. Morgagni pronounces the organ as the seat of disease, then proceeds brilliantly to link up changes in function to pathological changes, such as distention of blood vessels, and enlargements or indurations of the liver, heart and lungs.

Before *De Sedibus* made Europe's scientists call Morgagni "His Anatomical Majesty," a doctor who noticed a patient's abnormal heartbeat concerned himself almost exclusively with this phenomenon. He did not search for the actual cause of the disease. Morgagni revolutionized this superficial approach by showing through post mortem evidence the morbid changes of the heart's anatomy responsible for the patient's suffering.

Similarly he found that a patient's paralysis might be traced to a cerebral hemorrhage or other lesion of the brain.

Morgagni's erudite book established the high standards that made clinical pathology a leading discipline in the next century.

Leopold Auenbrugger's colleagues at the Spanish Hospital in Vienna thought him a little queer. They shook their heads when they saw this staff physician thumped the chests of patients suffering from thoracic trouble. The doctor used but one hand and drummed it over the patient's shirt. That a doctor in 1754 should thus use his hand in medical work seemed not only odd but showed a lack of dignity in a man of science.

From his youth Auenbrugger recalled that his father, a tavern keeper in Gratz, Austria, judged the amount of wine left in his casks by the way they sounded when he tapped on them. The young doctor had found that by thumping a patient's chest, somewhat as his father rapped on a cask, abnormal lesions in the lung, fluids in its cavities and the heart region produced a sound different from that given off by a healthy person. Auenbrugger continued for 7 years to test his patients' lungs by his experimental drumming. In 1761 he put before the medical profession the result of his experiments, his slim but basic *New Invention to Detect by Percussion Hidden Diseases in the Chest.*

His contemporaries pooh-poohed the idea of "that foolish drumming," but Auenbrugger gained immortality as the initiator of percussion after Corvisart, in 1808, saved the *"Inventum"* from oblivion with his translation and personal commentaries.

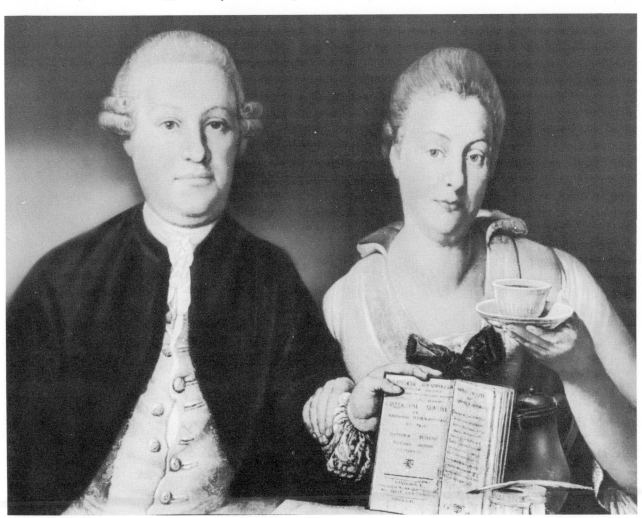

Auenbrugger, his handsome wife by his side, displays his magnum opus. Its nation wide lack of success bothered him little *for he led a pleasant life. His opera, The Chimney Sweep, earned him praise from the Empress Maria Theresa.*

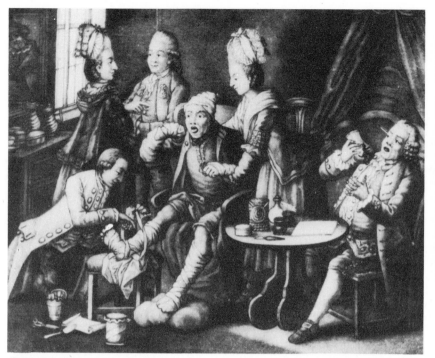

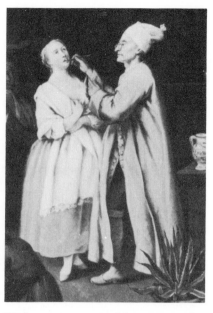

Oral examination in Venetian apothecary shop. (Painting by P. Longhi.)

Gouty patient visited by doctor who inspects urine while assistant binds legs. Devil in urine glass is premonition of surplus of uric acid, a feature of gout.

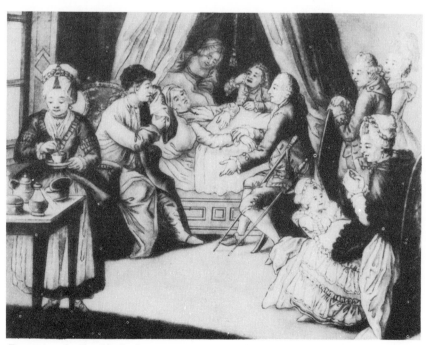

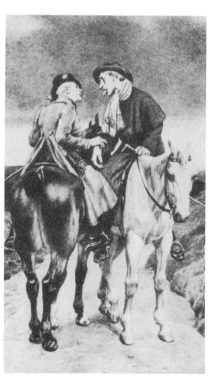

Doctor at the deathbed of a woman lectures on pulse beat while family resorts to prayer. Both illustrations by Johann Gottfried Haid, German etcher (1710-1776).

"Show me your tongue please," wayside diagnosis of country doctor.

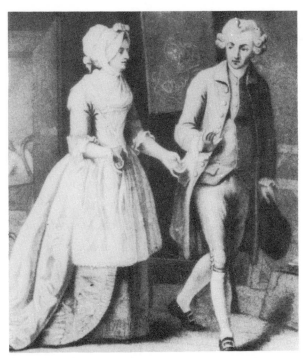

Benevolent physician refuses to accept payment from impecunious woman. (English mezzotint.)

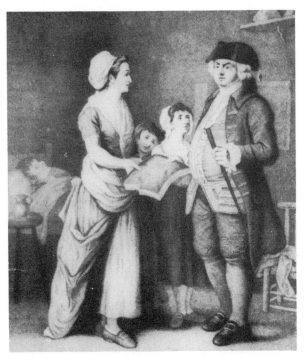

Rapacious doctor takes pay in form of much needed food from impoverished family. (English mezzotint.)

DOCTORS

"The physician is the only person with whom one dares to talk continually of oneself, without interruption, contradiction or censure."

Hannah Moore

"Whatever is good in medicine is to be found not in palaces but more often in the small unhealthy dwelling of the poor. To the praise of doctors be it said that no other citizens fulfill these splendid duties with so much zeal and courage."

Vicq-D'Azyr

"When I consider the assiduity of this profession, their benevolence amazes me. They use the most persuasive remonstrances to induce the sick to come and be cured."

Oliver Goldsmith

In this talkative age, much was said about medicine, the commonweal, and public hygiene. Most of it, although well meant, remained in the realm of theory. In the words of Defoe this was the "age of projects." Not till the second part of the 19th century were these ideas brought to practical fruition.

On the individual level, there was also much talk about the doctor's relation to his patients. Opinions on his attitude varied widely. Some praised him for his readiness to help, others thought that but a slim line divided medicine from quackery.

"A physician is one who pours drugs of which he knows little into a body of which he knows less."

Voltaire

"A doctor is a man who writes prescriptions till the patient either dies or is cured by nature."

John Taylor

"We may lay it down as an axiom that when a nation abounds in physicians it grows thin of people."

Joseph Addison

A wealthy doctor, who can help a poor man, and will not, without a fee, has less sense of humanity than a poor ruffian who kills a rich man to supply his necessities.

Tatler, Oct. 8, 1709

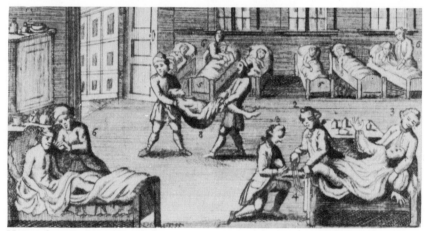

London surgeon explaining his private course in anatomy to a young candidate. Cheselden gave such courses. John Hunter was his star-pupil.

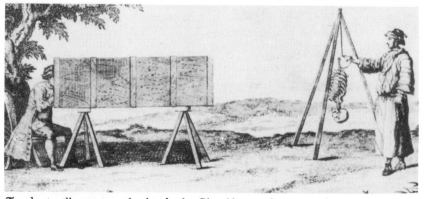

Hospitals, growing through humanitarian movement, gave surgeons opportunity to operate under controlled conditions, observe healing processes.

To obtain illustrations for his books Cheselden used camera obscura. His Osteographia, 1733, is one of the most beautiful medical atlases ever published.

SURGEONS BECOME GENTLEMEN

In Central Europe the strolling barber-surgeon did most of the surgery, sandwiched into his working-day between shaves and haircuts. Not so in England. Here, thanks to the Barber-Surgeons' Company, the medical activities of the tonsorialists were curtailed giving surgery a better chance to grow.

Then the hospitals of London, like St. Bartholomew, St. Thomas, Guy's and Chelsea Hospital, expanded and appointed young surgeons to their staffs. These clinics provided better opportunities for observation and supervision of cases.

At the same time the hospital surgeons set up special courses to teach pupils the surgical art and anatomy directly from life. This in turn enabled the surgeons to sever their connections with the Barber-Surgeons Company and establish a new and more professional association, The Commonalty of the Art and Science of Surgery — approved by Royal edict in 1745. The surgeon had outgrown his status as a craftsman and become a gentleman with a real profession.

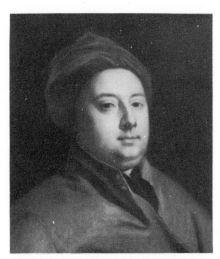

William Cheselden (1688-1752) wore silk turban during his operations, an elegant precursor of surgeon's cap.

The driving power behind these reforms was William Cheselden. His connections with the London hospitals had been a close one since his boyhood. At 15 he was apprenticed to a Mr. James Ferne of St. Thomas Hospital. (Surgeons were not called Doctor and still are not in England.) At 23 he started his own lecture course in anatomy, switching bodies away from the executioner and dissecting them in his own home. Cheselden's dexterity as a surgeon was based on sound anatomical insight. This enabled him to bring an operation like "cutting for the stone" to such a pitch of perfection that he could perform it in a record time of 53 seconds. The death rate, too, was amazingly low. He lost only 3 patients out of the first 53 cases.

In spite of his acknowledged mastery, Cheselden always tensed with fear before an operation — an experience probably shared by many of his confrères.

Cheselden attended Newton in his last sickness. He was surgeon to Queen Caroline until he lost favor due to an experimental ear operation performed on a criminal. The prisoner had been promised his freedom provided he let Cheselden perforate his ear drum. The Queen who had agreed to this arrangement was forced to dismiss her surgeon when the patient died.

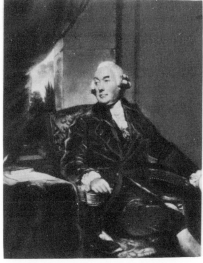

Percival Pott (1714-1788) of Pott's disease fame, a big surgeon but a small man, was an impeccable dresser.

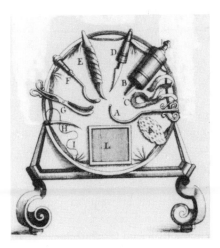

Dainty Percival Pott, an elegant gentleman and scholar, moved among London's aristocrats and intellectuals and showed that surgery had arrived. His sterling honesty, kindness of heart and great professional skill made him the head of the profession after Cheselden's death. The Royal Society recognized his scientific merits by electing him as a member. Many names familiar to the modern doctor keep his memory alive: Pott's disease (curvature of the spine caused by tubercular caries), Pott's puffy tumor and Pott's fracture.

Dr. Pott deepened his knowledge of fractures by his own sufferings. On a frosty January morning in 1756, his horse slipped as he was riding to Lock Hospital and the doctor was thrown to the ground. He suffered a compound fracture of the leg — not the fracture known by his own name, which is a fracture plus dislocation of the ankle joint.

To prevent aggravation of his injury Pott instructed his rescuers to carry him on "the door from a nearby house." The doctors who were quickly summoned to their colleague's bedside advised immediate amputation. While they were greasing their saw, Dr. Nourse, Pott's old master, arrived and pronounced that the limb could be saved. During his long recovery, Pott started his books on fracture, tumors and spinal curvature which are acknowledged as masterworks to this day.

Eighteenth century instrument table.   207

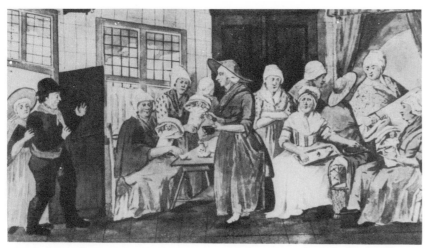

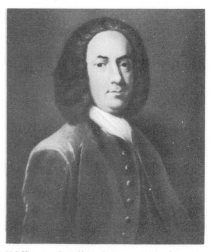

Midwives throng maternity chamber of Dutch farmhouse. Father is helped through door to see newly arrived quin-

tuplets. Babies (one dead) were exhibited for a fee. "Roads were black with carriages" (1719).

William Smellie (1697-1763) brought midwifery within the orbit of medicine.

RISE OF THE MALE - MIDWIFE

Just as surgery in the 18th century was groping for a scientific basis, so was obstetrics. Although midwives were ignorant, superstitious and on the whole unsanitary, prejudice against medical men assisting at childbirth was very strong. "True modesty," it was said, "is incompatible with the idea of employing a man midwife."

Despite tremendous opposition from midwives and prudes, William Smellie single-handedly brought obstetrics within the orbit of legitimate medicine. Without influence or the advantage of a hospital connection, he defied popular opinion, by practicing midwifery.

For 18 years Smellie was a country doctor in his native Lanark, Scotland. Like many another physician before and after his time, he yearned to try his luck in the city. After a short stay in Paris, he came to London in 1739. Although he was a complete stranger, he began to give courses for midwives in his own home. Smellie's classes were successful. The doctors became apprehensive. Dr. William Douglas, envied the meteoric rise of this country-come-to-town practitioner and asserted that Smellie displayed a paper lantern on his house inscribed "Midwifery taught for five shillings."

Smellie used a leather mannequin to demonstrate to his students the different positions of the foetus. He also took them along on his calls and instructed them in the use of obstetrical forceps. For years these instruments had been a closely guarded secret of the Chamberlen family.

Smellie probably had heard about them during his trip to Paris. He brought the forceps to England and became their staunch champion.

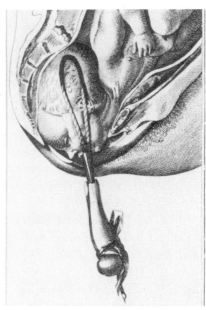

Method of child delivery with the aid of forceps. Smellie covered the wooden blades with leather to avoid alarming the mother by their ominous clanking. "He believed in forceps as firmly as he did in the Bible" (Thoms).

For his practice, this daring "male midwife" had to rely at first on the poor. In their homes, Smellie always gave his best. In one difficult labor case, he reported, "I sweated so much that I was obliged to throw off my waistcoat and wig and put on my nightgown with a thin napkin over my head."

Smellie's crusade for better obstetrics did a great deal to overcome public prejudices. Naturally, the midwives considered him an intruder in this field and, for once, found support among the fashionable doctors. One self-appointed warden of morality, disturbed by the thought that students assisting Smellie on one of his 1150 school cases touched the patients, exclaimed: "Pray sir, what is the use of such touching? These women are treated with less decency than a farmer would his cow!"

In spite of it all, Smellie forged ahead and in 1752 crowned his professional accomplishments with his *Treatise on Midwifery*, which Tobias Smollet, the writer, had helped to put into more readable form. It was this book, supplemented by other "common sense" treatises of the Dublin School that gradually brought midwifery into the orbit of legitimate medicine.

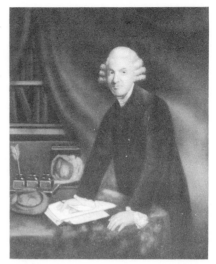

William Hunter published superb atlas on gravid human uterus in 1774.

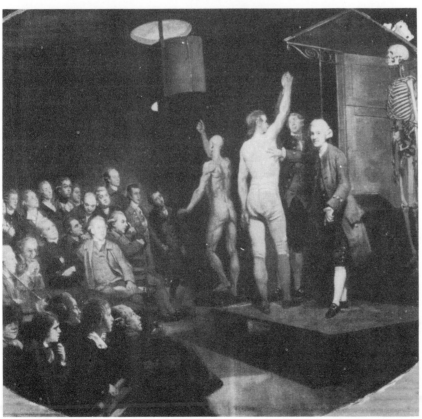

William Hunter (1718-1783) lecturing before Royal Academy. He supplemented discussion of skeletal anatomy by life demonstration. (Nat. Portrait Gallery.)

In 1741 a young Scottish doctor, William Hunter, came to live in Smellie's house in London. He had arrived from Glasgow, where the great Cullen had been his adored preceptor. Influenced no doubt by Smellie, Dr. Hunter established himself as an obstetrician. His courtly way and sagacious disposition gained him a wide practice, especially among the wealthy. Even Queen Charlotte sought his advice. Proudly and quaintly, Hunter could write to his teacher that he had assumed "the sole direction of her majesty's health as a child bearing lady."

As time went on, William Hunter made his Windmill School of Anatomy in London, a European center of medical study. It was in connection with his work as an anatomist that he came upon a "discovery" acclaimed as one of the most far-reaching in medical history: William Hunter discovered his brother John and developed his anatomical genius.

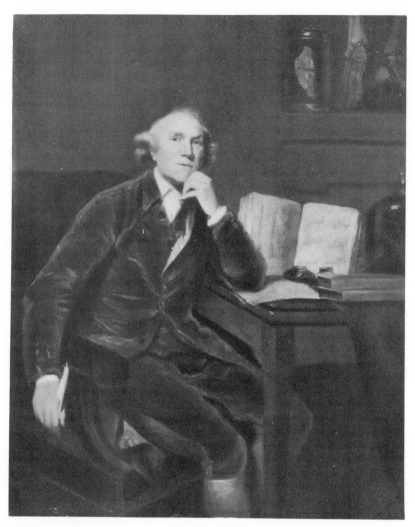

JOHN HUNTER

GIANT OF EXPERIMENTAL SURGERY

"To perform an operation is to mutilate a patient whom we are unable to cure — an acknowledgment of the imperfection of our art." This was the passionate belief of the world's first experimental surgeon, John Hunter.

In 1748, John Hunter, youngest brother of Dr. William Hunter, arrived in London. John was a thick-set, red-haired young man, unschooled and unpolished, straight from rural Scotland. He was put to work immediately in the dissecting room of William, who was ten years his senior. When John Hunter was asked to prepare an arm to lay bare its muscles, he did the job so skillfully that William decided to make him his assistant. He also sent John to Chelsea Hospital for training as a surgeon under William Cheselden. When John had acquired surgical skill and experience, William wished to give him an academic background. He sent him to Oxford. There all the well-

John Hunter (1728-1793). Painting by Joshua Reynolds (left). After the artist had complained of his inability to catch his subject in a telling pose, he observed Hunter one day in a profound reverie. The sketch he then made became the basis of this famed canvas in the National Portrait Gallery.

laid plans went wrong. John stayed at school for less than two months and accomplished nothing.

With his passion for exploring nature through original experiments, the classics appeared to him strictly a dead language. Even with his mother tongue he had great difficulty, and his grammar remained a social hazard throughout his life.

Such lack of polish and academic education, however, did not prevent John Hunter from becoming a real giant in biology and one of the most influential teachers of scientific surgery. When he first entered the medical world, surgery was changing over from a craft into a science. It was his life work to accelerate and complete that transformation. Even today medicine marches forward along the experimental path blazed by John Hunter.

Cheselden and Pott had done competent work and were creditable anatomists and operators. When they encountered atrophy in a leg or an aneurysm in an arm, they amputated skillfully and without hesitation.

In Hunter's opinion, these surgeons had been acting too quickly and without sufficient thought on the matter. Although he was an acknowledged virtuoso in surgery, Hunter did not believe in the expediency of operations. He warned the surgeon against acting like "an armed savage" and hacking away what he could not heal. An

operation according to Hunter was an admission of the physician's inability to heal by understanding nature's way.

Hunter was not satisfied merely to state a diagnosis. In his day to recognize and name a disease had been considered the aim of medicine; but to him diagnosis was only preliminary. "To know the effects of disease is to know very little," he kept hammering into his students during his lectures. "To know the cause of the effects is the important thing."

Hunter always wanted to know why the patient had become diseased — and what might have been done to prevent the ailment.

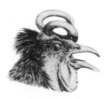

Cock's spur transplanted to comb — a famed Hunterian experiment.

For the answers he sought, he went directly to nature. His house overflowed with dogs, hedgehogs, leopards, eagles and every other creature he could collect by money, cunning or stealth. Carefully he observed them, drugged, operated or dissected them. Understanding the processes of diseases, he was sure, would offer the key to specific cures.

When Hunter himself accidentally ruptured the tendon of Achilles, he started to experiment on the dogs in his menagerie to observe the way these structures might heal. Based

on his observation, he developed the operation of tenotomy — a surgical procedure still in use today to relieve contracted and distorted joints. Probably his greatest triumph was the elimination of drastic surgery for aneurysm. In these cases the arterial walls distend and thus form blood-filled pouches. The doctor of Hunter's time gave the victim of aneurysm two dire alternatives: either he must submit to the amputation of the afflicted limb, or wait until the swelling burst, which inevitably meant death. By tireless experiments on the deer of Richmond Park, Hunter convinced himself that it was possible to ligate the artery feeding the aneurysmal sac. One day after he had blocked off the artery leading to a stag's antler he found that the horn was still warm to his touch. Checking further he discovered that the capillaries had expanded and were carrying the blood around the blocked artery in nature's attempt to keep the blood supply normal. From this observation Hunter worked out a successful technique for treating aneurysm in humans without amputation.

This highly practical kind of research helped to quiet Hunter's critics who had ridiculed his idea that surgery could benefit by studying deer, birds, fish, and other animal life ranging from flies to elephants. Of course not all of his experiments were equally successful. But he did show that the proper way to the operating room led through the laboratory. This was an enormously important new principle. Hunter applied it with signal success. Even when he failed and stumbled — "he stumbled in the right direction."

JOHN HUNTER
(Continued)

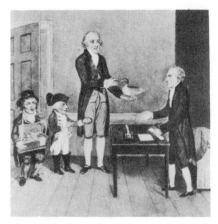

A live duck and a couple of dwarfs are welcomed by Hunter to his museum.

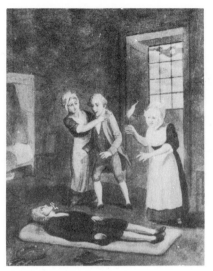

Severe attack of coronary thrombosis leaves Hunter's household stunned.

John Hunter did not shrink from using his own body to study the effects of disease. In 1767, he inoculated himself with what he believed to be gonococcal pus, in order to prove that syphilis and gonorrhea were identical. His deductions were fallacious because the man from whom he extracted the pus happened to have both syphilis and gonorrhea. This heroic experiment made Hunter a sick man for life. D'Arcy Power has shown that since undergoing this ordeal for science the famous surgeon suffered a permanent syphilitic affliction of his blood vessels.

Despite this drain on his health, Hunter kept up a large practice among patients of every class. In 1776 he was appointed surgeon-extraordinary to the king. The rich tolerated his rough manner in the hope of being cured, and the poor loved his straightforwardness. To be a practicing surgeon with hospital appointments was a taxing job in itself. Hospital visits occupied him in the afternoons until four o'clock. Then he took his first rest since the start of his working day before six o'clock in the morning. In the early evening he lectured and gave demonstrations.

Whenever Hunter was called away from his laboratory to attend a patient, he complained that those "damned guineas" were needed to keep his biological station afloat. Though highly successful in his private practice, he never denied that science was his true calling. He was not only a scientific genius blessed with a sure, acute instinct, but a real prodigy in his ability to work. In addition to operating, pioneering in science and teaching, he produced an actual cartload of manuscripts. He also left a museum with thousands of specimens.

"When I left him at midnight," a student reported, "it was with the lamp fresh trimmed for further study and with the usual appointment to meet him at six in the morning."

Shown below is the staggering collection that Hunter built up — the Hunterian Museum, as it appeared in the 1830s. During Hunter's lifetime his family was practically crowded out of its quarters by the ever-increasing influx of new specimen. Hunter invested all the earnings from his practice in this museum, where at one time he employed more than 40 helpers. The financial burden of this establishment nearly bankrupted him in 1790. After Hunter's death, Pitt rejected the acquisition of the Hunterian Museum by the British Government. "What! Buy specimens?" he exclaimed indignantly. "Why, I have not money enough to buy gunpowder!" In 1799, however, the government appropriated £15,000 with which to buy the museum and turned it over to the Royal College of Surgeons.

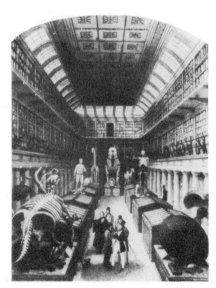

Hunterian Museum in 1830. At right, skeleton of the giant Bryn. Specimens were donated to College of Surgeons after Hunter's death. The London Blitz (1941) destroyed much of this invaluable collection.

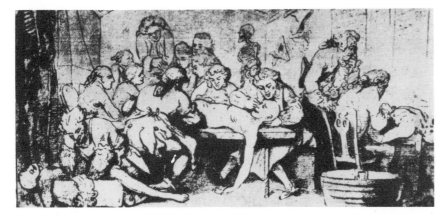

The Dissecting Room by Rowlandson. The figure standing above the rest is William Hunter; John stands at the right. Other onlookers are Hunter students who were to become leaders of early 19th century medicine.

HUNTERIAN SURGEONS

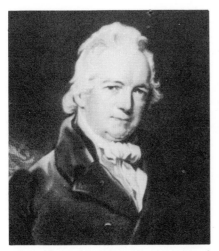

John Abernethy (1764-1831) improved on technique of ligating aneurysm.

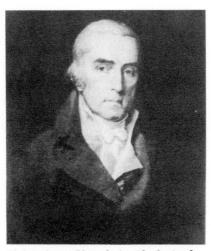

Philip Syng Physick (1768-1837), first to use animal tissues to sew up wounds.

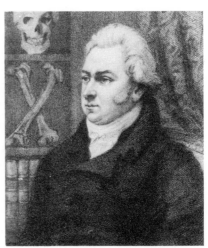

Sir Astley Cooper (1768-1841) described amputation of leg at hip joint.

Hunter trained a group of "thinking surgeons" who carried his gospel into practice. The outstanding representatives of his school were Abernethy and Cooper, both eminent as operators and teachers. Dr. Phil. Syng Physick, the master's favorite American student transferred the Hunterian science of surgery to the New World.

Of these post-Hunterian surgeons Abernethy was the most colourful.

Patients feared him for his gruffness. It was a practice with Abernethy not to be too sympathetic toward his patients. Women often found themselves shoved out of his office with a peppery remark. A young lady who became worried after swallowing a spider was quickly dispatched with the advice, "Put a fly in your mouth, madame, and the spider will come up to catch him."

Astley Cooper, anatomist and surgeon to Guy's Hospital was considerably more polished. His operative genius gained him perhaps the most remunerative practice ever achieved by a surgeon up to this time. Even his servant, Charles, is said to have made the not unconsiderable sum of £600 a year, just in tips from patients anxious to see the doctor without waiting their turn.

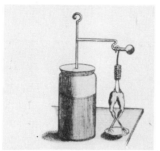

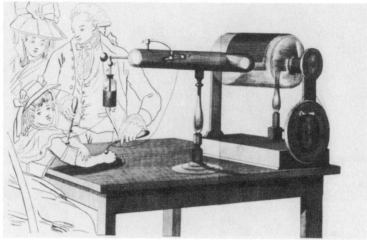

HEALING
ELECTRICALLY

Stimulating paralyzed muscle with the aid of a Leyden Jar.

Ever since Dr. William Gilbert had launched electricity on its way (in 1600) physicians had sought to apply it to medicine. Benjamin Franklin's *Experiments in Electricity*, sponsored by a doctor, John Fothergill, and published in 1753, gave new impetus to this trend. With Dr. John Pringle, noted hygienist and president of the Royal Society, Franklin discussed the possibility of using electric shock to cure palsy. Later, he conducted some experiments on paralyzed victims.

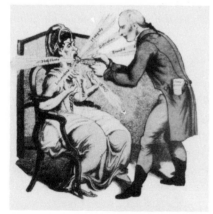

Elisha Perkins shown "extracting" malignity." (Gillray cartoon, 1801.)

Word spread that Franklin was able to cure blindness and dropsy. Since the public had heard of subtle nerve fluids and magnetic influences it was ready to hail a new "miracle". With typical honesty, however, Franklin admitted that no physical change was observed in the patient after electrical shock, though he thought there was some "lifting of the spirit."

When Luigi Galvani discovered "animal magnetism," the sufferers of palsy regained hope. His experiments seemed to prove that electrical currents in the body caused vital action, such as the contraction of muscles.

This work gained Galvani a place in the dictionary, and a distinctive nickname — "The Frog's Dancing Master." Thereafter, sufferers looked at electricity as a means to revive paralyzed muscles.

At this time, a number of doctors promised the public the electrical cures for which it had longed. Two of these men, Graham and Perkins, beguiled the people with melodramatic hocus-pocus. Mesmer, who had a more scientific grounding, also transgressed his bounds. Yet his teachings contained a kernel of truth that sprouted forth in the 19th century.

THE POWER OF HUMBUG: PERKINS

Dr. Elisha Perkins of Connecticut used in his cures electric tractors made of mysterious alloys. The sharp ends of these tractors were supposed "to draw out" disease wherever seated. Many patients were cured by Perkins — or at least they thought so. The public's enthusiasm was boundless. So was Perkins' business.

To test the effect of the mysterious rods, Dr. Haygarth of London made replicas of wood coated with metal. To his surprise he achieved the same "miraculous" effects. This demonstrated beyond a doubt that the curative mystery did not dwell in Perkins' metal but in the patient's mind. Perkinism disappeared — like so many other fads.

and even whole forests so patients exposed to the charged objects could regain their health. For one year of such magnetic showmanship, Mesmer received 400,000 francs in fees. But slowly the Parisians awoke from this trance. Franklin, Lavoisier, Guillotine and other members of the French Academy of Science issued a report showing that Mesmer's treatments resulted only in a powerful stimulus to the imagination.

Mesmer died in obscurity in 1815, but mesmerism lived on.

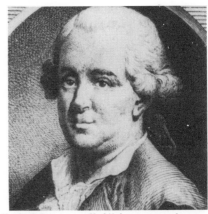

F. A. Mesmer, called "the great enchanter." He applied principle of "suggestibility."

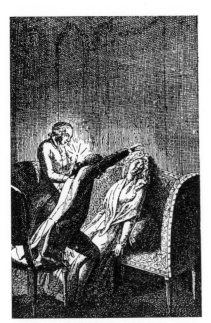

Magnetizer puts lady patient into mesmeric trance to effect cure.

Franz Anton Mesmer, a Viennese doctor, made "animal magnetism" a worldwide craze. A mysterious substance, magnetic fluid, pervades the universe and the human body, he asserted. Its proper flow means health. If the flow is interrupted, the resulting imbalance causes ailments. Dr. Mesmer claimed the power to correct this condition.

When Mesmer swept down on Paris in 1778 (the same year that Pinel settled there), his gospel was received with tremendous enthusiasm. The dynamic doctor's theories on electromagnetic influences sounded scientific enough to the layman, and his mere touch made women swoon. From the ensuing crisis they awoke, freed from their complaints, real or imagined. The rage for cures was so frantic that Mesmer soon started "mesmerizing" patients by remote control. He "magnetized" water basins, shrubs, parks

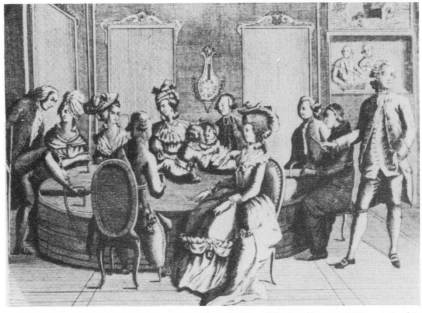

Visitors at a mesmeric séance grouped around a "baquet" containing a double series of bottles charged by Mesmer with his personal magnetic fluid.

A meeting with Benjamin Franklin in America inspired James Graham, an Edinburgh doctor, to create a colossal monument to charlatanry, an electro-therapeutical showplace, which he established in London under the name of "The Temple of Health." Its main attraction was the Celestial Bed. A night spent here, Graham promised, would rejuvenate the old.

The bed which soared above the floor on 40 magnetized pillars was available at a rate of 100 pounds a night with accompanying soft music and seductive shawl dancers such as the beauty who later won fame as Lady Hamilton. Graham called the state of medicine "inadequate, ineffectual, absurd, ridiculous." His words proved an apt verdict of his own efforts.

215

FOXGLOVE PLANT YIELDS STIMULANT

WITHERING TESTS DIGITALIS - INSISTS ON PROPER DOSAGE

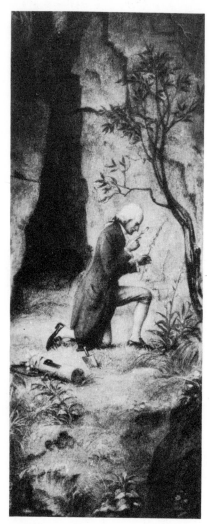

William Withering, (1741-1799) Doctor-Naturalist, studying digitalis.

Priestley (right) friend of Withering, chased from Birmingham by mob aroused by his sympathy with French Revolution (1791). (Birmingham Art Gallery.)

Up to this time the doctor still made use of a staggering number of traditional remedies. He knew little about the true effect of these substances and even less about the cause of the patient's trouble. Then in the second half of the 18th century, medical reformers subjected the pharmacopoeia to critical tests.

William Withering was outstanding in this group. Oddly, in his studies at Edinburgh the one subject he loathed was botany. But one of his first patients, Miss Helena Cooke, a talented flower painter, changed his loathing into love. She encouraged the young doctor to collect plants for her. After Withering had married Miss Cooke, he moved to Birmingham, a bustling industrial center, and the gathering point of much scientific talent. The young doctor's lively intellect was quickly recognized by the local luminaries. Dr. Erasmus Darwin, Charles Darwin's grandfather, sponsored him for a hospital appointment. Joseph Priestley, the chemist, Josiah Wedgwood of pottery fame, and James Watt became his friends. His practice flourished and world-wide fame came to him when his *Account of the Fox-Glove* appeared in 1785.

The plant foxglove had been known since antiquity and had been used by herb doctors and wise old women in multifarious concoctions. Subjecting such recipes to a critical test, Withering singled out digitalis as their most active ingredient. For nine years Withering experimented with the effect

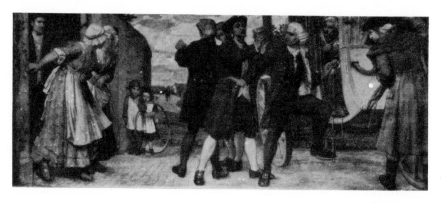

216

of decoctions or pills made from different parts of foxglove in various stages of growth. He found that a powder made from leaves just before the plant's blossoming time was highly efficacious. It brought relief to many of his patients who were suffering from dropsy, due to cardiac weakness. The powder acted as a diuretic effecting a draining of the surplus liquid accumulated in dropsical limbs. This in turn relieved the heart.

Withering kept experimenting tirelessly until he had clearly classified the various phases of the disease and defined the patient's physical makeup. Imbued with a spirit of scientific inquiry, like his friend the noted chemist, Priestley, Withering then set up dosages for cardiac disturbances. If Hunter, in Sir William Osler's words, "made all thinking physicians naturalists," Withering wanted to make physicians experts in scientific pharmacy. Yet the practitioners at large followed his precepts but slowly. Most of them administered digitalis "in doses very much too large." Dr. Lettsom, for instance, quickly lost eight cardiac patients after digitalis treatment. As Withering pointed out to Lettsom, the fault lay not in the medicine but in its improper use.

The higher Withering's fame rose as a doctor and an investigator in many fields of natural science, the lower his own health ebbed. Finally progressive pulmonary tuberculosis made him a chronic invalid. When death came in 1799, the century lost one of its greatest medical scientists.

Typical 18th century pharmacy. Suspended from ceiling is stuffed crocodile, symbol of the profession (right).

Scientific medication found another champion in William Heberden. This Cambridge scholar-physician cast a critical eye over the apothecary's shelves and pronounced them crammed with "remedies" whose medicinal value was exceedingly doubtful. His examinations proved the celebrated antidote, the theriac, a mixture of 70-odd useless ingredients. This exposure of a popular medicine was typical of Heberden's endless crusade against mystic and ridiculous remedies such as toad stones and "mummy powder."

Thanks to his efforts prescription writing was put on a more rational basis. As Garrison puts it, he "ridiculed the old nostrums out of existence." It was through the efforts of this inquiring, open-minded doctor that the 1788 edition of the London Pharmacopoeia excluded many noxious animal substances that had hampered rational therapeutics over the years.

As in his writings on medication, Heberden also was refreshingly critical in his appraisal of clinical medicine. During his more than 60 years of practice, he had made it his scientific

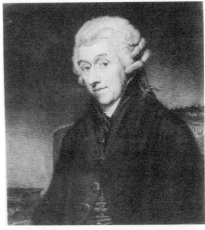

William Heberden fought for pharmacal reform — described angina pectoris, type of arthritis bearing his name.

habit to keep detailed records of all his observations. On these notebooks were based his famous *Commentaries* — compiled for the benefit of his son and published one year after Heberden's death at 91.

Heberden treated his colleague, John Hunter, during his attacks of angina pectoris, and he gave, if not the first, one of the first concise clinical pictures of this affliction.

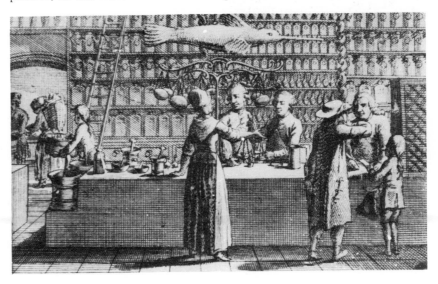

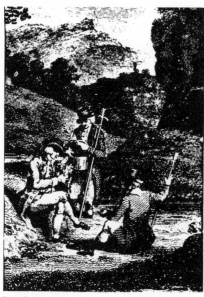

Dr. John Fothergill (1712-1780) deserved "esteem and veneration of all mankind" (Benjamin Franklin).

THE QUAKER DOCTORS OF LONDON

The age of reason and compassion found a representative of sterling quality in Dr. Fothergill of London. Rarely has there been a man who combined as he did the genuine warmth of the humanitarian with the mental acuteness of the scientist. This dynamic Quaker physician worked tirelessly and selflessly for the good of his patients — often 17 hours a day. In the words of his sister, "he was besieged by a perpetual clamour of people wanting him." In addition to his 36 years of work as one of the city's busiest practitioners he gained world renown as a pioneer in medical science. With Withering and Heberden, Fothergill helped to free the medical arts from the reign of polypharmacy.

Dr. Fothergill experimented extensively with medicinal plants. He wrote to all parts of the world for new specimens — and even requested rattlesnakes from a friend in the American Colonies. His botanical enthusiasm led him to found one of England's greatest flower gardens, a 35-acre tract at Upton in Essex. Anxious to keep in touch with this magnificent establishment despite his ever-growing practice, he is said to have gone there after dark to look at his treasures by the light of a lantern.

Guided by experience and his own original thinking, he applied his findings in research at the bedside and became one of the "best prescribers" in England. "I climbed on the backs of the poor to the pockets of the rich," Fothergill declared. But in reality medicine to him was a mission, and practicing "physick as a money-making trade" struck him as "a vice like intemperance." When economic hardship aggravated sickness, he pretended to feel the patient's pulse in order to slip into his hand a sum of money once, reportedly, as much as 150 £.

Beyond his care for the sick Fothergill had humanity's welfare at heart. He hated violence and injustice and staunchly backed the cause of freedom for which the American Colonies fought so valliantly.

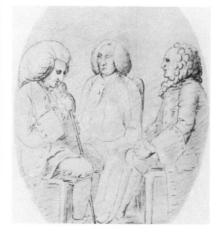

Weighty problems. Consultation of London physicians. Fothergill at right. (Caricature sketch by George Dance.)

London doctors on medico-botanical outing, instructed by Fothergill. He was called "England's best prescriber."

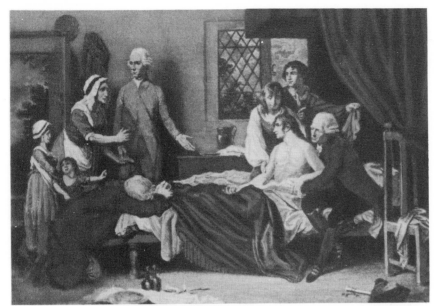

Mother rushes to bedside of son saved from drowning through aid of Royal Humane Society. Dr. Lettsom (left) supported this charitable group and countless others.

When Fothergill died in 1780 of a prostatic tumor, another Quaker physician assumed the leadership of the profession. John Coakley Lettsom, son of a West Indies cotton planter, had presented himself to Dr. Fothergill in 1769 after studies on the continent. Lettsom quickly won Fothergill's friendship and professional backing.

In interests and humanitarian views, these men had much in common; in temperament, they differed widely. Fothergill was a restrained introvert. Lettsom was "the volatile creole" — sociable, quick-witted, a ready talker and booster of professional and humanitarian causes. In no way a scholar, he owed his unequaled popularity to his good fellowship and a rare diagnostic instinct that can never be learned at a university. Quick and resourceful, he found it easy to see 50 cases before breakfast and was said to have seen 82,000 patients during 1795 alone. Lettsom was so busy that he found time to dine with his wife only once a week. "I live with my patients," he declared. "I love my profession and it loves me."

Such mutual devotion paid off handsomely. His income rose to £ 12,000 a year — equivalent to about $100,000 today. When he had time, he entertained like a lord at Grove Hill, his beautiful country estate. The rural fêtes he gave here to as many as 500 fashionable guests created a stir in the society columns of the time.

Like Fothergill, Lettsom was an ardent supporter of the Colonies and because of his birth in the West Indies proudly considered himself an American. In 1788, he became a member of the New York Medical Society, and Harvard honored him with a LL.D. degree. His strongest tie with America, however, was the New World's medical center at Philadelphia, which he helped with counsel, money and books.

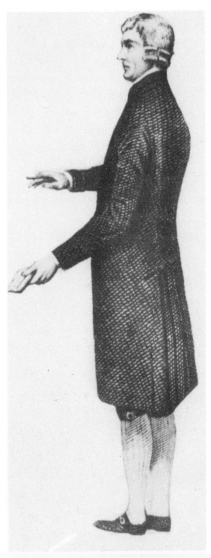

Dr. John Coakley Lettsom (1744-1815) thought many patients could be cured "by money rather than physick."

219

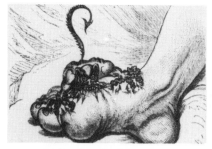

THE GOUT (GILLRAY)

LAUGHTER SHOOS
DEVILS OF PAIN

Got a twinge of pain? It's the Satan in your system just raising a little hell — or so they believed in medieval times and later. The devil's demoniacal helpers were blamed for illness of body and mind.

Laughter does not kill the little demons of agony, but it brings relief by deriding their mal-doings. It is in this sense that England's great caricaturists of the late 18th century, such as Gillray and Rowlandson, brought the solace of laughter to the suffering.

Gout, a mainstay of the fashionable practitioner among the overfed rich was caricatured by Gillray as a fire-spitting foot-eating devil (above). In *The Cow Pock* he showed Dr. Jenner inoculating his patients with "vaccine pock hot from ye cow" while little cows burst out from all parts of the patient's body.

As for the sickness in general, the doctors did their best to cure the patient, but in most cases, the best wasn't quite good enough. In this situation caricature offered a welcome opiate. These hilarious prints showed medicine as the patient saw it. If he wasn't cured, the erstwhile admiration for his doctor changed into spite — and even if the doctor wasn't to blame, the sick felt a sense of relief by blaming the doctor.

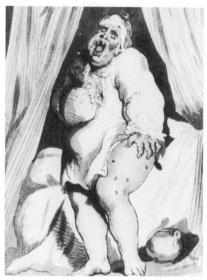

THE ITCH (ROWLANDSON)

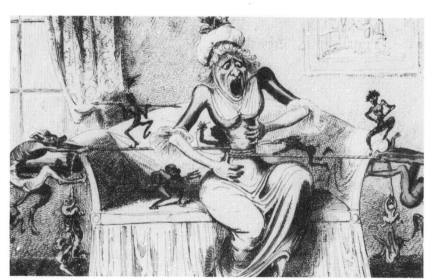

LADY RECOILS FROM GASTRIC PAIN (CRUIKSHANK)

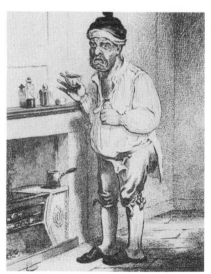

TAKING A PHYSICK

220

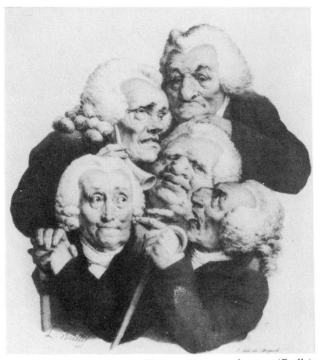

Doctors in consultation (Boilly).

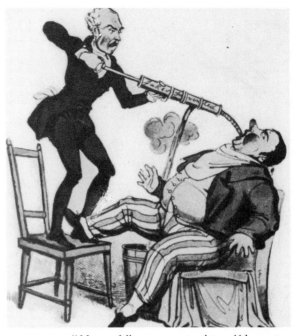

"Now a fellow may enjoy himself by eating three dinners." Stomach pump in action.

Below (left to right): Gillray's cartoon of doctor and patient.

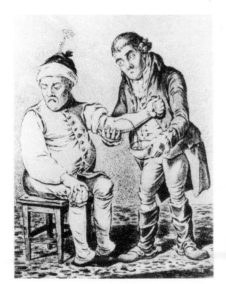

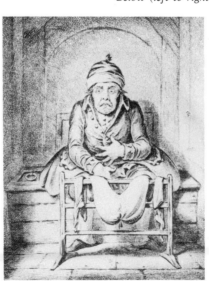

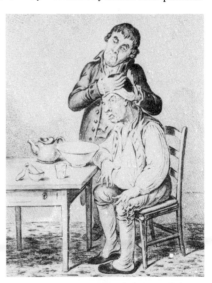

BREATHING A VEIN **BRISK CATHARTIC** **GENTLE EMETIC** 221

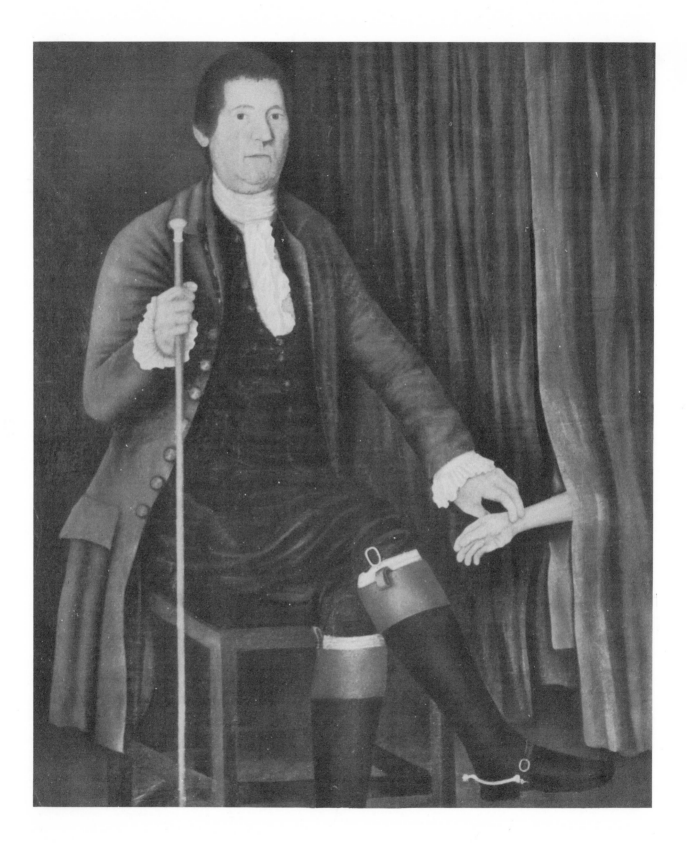

FROM STABLE BOY TO SURGEON

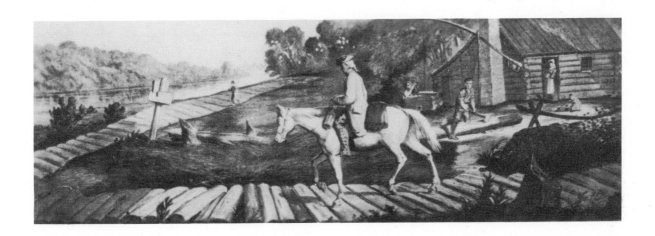

Today the doctors of American rank with the best in the world, but during America's first hundred years her total contribution to scientific medicine could be summed up in a single word — nothing.

Books were scarce. Daily medical emergencies did not permit the colonial doctor to pioneer in science. Europe's medical centers were too far away and only a few sons of the rich could afford a continental education.

These shortcomings, however, eventually worked in favor of the American physician. Out of the wilderness emerged a new type of doctor who in acumen and resourcefulness measured up to his more learned, socially more polished colleague abroad. Also, fron-

Dr. William Glysson of Woodstock, Connecticut (left) discreetly feels a lady's pulse outside a canopied bed. Painting by Winthrop Chandler, 1785.

tier conditions did away with the old separation between surgeon and physician and rounded out the doctor as a highly practical man. That trait, in the words of Baas, the medical historian, was to become "in recent times the chief glory of American medicine."

Bleeding and purging were practiced with the same abandon in the New World as in the Old. Yet polypharmacy had no chance to develop in the Colonies, since the doctor was compelled to stick to the simple, homely remedies that were available.

Without the benefit of medical schools, doctors were trained by the apprentice system. A lad anxious to learn the healing arts entered the services of an acknowledged practitioner. In his house the apprentice doubled as stable boy and personal servant, but did gain at the same time a knowledge of prevailing practices by watching the doctor at work.

After this an apprentice was "graduated" into practice for himself by receiving a certificate that he had successfully served his master.

It has been estimated that of the 3500 doctors practicing at the outbreak of the American Revolution, less than 400 held university degrees. All others were graduates of the stableboy-to-surgeon-school.

While in training the medical hopefuls were permitted to use the preceptor's library. They also received some private tuition. Yet the need for a systematic training of the medical aspirant was felt acutely. In the 1750's three young men who had served their apprenticeship, Shippen and Morgan from Philadelphia and Sam Bard from New York, went to Europe to obtain their degrees at Edinburgh. They turned home with plans for a medical school in the Colonies on par with those of the Continent.

FIRST
MEDICAL
SCHOOL

PHILADELPHIA 1765

When William Shippen returned to his native Philadelphia in November 1762 with an M.D. from Edinburgh, he began a course in anatomy and midwifery at the State House (later Independence Hall). Life-sized anatomical drawings, donated by Dr. Fothergill (below), enlivened the discourse on anatomy, and gypsum cast models helped to demonstrate the mechanics of child-birth. Some Philadelphians became suspicious when Shippen showed specimens from human dissections. One day a mob gathered incited by the belief that the anatomist had obtained his specimen via grave robbing. Dr. Shippen had to run for his life. But the uproar soon subsided.

Meanwhile, John Morgan, another medical student from the Colonies who had obtained his degree in Europe and had met Voltaire and Morgagni in a postgraduate Grand Tour of the Continent, put on paper his ideas for the establishment of an American medical school. Sparkling with enthusiasm, the dynamic young doctor set to work immediately upon his return to Philadelphia to establish a medical college modeled after the Edinburgh school. Trustees of the College of Philadelphia received his plan favorably and on May 13, 1765, appointed him Professor of Theory and Practice of Physick. His pungent, two-day inaugural address, "Discourse upon the Institution of Medical Schools in America," served as the Magna Charta of medical education and Philadelphia's College of Physick became the first School of Medicine in the New World.

Shippen soon joined Morgan as Professor of Anatomy. The question of who had originated the idea of a school of scientific standing seems to have embroiled the two men in a dispute bringing them to blows during the Revolution. At that time, Shippen had his adversary Morgan thrown out of his job as Director General of Hospitals and took over the Medical Department himself. Dr. John Morgan, whose career had begun so auspiciously, died in 1789 — a broken man.

Pennsylvania Hospital, 1751.

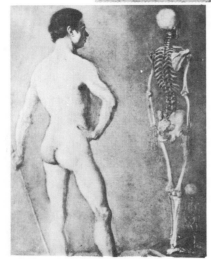

One of 18 carbon drawings presented by Dr. Fothergill to Pennsylvania Hospital for use in anatomy classes.

In his *Discourse*, Morgan had postulated that students be trained both in medical theory and at the bedside. No town in America possessed better facilities than Philadelphia to fulfill this requirement. The Pennsylvania Hospital, the oldest hospital in the United States had been initiated in 1751 by Dr. Thomas Bond with the aid of Franklin. The teachers of the College and the town's leading doctors volunteered as the hospital's consultants. Students had "to walk the ward" before they were admitted as candidates for a degree. In time Pennsylvania Hospital grew into an educational center of vast importance.

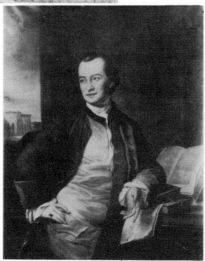

Dr. John Morgan painted by Angelica Kauffmann in gratitude for Morgan's medical services during his stay in Rome.

224

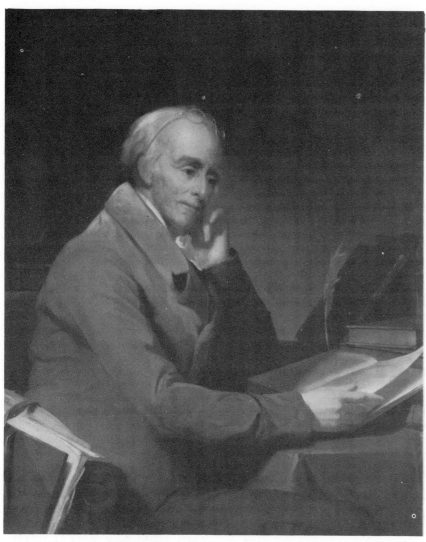

Dr. Benjamin Rush (1745-1813). Painting by Thomas Sully.

Benjamin Rush's background was similar to that of Shippen and Morgan; he was Philadelphia born, apprentice to Dr. John Redman and an M.D. from Edinburgh. With his colleagues, Shippen and Morgan, he was the third man in a Philadelphia medical triumvirate that was formidable but far from peaceable.

Rush had a genius for stepping on the feet of his colleagues. He had pronounced, it the physician's duty "to endure the patient's temper and bear his irritability and his reproaches with meekness and silence." But Rush himself was neither meek nor silent.

From the moment Rush hung out his shingle in 1769, bitter controversy swirled about him. Incapable of working in harmony with others, he would not "yield an inch to gain a foot." In spite of his quarrelsome nature, he became an overpowering figure in American medicine.

To the 3,000 doctors whom he trained, he remained an inspiring example. To the English, less exposed to his upsetting antics, he was "the American Sydenham."

Because of his unflagging belief in bloodletting, this "sanguinary moloch" tapped off the blood of sick Philadelphians by the gallon. Withdrawal of 40 to 50 ounces would save an apoplectic patient's life, he firmly believed. Often he favored further evacuation by physicking, sweating, diuretics, vomiting and blisters. During the yellow fever panic in Philadelphia in 1793 he was accused of killing more people than the scourge itself. He noted that in this "sickly autumn . . . mosquitoes were numerous" but ascribed the disease to a miasma created by dumped coffee rotting in the city harbor.

His treatment was little better than his theory on yellow fever: bloodletting — more bloodletting — "mercurial thunderbolts" (calomel). Yet this reign of blood did not cost Rush his popularity. People recognized that he was selfless in his devotion to the sick. He visited Pennsylvania Hospital daily for 43 years and humanely crusaded to better the lot of the insane. Even these unfortunates were bled by him to exhaustion. The harm he did, however, was outweighed by the reforms he brought about in introducing occupational therapy for the demented. Also, he urged his mental patients to write down their symptoms and suggested that doctors listen to their talk — a pioneer application of Freud's idea of "mental catharsis." All in all Rush was a physician of great intellectual stature and the first American doctor to gain world repute.

225

NEW YORK AWARDS A FIRST M.D.

"I wish with all my heart that I might assist in founding the first medical college in America," Samuel Bard wrote to his father during his studies in Edinburgh in the early 1760's. Young Bard had been listening to the plans of his fellow students, Morgan and Shippen, intent on founding a school of medicine in the colonies.

Sam's father, Dr. John Bard, a native Philadelphian, had become a prominent New York practitioner. Naturally the son hated to see the City of Brotherly Love outdistance his own Gotham, but studies kept him abroad. Bard pursued his idea for a school similar to the Philadelphia College of Physick after he returned home and joined his father in practice. The young doctor interested the trustees of King's College — later Columbia University — in his plan, and in 1768, New York's medical school was officially opened.

Its first Professor of Physick was, of course, no other than Samuel Bard. Five outstanding practitioners in the city completed the faculty. The school had fewer students than the Philadelphia college but offered a more comprehensive course, including anatomy, physiology, pathology, surgery, chemistry, materia medica and midwifery.

In 1770 New York achieved an added distinction. It conferred upon one Samuel Kissam the first legitimate M. D. degree awarded in America.

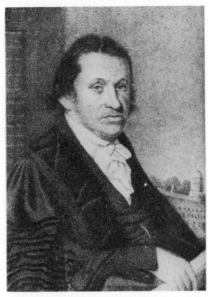

Dr. Samuel Bard was moving spirit in founding of New York's first medical school and hospital (1767-1773).

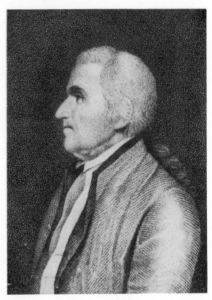

Dr. John Bard, father, tutor and partner of Dr. Samuel Bard, was a close friend of Benjamin Franklin.

In 1744, Yale College, though lacking a medical department, had given a doctor's degree of sorts to one Daniel Turner, a London practitioner at odds with the local College of Physicians. In return for a gift of books to Yale's "infantile library," Turner received official recognition as an M.D. — humorously interpreted as "multum donavit" (gave plenty). Naturally, that M.D. takes no glory away from New York's "first."

Dr. Samuel Bard also helped to found New York Hospital in 1771 and was the moving spirit in many other benevolent undertakings. In the next decade he became the city's best loved physician.

On June 17, 1789, six weeks after George Washington's inaugural, Bard operated on the first President for a carbuncle on the left thigh. Dr. Bard's father, who assisted, kept urging his son "to cut away — deeper, deeper still" to extirpate the infected area. The president's recovery was slow.

Unlike most successful doctors, Dr. Bard was wise enough to know when to retire and enjoy life. At 56 he turned over his large practice to his pupil and partner Dr. David Hosack, and moved to his country estate at Hyde Park. Though he did not give up his interest in the profession, he lived more than 20 happy years as a country squire. He died in 1821 at 79.

The most dramatic event in Dr. Bard's lifetime was probably New York's "Doctors Riot." On April 13, 1788, a group of boys climbed a painter's ladder in front of New York Hospital and peeked into a window. There they purportedly saw four medical men dissecting a corpse. A rabble, furious over the rumors of grave robbings, surged into the hospital and seized the four anatomists. Luckily they were rescued. All other doctors also escaped unmolested. Some of them fled from town, others crawled into bean barrels, or hid in chimneys.

Not so Dr. Bard. When the rioters, torches in hand, peeked into his study, they saw a man in long dressing gown pacing the floor studying a book in olympic tranquility. Taken aback by Dr. Bard's defiance, the mob retired.

Dr. David Hosack (right) successor to Dr. Bard, developed botanical garden, now the site of Rockefeller Center. Dr. Valentine Seaman (far right) trained midwives at New York Hospital.

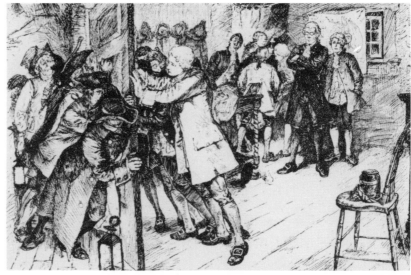

New York doctors during secret dissection, dodge searchers, Drs. Bard, Sr. and Middleton held first "anatomy" in 1750.

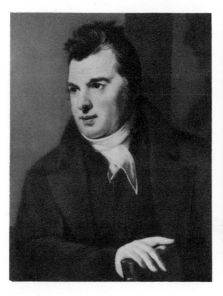

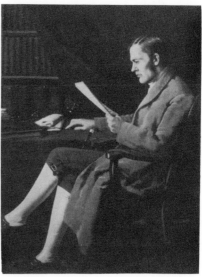

Elgin Botanical Garden at Bloomingdale Road, New York was bought by Dr. David Hosack in 1801 for $5,000. After spending $100,000 on it, he sold it to the city for $80,000. In 1814, Columbia accepted the city's gift of the land "with apprehension." Today it is the most valuable site in the world — Rockefeller Center.

227

PINEL UNSHACKLES THE INSANE

Much had been achieved by the humanitarians of this age to lighten the burden of the oppressed and the poor. But for the most unfortunate people of all, the insane, little had been done. They continued to live without hope in filthy asylums or pined away in private homes. The public's superstitions, barred their liberation.

Though individual physicians sometimes showed sympathy and understanding for the demented, the medical fraternity had made only feeble attempts to improve their lot. Most doctors adhered to the comfortable belief that the insane were incurable and insensible to pain. Insanity, then, was considered merely an administrative problem, not a medical one. The doctors held that to handle these "wild beasts" was not the physician's duty but the job of the prison keeper.

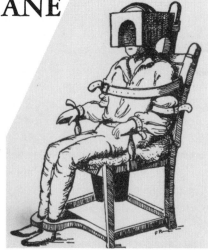

Benjamin Rush suggested use of "tranquilizer" to restrain unmanageable cases.

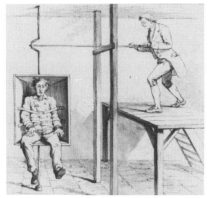

Gyrator (100 rounds a minute) a device "to calm cases of torpid madness."

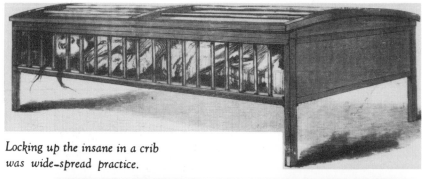

Locking up the insane in a crib was wide-spread practice.

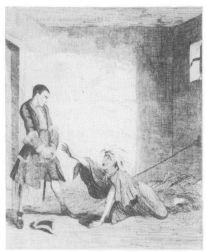

Waning away in dungeon, Bedlam inmate pleads for mercy. (Cruikshank.)

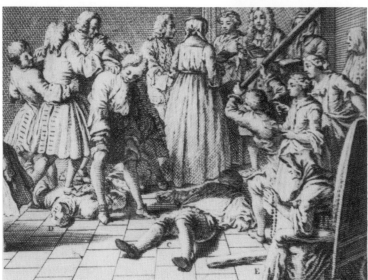

Patients suffering from convulsions beaten at St. Médard near Paris.

228

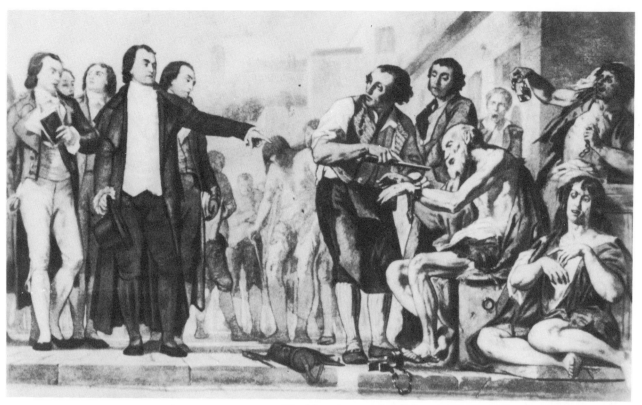

Pinel has chains removed from insane at Bicêtre Hospital (Paris 1793).

What "the wild beasts" needed was a doctor who would understand them and treat them as patients. This mission was fulfilled by Philippe Pinel. When Pinel came to Paris in 1778 he had difficulty in adjusting himself. Due to his shy and retiring nature, he did not go into practice, but supported himself by literary work and teaching.

A deep personal experience, it is said, prompted him to take up psychiatry in the 1780's. One of Pinel's friends became insane, ran into the woods and was devoured by wolves. As a result of Pinel's studies of mental diseases he brought out a book in 1791 advocating a more humane treatment of the insane. Though Pinel was not the first to voice these ideas, it was he who dramatized the desperate plight of the insane and effected their liberation.

When Pinel became chief physician at the Bicêtre in 1793, he introduced a new principle: He looked at the insane — and taught his contemporaries to look at them as victims of specific diseases.

Like other afflictions, he argued, insanity must have organic causes, and he sought to find the bodily changes that caused deranged minds. Pinel analyzed the various aberrations, distinguished between the "lunatics" and the "depraved," and worked out methods to improve their lot.

When Pinel asked permission to unchain the patients under his care, the Commissioner of Hospitals exclaimed: "Are you crazy yourself, wanting to liberate those ferocious beasts?" However, when Pinel unshacked his patients at the Bicêtre and later those at the Salpêtrière (May 24, 1798), no outburst ensued. The "maniacs" proved exceedingly docile.

A cardinal point in the program of this great doctor and able administrator was to give useful employment to every inmate able to work. Pinel's idea of recording the patient's case history was another vital contribution toward systematic research into the causes and treatment of insanity. He transformed the asylum into a hospital and linked psychiatry to medicine. His work paved the way for the rise of French clinical neurology.

229

VACCINATION WORKS

JENNER PREVENTS SMALLPOX

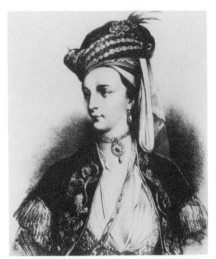

Lady Montagu, brilliant wife of British ambassador to Turkey, popularized inoculation in England (1721).

Smallpox filled the churchyard with corpses and left hideous traces of its passage among the living. In the early 1700s the disease pockmarked the faces of more than half the population of Europe. No medical triumph in the 18th century bestowed a greater boon on mankind than did Edward Jenner's discovery of the prevention of smallpox through vaccination.

The basic facts of immunization had been well known in the East for centuries. Noting that patients recovering from smallpox seldom contracted it again prompted the people of China and Turkey to produce smallpox in a mild form — by direct inoculation. They scratched the person wanting to be variolated (variola — smallpox) with exudate matter of a smallpox victim. If these patients survived the disease, they had little to fear from an approaching epidemic.

In America the Reverend Cotton Mather spread the news of this important phenomenon. He found that his slave was immune to the disease because of a previous inoculation in his native Africa. After reading about Turkish inoculation in the Reports of the Royal Society, Mather sought to interest the Boston doctors in this startling counter-measure. He was unsuccessful. Only a homespun practitioner in rural Brooklyne, Zabdiel Boylston, took the hint. In June 1721, he inoculated his son and two slaves. Though he roused much opposition, his pioneering in "direct inoculation" finally won him recognition and membership in the Royal Society. Later Washington had his household, then his army, inoculated. Franklin, too, became an advocate of the idea after the pox had killed his youngest son.

"I cannot take the smallpox, since I have had the cowpox." Edward Jenner had heard this remark from the mouth of a dairy maid — and it had stuck in his mind.

For years he wrestled with this problem, conducting a series of experiments to test the relation between smallpox and cowpox. As a busy country doctor in Gloucestershire, he performed inoculations to protect people from the smallpox epidemics which usually appeared in a virulent form. Whenever he found a mild case

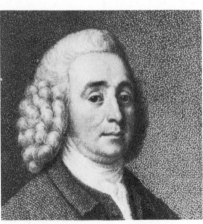

Dr. Thomas Dimsdale of London, inoculated Catherine the Great, received £12,000 and lifetime annuity of £500.

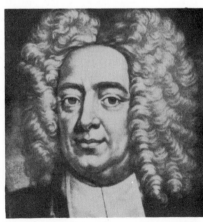

Cotton Mather, Boston divine, first to advocate inoculation in America. found scant response among doctors.

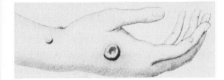

The hand that made history: Cowpox pustules of Sarah Nelmes. Jenner used them as source of protective lymph.

230

of the disease, he extracted lymph matter from the patient's pustules. This liquid he scratched into the skin of anyone who wished to be inoculated. If everything went well, a harmless smallpox infection followed. After recovery the patient could be considered immune.

Unfortunately, variolation was wrought with dangers. Often the disease "took" too violently. Ugly pustules appeared, and now and then the inoculated patient died. Another shortcoming of this method was the danger of spreading the disease. The rich undergoing this ordeal went to special smallpox hospitals so that other members of their family would not be infected.

After 28 years of observation however, Jenner found that the dairymaid's remark offered the clue for the solution of all these problems. Liquid of the pustules taken from a patient suffering from cowpox (vaccinae) had the power to protect others from smallpox (variolae). After he had checked all his observations carefully, he undertook the experiment that made him a medical immortal. On May 14, 1796, Jenner vaccinated the arm of a boy, John James Phipps, with the lymph taken from a cowpox pustule on

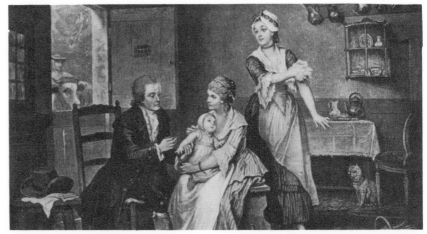

Jenner vaccinated baby with the lymph from a cowpox-infected dairymaid. He also used lymph from sores on cows teats — found it equally effective.

the infected hand of the dairymaid, Sarah Nelmes. Then six weeks later, young Phipps was inoculated with smallpox. No trace of infection appeared. Further tests proved conclusively that vaccination acted as an effective, easily applied preventive against smallpox.

Jenner's epochal paper on his vaccination experiments received only a

rejection slip from the Royal Society — on the ground that its contents would spoil the good name that he had gained by his previous researches on the cuckoo. Still he won world fame when he did publish his findings in 1798. Jenner provided the foundation stone for the triumphal arch of preventive medicine, which the 19th century was to erect.

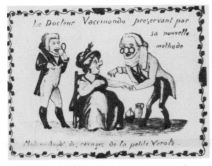

Doctors tried to preserve secret of vaccination — resented spying colleagues.

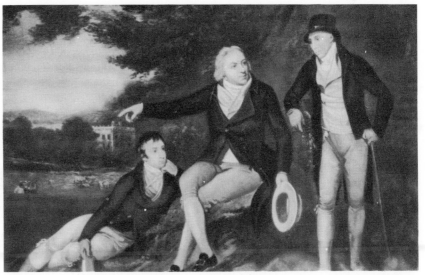

Dr. Jenner remained country practitioner in spite of world wide fame. Here he explains to his neighbors, fearful of small pox, how vaccination works.

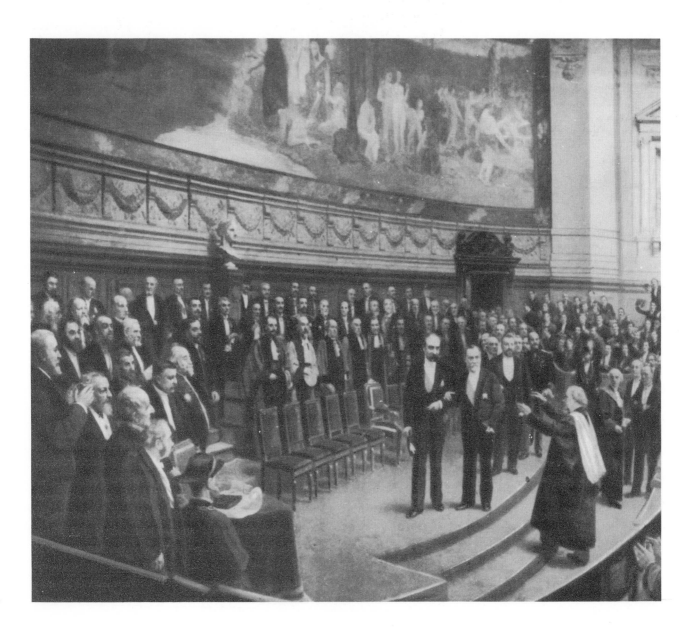

"For countless generations the prophets and kings of humanity have desired to see the things which men have seen . . . in the course of the wonderful nine-teenth century. In the fulness of time, long expected, long delayed, at last Science emptied from the horn of Amalthea blessings which can not be enumerated, blessings which have made the century forever memorable; . . . To us in the medical profession . . . whose work is with the sick and suffering, the great boon of this wonderful century . . . is the fact that the leaves of the tree of Science have been for the healing of the nations. This is the Promethean gift of the century to man."

Sir William Osler

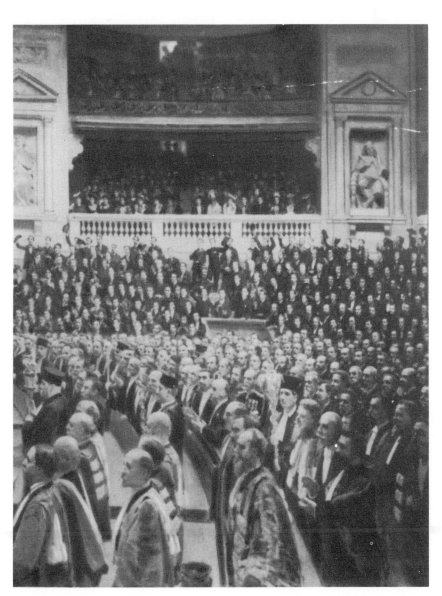

On December 27, 1892 Pasteur cele-brated his 70th birthday. When he entered the assembly hall of the Sorbonne on the arm of Carnot, the President of the French Republic, the audience — more than 2500 persons from all corners of the world — gave him a rousing ovation. Overwhelmed by emotion, Lord Lister moved forward to embrace Pasteur. In the course of this ceremony, Lister was to give a memorable address in which he eulogized the fraternity of science and medicine. It was under the auspices of this fraternity that the century's great contributions to human welfare were made.

MEDICINE MARCHES ON WITH NAPOLEON

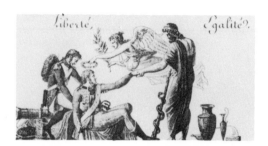

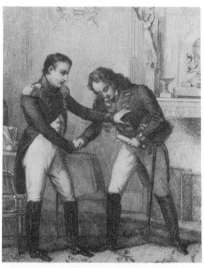

Napoleon and Larrey, his trusted surgeon, who also was loved by troops.

During the French Revolution, the tribunal boasted that scientists were unnecessary in the Age of Reason. Then it proceeded, quite "rationally," to lop off scientific heads. But Napoleon knew better. He recognized the importance of engineers, chemists and physicists. If he had no use for their windy debates, he could and did use them to develop and exploit the resources of conquered countries.

Medicine was subjected to the same rigorous test. For his campaigns, Napoleon wanted practical surgeons instead of heady medical philosophers. His armies had to fight under ever-changing climatic conditions. They were exposed to heat in Egypt, to epidemics in the marshy sections of Italy, and to frostbite on the Russian steppes. The brilliant general recognized that doctors would be vital in this scheme of things — and the doctors allied themselves more closely with science under the stimulus of Napoleon's campaigns and the force of his dicta.

This development was also supported by legislation. The medical regulations law of 1803 provided that only university-trained doctors, surgeons, and health officers could be licensed to practice medicine in France. Moreover, prescribed courses of study, plus extensive examinations, were outlined and enforced. A prospective doctor was obliged to spend four years at a state medical school (in Paris, Montpellier, Strassburg, Mainz or

Turin). Then he had to pass examinations covering anatomy, physiology, pathology, nosology, materia medica, chemistry, pharmacy, hygiene, and forensic and clinical medicine. Future health officers were put through similar paces. And in all phases of training, practical demonstrations, by professors and students, were heavily emphasized. Such measures sped medical progress

But the decisive advances were made

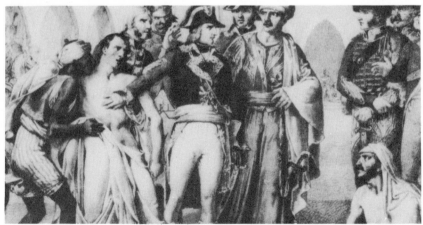

Reviving age-old magic of king's touch, Napoleon strokes plague victims in hospital at Jaffa. He forbade use of word "plague" for fear of panic among his soldiers.

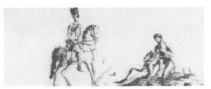

during the campaigns. One of these sorties, against Egypt in 1798, served as a test for Napoleon's future pattern of world conquest. The venture was prepared with great attention to detail. Sanitary problems for 35,000 troops were anticipated, and a shipload of medicines, bandages and other surgical supplies were dispatched to Egypt. But the English captured the supply ship, and the medical men were forced to battle as best they could against such nemeses as ophthalmia, dysentery and tetanus. When the plague broke out in Jaffa, Napoleon's surgeon, Desgenettes, tried to calm the soldiers by inoculating himself with the pus from a sufferer. Napoleon himself comforted the victims, and touched their buboes to dispell all fears. He also gave orders that the plague should not be mentioned by name.

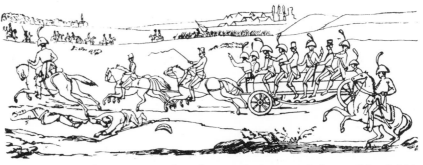

Army doctors atop medicine-box-on-wheels are rushed toward battlefield.

Such catastrophes were always met with a centralized approach, and medical strategists inevitably achieved enormous importance within the military hierarchy.

Among them, the surgeon Dominique Jean Larrey was held in highest esteem, both by Napoleon and his soldiers. Larrey served the emperor with unflagging devotion from the first campaign to the last. When his name was mentioned, Napoleon once exclaimed: "What a brave man; what a brave and worthy man" — a rare compliment from the emperor. He left Larrey 100,000 francs in his will, and called him "the most virtuous man I've ever known."

Larrey was indeed a devoted and humane doctor. He introduced many new measures to aid the wounded on the battlefield. The most important of these were the "flying ambulances" — maneuverable horse-drawn vehicles in which the wounded could be conveyed speedily to the nearest field hospitals. According to Larrey, only one hour elapsed in many cases between the infliction of a wound and the soldier's arrival at a hospital tent. This efficient service resulted in the saving of thousands of lives.

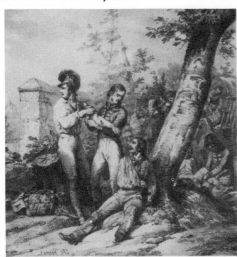

Larrey kept close to field of battle; he often operated as shells burst around him. He was wounded three times.

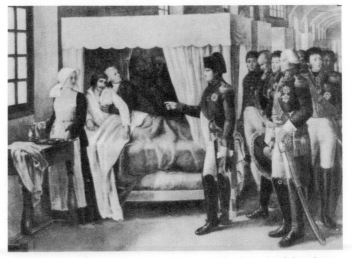

Napoleon inspects veterans' hospital. His farsighted legislation helped in development of up-to-date medical centers in Paris and the provinces.

235

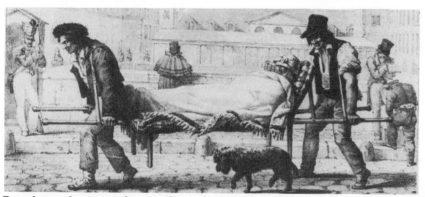

Foundling Home in Paris with baby cribs arranged in neat military order.

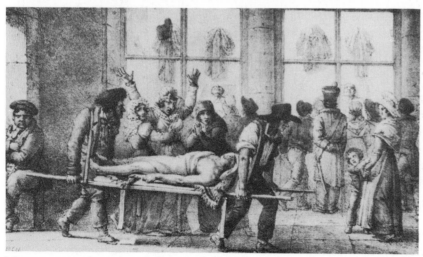

Paris hospitals were ready to render medical services to expanding populace.

Morgue attracted sensation-seekers, gave doctors ample autopsy material.

PARIS . . .

BEDSIDE-STUDY . . .

In the words of Sir William Osler, "Minerva Medica lived in France during the first four decades of the 19th century." By a fortunate combination of social, political and intellectual circumstances, and thanks to Napoleon's patronage, Paris had become the scientific capital of Europe. This bustling urban center now attracted the best minds in medicine and in other fields of research.

Its populace had expanded rapidly, and with this expansion came an all-too-disproportionate rise in the number of sick. But from a coldly scientific standpoint, here was an abundance of material for clinical and post mortem observation. Moreover, Napoleon had provided facilities for the care of the sick, foundlings, and veterans. In 1830, Paris had 30 hospitals geared to accommodate 20,000 patients. So on the one hand, the city could boast of a vast "arsenal" of facilities and medical talent, and on the other, it could refer to ample opportunities for research. Moreover, in France, there were no laws or moral prejudices against the use of corpses in the pursuit of pathological studies.

During the late 18th century, medicine had been slow to catch up with the new standards of exact observation achieved by such disciplines as chemistry and astronomy.

NEW CENTER OF SCIENCE

CORRELATED WITH POST-MORTEM RESEARCH

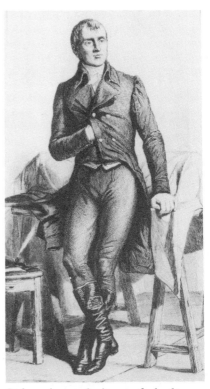

But the way for rejuvenation was now clear with the aid of mathematics, a science in which France had always excelled. It is in this period that French doctors learned exact methods of observation, both at the bedside and at the dissecting table. More important, they learned to merge their findings in each of these fields. This was a revolutionary step, since clinical and pathological research had hitherto followed independent paths. From now on, medicine would profit by the follow-up from hospital ward to death house.

Marie Francois Bichat was foremost among the pioneers in this type of co-related research. At the age of 28, this prodigious anatomist embarked on a tour de force: He performed in six months' time 600 autopsies in the Hôtel-Dieu in Paris. At times he even slept in the morgue. Overwork weakened his frail constitution and he died at 31 years of age. "That battlefield on which he fell," wrote Corvisart to Napoleon, "is one which demands courage and claims many victims . . . No one at his age has done so much so well."

What Bichat had done so well was to direct attention to the structural changes wrought by disease. Until then, Morgagni's theory — that the individual organs were the seats of disease — had prevailed. But Bichat demonstrated that disease affected the structure and vital properties of body *tissues* themselves. His powers of observation were so keen that he could distinguish 21 tissue structures without the aid of a microscope. By expressing his ideas eloquently in his five-volume *Traité d' Anatomie Descriptive*, he became the founder of modern histology — and one of the pioneers in pathology to fulfill the famous inscription over the entrance of a Paris dissecting-room: "Death comes to the aid of life."

Bichat (1771-1802) ascribed diseases to organic changes in the tissues.

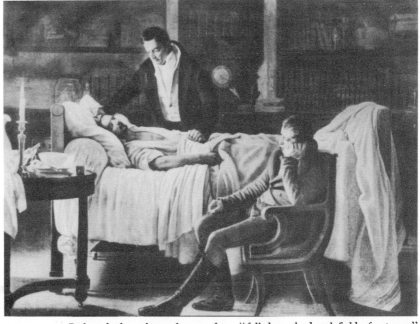

Bichat died at the early age of 31, "felled on the battlefield of science."

THE FIRST STETHOSCOPE

CORVISART AND LAËNNEC

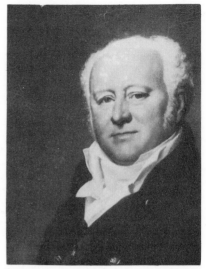

Corvisart re-introduced auscultation, made it basic diagnostic technique.

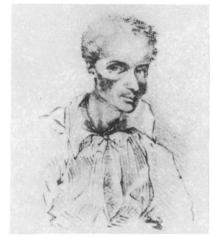

Laennec suffered from tuberculosis, described it in detail. Selfportrait, 1820.

A student once asked Dr. Jean Nicolas Corvisart, chief physician at La Charité in Paris, what books he should read. Corvisart turned to his ward-patients and observed sharply: "There are your books, read them, but you will find them more difficult than the printed ones."

The problem of "reading" patients obsessed this generation of French doctors. They wanted to get at the physical root of disease instead of passively observing its course, as their forebears had done. Following Corvisart's example, they began to make intensive clinical examinations. "A patient is a mobile painting," Corvisart reminded them, "which must be forever observed." He himself pioneered in the accurate diagnosis of heart and lung diseases, and may be considered rightfully as the first cardiologist.

Corvisart was also the first to direct attention to the "chest-thumping" techniques of Auenbrugger. His translation of Auenbrugger's treatise on percussion together with his own comments led to a revival of interest in accoustical methods of diagnosis.

It was in this connection that Corvisart influenced his most famous student, René Théophile Laennec, the inventor of the stethoscope. Laennec made his famous discovery in 1816, while examining a young woman whose complaints indicated a heart affliction. Modesty and the patient's stoutness prevented him from putting his ear close to her chest to detect the heartbeat. But the resourceful Laennec then recalled a well-known phenomenon: that sounds are magnified when heard through a hollow beam. Accordingly, he fashioned a makeshift tube from a piece of paper, placed one end over the woman's precordial region, and tuned in on the other: "I was both surprised and gratified," he wrote, "at being able to hear the beating of the heart with much greater clearness than I had ever done before."

Later on, Laennec constructed a wooden stethoscope, and the instrument soon became the very symbol of pulmonary diagnosis. When Laennec's masterwork, *De l'Auscultation*, appeared in 1819, the publisher gave a stethoscope with each copy of the book. In this work Laennec had included an enormous amount of information on the rales and rhonchi — all the cardiac and pulmonary sounds heard through the stethoscope. He classified them with great care and explained their significance.

Laennec was an incurable consumptive when he conducted his epochal research. This makes his accomplishment seem all the more remarkable. He died in 1826, after a few decades of voracious work in clinics and dissecting rooms. But his influence lives on, for, as Létulle says, "Every physician . . . who auscultates is, by this act, a disciple of Laennec."

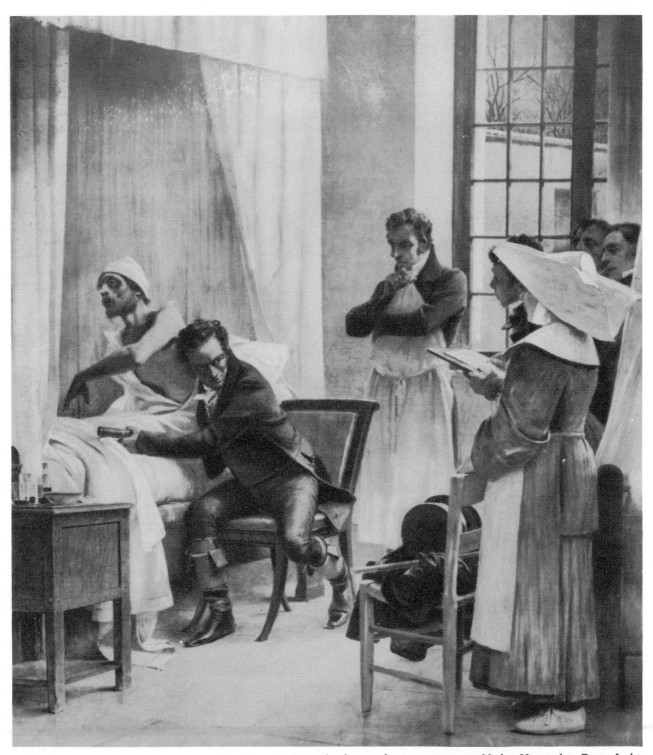

Laennec examining the thorax of a consumptive at Necker Hospital in Paris. In his left hand he holds the stethoscope, a simple wooden tube about one foot in length.

239

RISING
SPECIALISM

PARIS 1820-1830

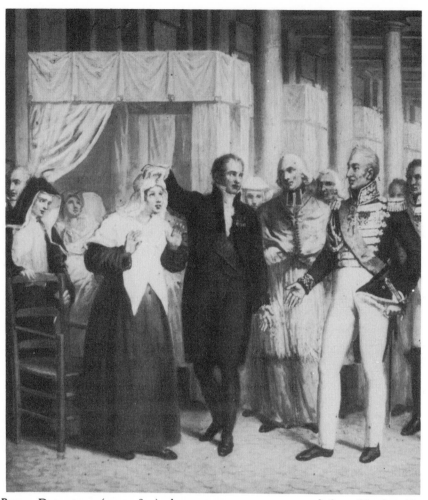

Baron Dupuytren (1777-1835) demonstrates cataract case before Charles X.

Paris boasted of brillant doctors in other than clinical fields. The Napoleonic wars had bred a large number of dashing surgeons, who returned home with much practical experience. They were quick to profit by the insights into morbid anatomy which Bichat and his school had gained in their absence. Moreover, the usual gulf between medicine and surgery was hardly noticeable in France. Surgery had been recognized as a legitimate medical specialty in the Napoleonic code, and scientific training had been instituted for doctor and surgeon alike.

The most brilliant leader of surgery in the Empire was Baron Dupuytren. As a medical student, he had experienced utter poverty. According to one report, he once lived for six weeks on bread and cheese, and used the fat from bodies in the dissecting room to make oil for his lamp. But thirty years' toil at the Hôtel-Dieu gave him discernment as a pathologist, and exceptional skill as a surgeon. Aided by an imposing personality, he gained an immense practice. His lectures thrilled students from all nations. Consequently, he was able to amass a fortune of three million francs.

A man of such prominence was quite naturally exposed to both accolades and sneers. His self-control and aplomb during difficult operations earned him high praise as "the Napoleon of Surgery." But since he tolerated no rivals, he was also accused of aloofness. His colleagues therefore coined the bon mot: "Dupuytren, first of surgeons but least of men." Yet he could always disarm his critics when it came to surgery. "I have been mistaken," he would admit, "but I have been mistaken less than other surgeons." And he probably did make fewer mistakes, since he was so thoroughly grounded in pathological anatomy.

With all his activities, Dupuytren still found time to study the structure of bone, muscle and sinew. His written summary of the pathology of luxations has never been outdated. He also devised a great many novel operations which, if taken by themselves, would still secure his name in the galaxy of great surgeons.

240

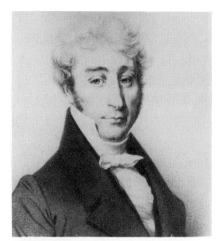

Delpech (1777-1832) founder of orthopedics was murdered by patient.

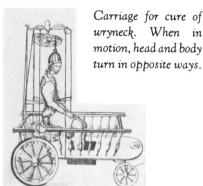

Carriage for cure of wryneck. When in motion, head and body turn in opposite ways.

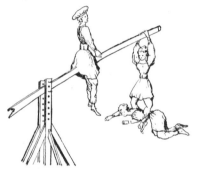

Graded exercise to strengthen muscles, prevent and also cure scoliosis.

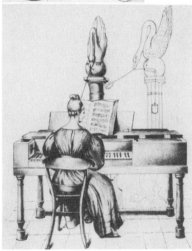

Proper posture insured by weighted cord tied to piano player's forehead.

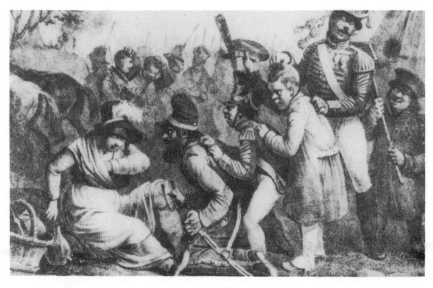

Skin afflictions caused by army life accelerated emergence of dermatology.

ORTHOPEDICS

Like surgery, orthopedics made great advances in the early 1800's. The new science owed much to the work of Jacques Mathieu Delpech. His *Orthomorphie* (1828) gave the first comprehensive descriptions of bone and joint deformities based on pathological findings. He also set up an orthopedic sanitarium in an attractive pastoral setting outside Montpellier. There were playgrounds and exercise areas for the patients, since Delpech firmly believed that deformities could be redressed, or prevented, by the development of muscular balance. Unfortunately, he was killed in 1832 by a disgruntled patient from his own institution.

DERMATOLOGY

Dermatology came into its own through the efforts of Baron Jean-Louis d'Alibert. A diligent if superficial classifier of skin lesions, the benevolent baron spent 300,000 francs to publish his splendidly illustrated *Description des Maladies de la Peau* (12 vols.). He gave his lectures to overflow audiences in the courtyard of the Hospital St. Louis in Paris — with pictures of skin diseases dangling from the trees.

A decade later, Philippe Ricord, a Baltimore-born Frenchman removed one of the obstacles that had blocked dermatological advance for decades. He disproved Hunter's contention that gonorrhoeal pus could cause syphilis.

241

THE BELLS OF SCOTLAND

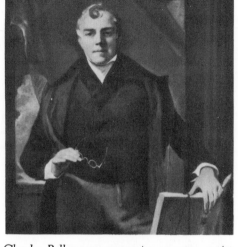

Charles Bell neuro-anatomist, surgeon, artist.

Great strides in medicine usually follow a period of intensive anatomical research. French medicine, for example, developed rapidly after the work of Bichat in the early 1800's. Now the English doctors received the same stimulus from the dissecting room. Once more, as in the days of the Hunter brothers, two Scotchmen — brothers, surgeons and anatomists — paved the way for medical advance. And once more the stream of influence fluctuated between London and Edinburgh.

In the latter city, John Bell had attained a great reputation as a surgeon, anatomist and obstetrician. He was to be remembered, in America, as the teacher of surgeon Ephraim McDowell. But it was Charles Bell, his younger brother, who made the greater contribution to medicine. Both brothers were fine artists, and it was as an artist-anatomist that Charles Bell achieved his first success.

When the younger Bell came to London in 1805, with £12 in his pocket, he set up a course in anatomy designed especially for artists. In his spare time, he composed his classic treatise on the relation between muscular actions and emotions (such as fear, joy, etc.). He illustrated it with the works of great artists. When the *Essay on the Anatomy of Expression in Painting* was published in 1806, Bell became famous almost overnight. His lectures were swamped, and in 1812 he was appointed surgeon to Middlesex Hospital.

Bell's most significant work was done in the field of neuro-anatomy. His discovery that the nerves in the human body consist of two distinct classes, motor and sensory, has been compared in importance with Harvey's theory of circulation. Phrenology, neurology, and the triumphs of modern nerve and brain surgery all developed from Bell's important research. The validity of his findings was demonstrated by surgeon Astley Cooper. Cooper presented to Bell a woman patient whose facial muscles had been paralyzed following an ear operation. The seventh nerve in the rear of her ear had been inadvertently divided. This paralyzed all muscular action on one side of her face, but her sensory nerves were obviously intact — she could still feel a touch or a pin prick. The case proved Bell's theory, and the lesion became known as "Bell's Palsy."

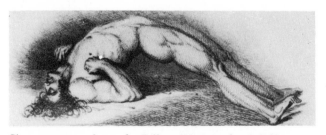

Tetanic spasm, drawn by Bell on Waterloo battlefield.

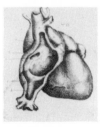

Heart structure.

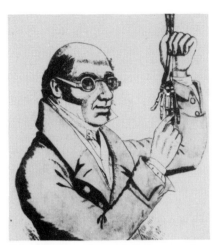

John Knox, client of body snatchers had to leave Edinburgh after exposure.

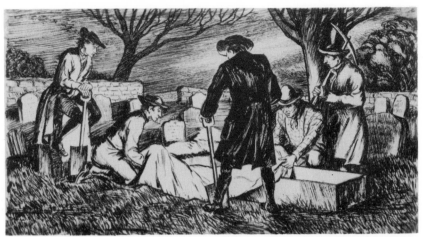

Body snatchers worked with split-second efficiency, prying coffin open with heavy grapple, roping out corpse. They left shrouds to avoid arrest for theft.

THE SACK-THEM-UP MEN

As interest in anatomy increased, a critical shortage of dead bodies developed. Students flocking to anatomy schools were required to perform dissections. But the law forbade all trade in corpses. As a result, a thriving black market sprang up to accommodate the anatomists. Resourceful "sack-them-up men" robbed funeral parlors and pillaged cemeteries. They stripped off shrouds to avoid prosecution for theft — corpses were not considered property, but their garments were.

Since corpses were in such great demand, prices skyrocketed and extortion was common. To obtain an adequate supply of bodies, teachers had to pay "opening money" as the school year began, and sustenance fees during vacations or the grave robbers' prison terms. The body snatchers also resorted to gang warfare; to stealing bodies from one school and selling them to another; and eventually, to murder.

In 1829, Dr. Robert Knox of Edinburgh began to buy bodies from one William Hare, who ran a cheap lodging house in Tanner's Row, Edinburgh. When Hare's roomers died, he "cashed in" their bodies for back rent. But they didn't die fast enough, so Hare, his wife, his friend Burke and Burke's mistress decided to speed up the process. They placed their victim's head down on a bed; then Hare sat on them while Burke smothered them — a process now known as "burking."

Suspicions were aroused when well-known Edinburgh characters like Daft Jamie and prostitute Mary Patterson disappeared. When the latter was found in Knox's anatomical theatre, the culprits were prosecuted to the tune:

*"Burke's the butcher, Hare's the thief,
Knox the man that buys the beef."*

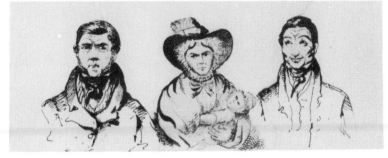

Anatomy Murder Inc. in the dock: Hare, his wife (baby had whooping cough), and Burke, who purveyed murdered bodies to the Edinburgh School of Anatomy.

243

PIONEER INTERLUDE

McDOWELL PERFORMS OVARIOTOMY

In the early 1800's, medical students received excellent training in Paris, London or Edinburgh. In wards and dissecting rooms they gained practical experience, and they profited, spiritually, from the example of great physician-teachers.

But America was then still a back-woods country. This was especially true with regard to medical education. The schools in the South and West were pitifully short in facilities. Most doctors served an apprenticeship, in the approved from-stable-boy-to-surgeon tradition. Medicine did not rank very highly. No wonder, then, that the remark was made: "The boy who goes into medicine is too lazy for farm or shop, too stupid for the bar and too immoral for the pulpit." Yet in spite of all handicaps, America produced two outstanding figures in the world of medicine.

In December 1809, Dr. McDowell of Danville, Kentucky, was called 60 miles across country to deliver a Mrs. Jane Todd Crawford of "twins." McDowell soon found that Mrs. Crawford had a large ovarian tumor, not twins. To wait meant certain death; to operate, according to the best medical opinion in Europe, meant certain death through peritonitis. Nevertheless, McDowell offered to operate. Mrs. Crawford assented. Lifted carefully on a horse she was taken to the doctor's house in Danville.

To be sure of heavenly guidance, McDowell waited to perform the operation until Christmas Day, a

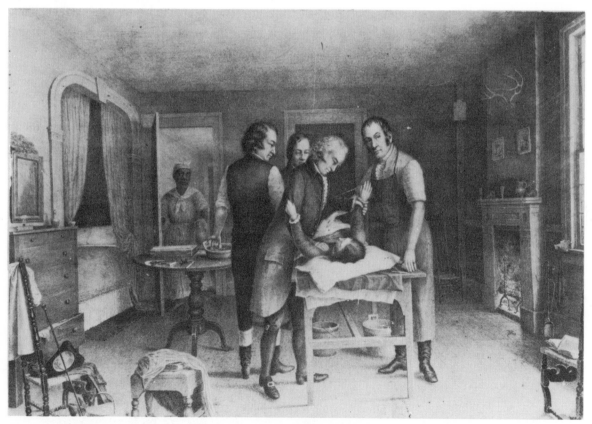

First ovariotomy performed by Dr. McDowell (in apron right) at Danville, Ky., December, 1809. Patient was strapped to kitchen table, sang hymns to counteract pain. Operation took 30 minutes — was complete success.

DR. WILLIAM BEAUMONT PEEKS INTO HUMAN STOMACH

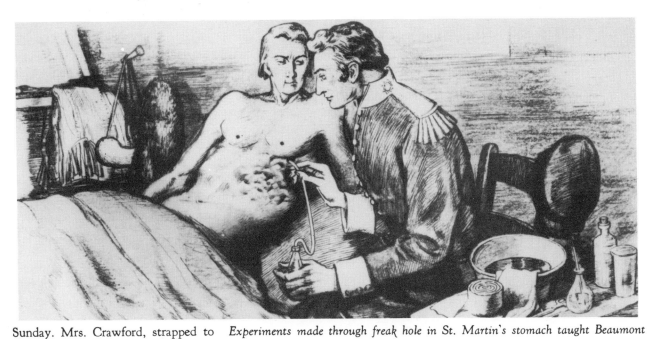

Experiments made through freak hole in St. Martin's stomach taught Beaumont how digestion works. Investigations took 7 years, resulted in classic book.

Sunday. Mrs. Crawford, strapped to a wooden table in his office, sang hymns as the surgeon cut into her side. Her intestines cooled on the table as McDowell snipped out the ovaries and tossed them into a bucket (before sewing her up, he bathed the intestines in tepid water). The operation was performed in about 30 minutes.

Twenty-five days later Mrs. Crawford was back at her home, fully recovered. She lived to be 78.

McDowell had studied for two terms in Edinburgh, but Dr. William Beaumont, Surgeon, U. S. Army, had never gone to medical school. On June 6, 1822, he entered into one of the strangest doctor-patient relationships in history. On that day, a young Canadian voyageur, Alexis St. Martin, was accidentally wounded by a shotgun blast in the trading post on Mackinaw Island. Beaumont, the fort surgeon, was quickly called to the scene. One look convinced him that

St. Martin would not last more than 36 hours. But the surgeon bound up his patient, pressed his protruding lung back into position and placed a compress over the stomach, which, in Beaumont's words, "showed a puncture large enough to hold my forefinger."

St. Martin's good constitution helped him to survive all complications. Two years later he had completely recovered except for one important defect: the lips of his stomach wound would not close. He placed a compress over the hole while eating, though he ate and digested normally. By May 1825, Beaumont's curiosity was aroused since he could "almost see the process of digestion" while looking into St. Martin's stomach. He decided to conduct some experiments on his "living laboratory." Suspending meat, raw and roasted, on silk threads, he sunk

them into the stomach. Then he carefully studied the time needed for digestion, the influence of temperature, and the patient's reactions.

These experiments extended over a period of seven years, with many interruptions caused by the patient's repeated return trips to Canada. But Beaumont was finally able to publish, at his own expense, *Observations on the Gastric Juice and the Physiology of Digestion* (Plattsburg, 1833). Though his methods had been crude, he was able to show that gastric juice is the active principle in digestion. His 51 modest inferences were astoundingly to the point (as Dr. John Fulton of Yale has demonstrated), and most of them are still acceptable. Through his classic book, the wilderness surgeon became one of the founding fathers of modern physiology.

PHLEBOTOMY KILLED BY STATISTICS

The medical torch still flared brightly in the Paris of the 1830's. Young men assembled there from every land. They scrambled from one hospital to another, from La Pieté to La Sâlpetrière to La Charité. They attended demonstrations, seminars, autopsies. For the first time, in the Paris of this period, one could identify the modern medical student.

This atmosphere was largely the work of a group of brilliant teachers. Contemporary reports speak in glowing terms of such men as Andral, Chomel and Bretonneau. In contrast, P. C. A. Louis appeared grave and aloof — a plodding and awkward speaker. Yet it was Louis who exerted the most deep-felt influence on medicine through his new method of clinical investigation. Like other contemporaries, he tirelessly correlated bedside observations with

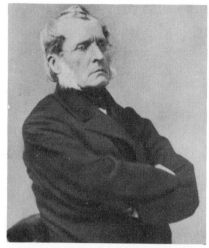

P. C. A. Louis (1787-1872) was the guiding spirit of Paris clinical school.

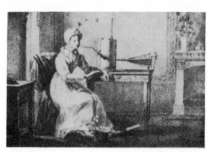

Steam inhalation to cure tuberculosis. Louis introduced far saner methods.

autopsy findings, but his work was much more scientific, since he interpreted it with the aid of statistics.

After his studies in Paris, Louis had practiced in Russia. When a diphtheria epidemic broke out in Odessa, he became painfully aware of the gaps in his medical knowledge. Dissatisfied with current therapies, he gave up his practice and returned to Paris. For the next six years he worked steadily at La Charité, gathering material for his famous book on phthisis (1825). In this work he reported with meticulous detail on 123 clinical cases and autopsies. (Tragically, his own son died of tuberculosis.) Ten years later, in *Effects of Bloodletting*, Louis added further numerical proof that venesection was useless, if not harmful, in most inflammatory diseases. This book was epoch-making for medical methodology.

It was this numerical approach which opened up new possibilities for research. As his disciple Henry P. Bowditch put it, "Louis showed us the habit of passionless listening to the teachings of nature . . . and the sure means of getting at results by accurate tabulation." Louis also convinced his students that no man could become a good doctor without what we now call "postgraduate research."

BROUSSAIS THE BRUSQUE

F. J. V. Broussais advised his colleague Louis not to spend time on post mortems, but rather to prevent them. The best way to do this he said, was through "physiological medicine." By this he meant merciless bloodletting and a starvation diet. This former

razzle-dazzle surgeon with Napoleon's armies was responsible for a boom in the leech trade by setting suckers all over his patients' bodies. The influence of this "most sanguinary doctor in history" declined, however, when Louis proved bloodletting harmful.

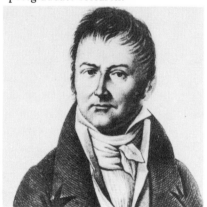

Broussais: a boom in leeches followed his plea for relentless bloodletting.

THE ARGONAUTS

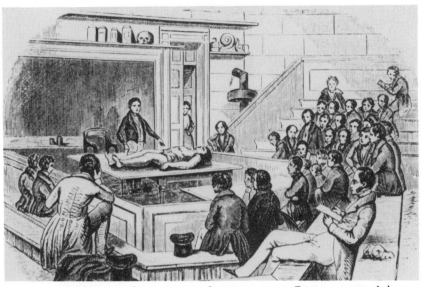

Students watch postmortem demonstration in Paris anatomical theatre.

Since facilities for medical education were notoriously poor in America, the more well-to-do students gravitated towards Paris for additional training. P. C. A. Louis took many of these "argonauts" under his wing. He attracted them from all parts of America; probably because he was a type of scientific thinker as yet unknown in the New World. The impressions he left on their minds were deep and lasting.

Louis did three important things for his American students: first, he made them see the connection between bedside observation and post mortem research; second, he kept them at work in the hospitals (and thanks to Louis, hospital work has since become an integral part of every doctor's career); and third, he made them research-conscious, so they could at last take their place beside their European brethren. By pursuing his methods, Americans made lasting contributions to our knowledge of typhus, tuberculosis and cardiac diseases.

When the argonauts returned, they made short shrift of the theories of the local dogmatists. Elisha Bartlett, one of Louis' earliest American adherents, bore down particularly hard upon the theories of Benjamin Rush. While the "Philadelphia Moloch" had passed on — his teachings still held sway. Rush had attempted to cure all disease by one remedy — bleeding. This approach was diametrically opposed to that of the Paris school, which aimed at a much more accurate differentiation of morbid phenomena. So Bartlett gave Rush's work the verbal coup de grace in 1844, when he said in his *Philosophy of Medical Science:* "In the whole vast compass of medical literature, there cannot be found an equal number of pages containing a greater amount and variety of utter nonsense and unqualified absurdity." (Quoted by Shryock: *Dev. of Modern Medicine,* p. 4.)

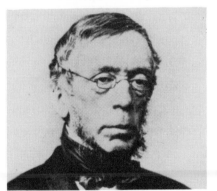

Gerhard of Philadelphia showed difference between typhoid and typhus.

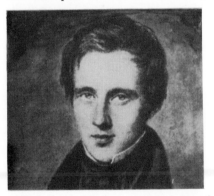

Bowditch of Boston introduced Louis' method of diagnosing lung trouble.

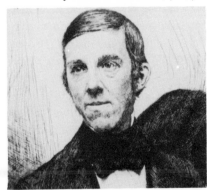

O. W. Holmes, author-anatomist, eloquently described medical Paris in 1830's.

247

THE ENGLISH AND IRISH CLINICIANS

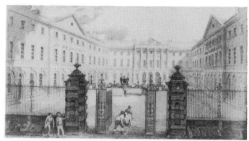

Guy's Hospital in London produced great diagnosticians.

As in France, a great many brilliant physicians appeared in England, each one focussing attention upon a specific disease group. Painstaking research by the doctors at Guy's Hospital, London, clarified the various forms of kidney afflictions, heart lesions and other organic changes. Most of these ills were named after the men who had observed them at the bedside, then had traced their inner causes at the dissecting table. Their attempt to localize disease was extremely important, though it increased the danger of over-specialization.

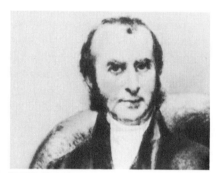

HODGKIN

Hodgkin's disease: Enlargement of the lymph nodes and spleen accompanied by anemia.

Although Malpighi first observed this disease, Thomas Hodgkin clearly recorded it as a clinical entity when he was a physician at Guy's Hospital (1825-1837). Hodgkin helped to introduce at this institution the use of the stethoscope. In his later years, he abandoned medicine to devote himself to philanthropic work. He travelled in the East as companion to Sir Moses Montefiore, and died of dysentery in Palestine on one of Montefiore's journeys undertaken to help the Jews (April 5, 1866).

ADDISON

Addison's disease: A form of anemia caused by the malfunction of the suprarenal glands.

When Thomas Addison published his paper on anemia in 1849, he unknowingly founded the science of endocrinology. It was he who first formulated the importance of suprarenal secretion for the sustenance of life. This physician was passionately interested in diagnosis. He would rise in the middle of the night and rush to the hospital to clear up some "important detail bearing upon a case." But once he had tracked down the origin of a disease, he was said to have lost interest in curing the patient.

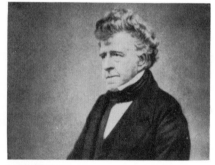

BRIGHT

Bright's disease: Chronic nephritis (inflammation of the kidney) resulting in albuminous urine.

Richard Bright (1789-1858) was probably the most renowned physician on the staff at Guy's Hospital. In contrast to Addison, whose origins were humble, Bright came from a wealthy family of bankers. Frequent travel on the continent made him an affable, polished man of the world. Though an avid classifier and interpreter of renal disease, he did not let such interests overshadow his duties as a doctor. Humane yet critical, he belongs to the group of truly great English physicians.

At this same time, the Irish school of medicine at Dublin University and Meath Hospital developed several great diagnosticians, most of whom had studied at Edinburgh and Glasgow. Their relation to the French school also was intimate. From Laennec, they derived their keen interest in cardiac disturbances. Their cooperative spirit, so important in medical research, was particularly evident, fostered perhaps by their extreme youth — all of them did their best work before they were 30 years old.

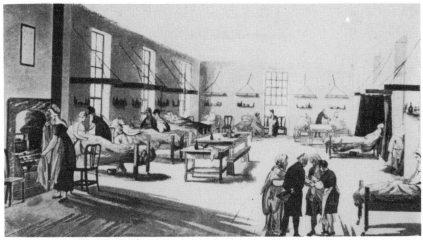

Studies in hospital wards yielded new classification of heart diseases.

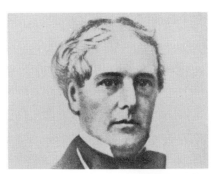

CORRIGAN

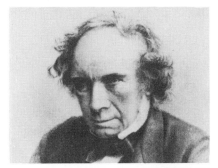

STOKES

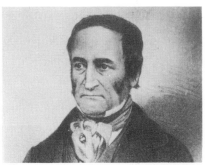

GRAVES

Corrigan's pulse: Visible pulsations of the arteries due to insufficiency of the aortic valve.

Picturesque Sir Dominic John Corrigan (1802-1880) graduated from Edinburgh and worked at the Jervis Street Hospital in Dublin. Here he observed that in certain cardiac cases the pulse is "thrown out on the surface in the strongest relief." In the pathological laboratory, he traced this "water hammer pulse" to a malfunction of the aortic valve. Though too outspoken, at first, to be liked by his colleagues, he later became the most popular and highly-paid doctor in all of Ireland. His works rank as cardiac classics.

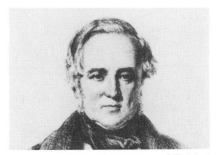

ADAMS

Stokes-Adams syndrome: A slowed pulse accompanied with fainting or convulsive seizures.

Robert Adams (1791-1875) wrote the classic account of essential heart-block; William Stokes (1804-1878) was Laennec's disciple.

Graves disease: Goiter indicated by an extraordinary protrusion of the eyeballs from orbit.

Robert James Graves (1797-1853) was thoroughly trained in clinical medicine on the continent. Upon his return to Ireland, he instituted at Meath Hospital clinics after the European plan. He also placed senior students in charge of patients. But his most far-reaching reform concerned fever. In Dublin fever patients were starved. Graves thought they would recover faster if their resistance was built up. The success of this method made him suggest his own epitaph: "He Fed Fevers."

249

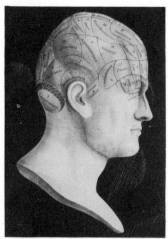

Head chart with talent areas.

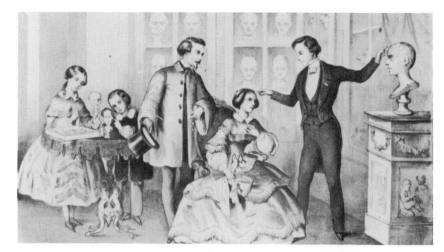

Phrenologists diagnosed bumps, gave character analyses, read future.

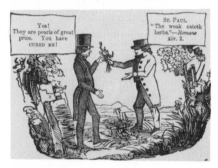

Thomsonian therapy made doctors furious and Dr. Thomson a millionaire.

FADS OF THE THIRTIES

In spite of great bursts of clinical activity in England and France, the average doctor still moved along the old ruts, with bloodletting and heavy doses of drugs as his therapeutic mainstays. In Germany, "Natur-Philosophie" reigned supreme, though later on, her scientists would take the lead in laboratory medicine. On the whole, the profession floundered, and quacks and cultists flourished in every land.

In Vienna, for instance, Dr. Franz Joseph Gall persuaded the local aristocrats to have their heads examined. They did so in droves, believing that the learned doctor could detect mental power, character and future prospects from the bumps on their heads. To support his theory, he filled a phrenological museum with plaster casts and charts of the brains of great men, eccentric ones, or criminals. Gall's disciple, J. C. Spurzheim, brought the gospel to America, where he was welcomed by such leading scientists as Drs. Nathaniel Bowditch and Benjamin Silliman. Phrenology soon became intermingled with medical practice. But palpating a patient's head was, in the long run, a poor substitute for auscultating his lungs.

In this period the United States was a fertile breeding ground for medical cults. Although schools had sprung up all over the country, their courses were superficial, and their graduates favored harsh doses of calomel as therapy. But people looked for simpler purgatives than calomel; and the cultists were ready to oblige.

"Thomsonian medicine" swept through the western states. Dr. Sam Thomson and his adherents swore by vegetable compounds which had been endorsed both by God *and* the President of the United States (some of the medicines were patented). Indian plantlore tradition helped to make these remedies more plausible. Consequently, there were Thomsonian Hospitals and "Botanical Conventions" in the 1830's. Thomspon's $20 *New Guide to Health* became a best seller.

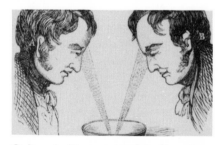

Cult of "impressionability": operators on receiving end of patient's brain wave considered themselves better diagnosticians than the doctors.

WATER DOES IT

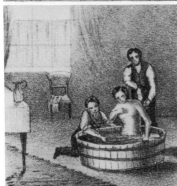

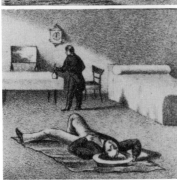

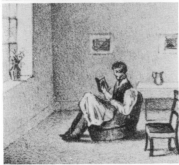

Hydropathic Institute of 1840's. Luxuriously furnished, it offered showers, hot packs, massage. Walls often showed sylvan murals. Patients lived here too.

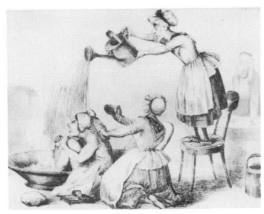

Double treat: Cold shower with rubdown.

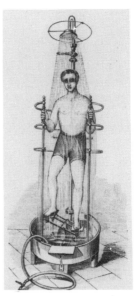

Pedal-powered shower

At bottom, a medical vacuum existed in this period. The academic clinicians were busy diagnosing diseases. Working in ward and dissecting room, they had little time for therapy. But a simple Silesian peasant, Vincenz Priessnitz, had plenty of time, and plenty of water. With plain well water, "Doctor" Priessnitz proclaimed that it was possible to bathe oneself back to health. To this end, he set up outdoor baths in an arcadian setting, and placed his fashionable customers on a strong regimen: cold douches, massage, and chopping wood.

Though he could not read nor write, Priessnitz was a shrewd judge of human nature. He relieved his patients of non-existent diseases. In 1829 he treated only 45 patients, but by 1843 he averaged 1500 a year. In the meantime, the medical profession tried to stop the craze. They cut open his sponges in search of some hidden panacea, but all they found was water. From then on, powerful friends shielded Priessnitz and the Austrian Government endorsed his system.

In America, Dr. Joel Shew developed a more systematic water cure. His hydropathic establishment at 47 Bond Street, New York City, was geared to cope with any complaint. There were tub, shower and sitz baths. But the wet sheet was the mainstay of therapy, since "water administered through subcutaneous absorption coupled with exosmosis or transudation" was obviously health-giving. Thus, women were advised to wear under their clothes wet girdles, to be changed every three hours. The main thing, obviously, was to get wet and stay wet. It was best, however, not to drink water "unthinkingly," but only in specified doses. Bleeding ulcers? Swallow ice-cubes, said Shew. He and his aides were always ready to lull pain, cure fever, and "wrap watchfulness in slumber" — with water.

251

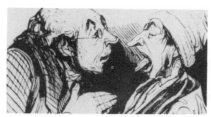

A case of gastritis.

To the critical outsider, the medical scene of the 1840's must have seemed hopelessly mad. There were 20-odd systems going full blast. Each of them coated its kernel of truth with unadulterated nonsense, then fed it to the patient. Obviously, the cartoons which attacked these medicasters were not entirely anti-medical. Daumier, for instance, did not hate doctors. But he did hate fakers, frauds and faddists. He purged them with humor (see cartoons on this page), and thus upheld the good physician.

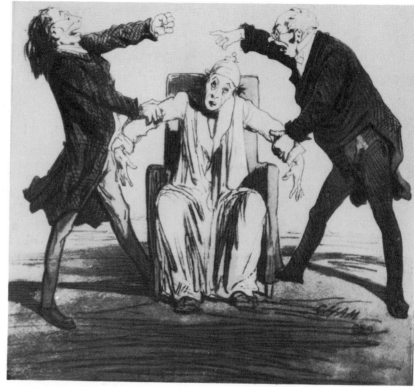

Homeopath: If you take me you'll die of the disease. Allopath: If you take me you'll die of the cure. Patient: It's all the same to me.

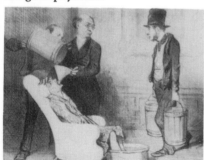

A cold shower for the stomach.

DAUMIER
AND THE DOCTORS

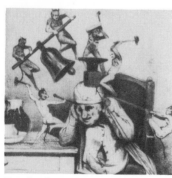

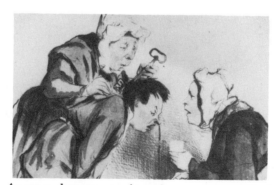

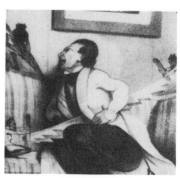

Devils of pain cause headache.   *Amateur doctress uses house-key to stop nosebleed*   *A seesaw stomach ache (Traviés).*

The wry smiles provoked by Daumier's art could not be compared with the wholesale laughter produced by a whiff of nitrous oxide. First explored scientifically by Humphry Davy in 1799, "laughing gas" provoked ecstatic comments. Poet Samuel Coleridge said: "I had the most entrancing visions." Poet Robert Southey said: "The atmosphere of the . . . heavens must be composed of this gas."

Laughing gas soon led to a new form of entertainment. There were frolics in college dormitories and private homes.

Itinerant entertainers, like Samuel Colt (of revolver fame) used the gas to stage hilarious shows.

The public refused to take these freakish fumes seriously. But a few wise men foresaw their possible use in the alleviation of pain. Finally, in the 1840s, nitrous oxide proved its worth in dentistry, and that blessed innovation — anesthesia — came to pass.

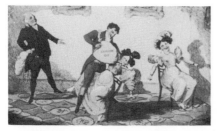

Laughing gas to sooth scolding wives.

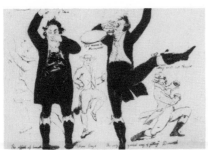

Effects of nitrous oxide, from 1808 Univ. of Penn. thesis. At right: Poster, New York Academy of Medicine.

Let those now laugh, who never laugh'd before,
And those who always laugh, now laugh the more.

A GRAND
EXHIBITION

OF THE EFFECTS PRODUCED BY INHALING

NITROUS OXIDE, EXHILERATING, OR

LAUGHING GAS!

WILL BE GIVEN AT *The Masonic Hall*

Saturday EVENING, *15 th*   1845.

30 GALLONS OF GAS will be prepared and administered to all in the audience who desire to inhale it.

MEN will be invited from the audience, to protect those under the influence of the Gas from injuring themselves or others. This course is adopted that no apprehension of danger may be entertained. Probably no one will attempt to fight.

THE EFFECT OF THE GAS is to make those who inhale it, either

LAUGH, SING, DANCE, SPEAK OR FIGHT, &c. &c.

according to the leading trait of their character. They seem to retain consciousness enough not to say or do that which they would have occasion to regret.

N. B. The Gas will be administered only to gentlemen of the first respectability. The object is to make the entertainment in every respect, a genteel affair.

Those who inhale the Gas once, are always anxious to inhale it the second time. There is not an exception to this rule.

No language can describe the delightful sensation produced. Robert Southey, (poet) once said that "the atmosphere of the highest of all possible heavens must be composed of this Gas."

For a full account of the effect produced upon some of the most distinguished men of Europe, see Hooper's Medical Dictionary, under the head of Nitrogen.

The History and properties of the Gas will be explained at the commencement of the entertainment.

The entertainment will be accompanied by experiments in

ELECTRICITY.

ENTERTAINMENT TO COMMENCE AT 7 O'CLOCK.

TICKETS *12½* CENTS,

For sale at the principal Bookstores, and at the Door.

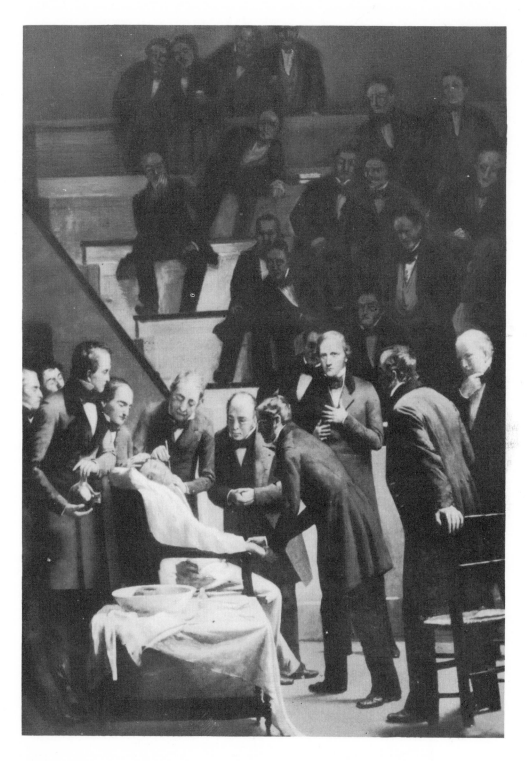

Original Ether Day, Boston, October 16, 1846. Dr. Morton (left) holds inhaler while Dr. J. C. Warren excises tumor on the jaw of Gilbert Abbott.

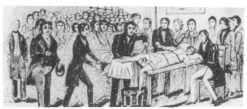

Operating theatre in pre-anesthesia days.

PAIN PUT TO SLEEP

ETHER USED IN SURGERY

On December 10, 1844, Professor Gardner Colton displayed the wonders of laughing gas at Union Hall, Hartford, Connecticut. As his show progressed, a man who had inhaled the gas rushed through the hall pursued by another "volunteer." The pursuer tripped; he fell to the floor and hurt his leg, but obviously felt no pain.

This incident deeply impressed one member of the audience, Dr. Horace Wells, an ingenious local dentist. After the show, Dr. Wells asked exhibitor Colton to visit his office with a supply of nitrous oxide. Colton complied. The next day at the appointed hour he administered laughing gas to Dr. Wells; then Dr. John Riggs, one of Wells' students, extracted a bad molar tooth. Wells had been completely quiet during the operation. As he came to, he excitedly proclaimed " . . . a new era of toothpulling."

It proved to be considerably more than the beginning of a new era of toothpulling. Wells went to Boston and approached his former partner, Dr. William Morton. Through Morton's intercession he received permission from Dr. John Collins Warren to conduct a "painless" tooth extraction before his class at Cambridge College. But at the moment of extraction the patient screamed, and Wells was hissed from the auditorium by the hardboiled students. During the next few years he performed many painless extractions. But he was unable to gain public recognition for his work.

His erstwhile partner, Morton, was more successful. At the suggestion of Dr. Charles T. Jackson, a chemist, he decided to replace nitrous oxide with ether. On September 30, 1846, he put Eben H. Frost under ether, then freed him painlessly of an abscessed tooth. Morton was quick to publicize his feat. Two weeks later he appeared in the same amphitheatre where Wells had fared so poorly. Dr. Warren had agreed to another try.

The events which took place in Boston on Friday morning, October 16, 1846, were well staged for dramatic suspense. The scene has been described innumerable times: Dr. Morton's delay; Dr. Warren's dry cough and his slight sarcasm — "Since Dr. Morton has not arrived I presume he is otherwise engaged"; the burst of laughter from the gallery; Morton's entrance at this juncture; the strapping down (just in case) of patient Gilbert Abbott; the long (three-minute) dose of ether; and then Morton's momentous announcement to Warren: "Sir, your patient is ready." And at that point, Warren's first incision; his steeling himself against expected screams; and his calm manner when only silence followed. Then, when the operation was over, his historic words: "Gentlemen, this is no humbug."

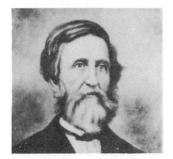

Dr. Crawford Long used ether in 1842, but did not put in claim as originator of anesthesia until 1849.

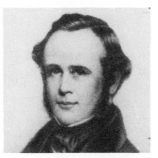

Dentist Horace Wells used nitrous oxide in tooth extractions, 1844, but bungled demonstration before surgery class.

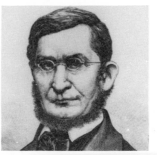

Chemist Jackson suggested use of ether to Dr. Morton, who gave successful demonstration in Boston General Hospital.

255

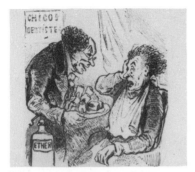

Having teeth pulled a pleasure.

BLISSFUL

INSENSIBILITY

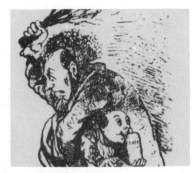

Being spanked — a joyride.

The reverberations of Ether Day are difficult to assess. Before anesthesia, patients faced an operation as if it were an execution. Sensitive surgeons found their work revolting. Cheselden had sleepless nights; Astley Cooper confessed that it turned his stomach. Conversely, some doctors saw pain as a "providential" concomitant of disease, and refused to adopt "this highest mercy brought from man to man." At first, Velpeau was sure the idea was not feasible, but once anesthesia had been demonstrated, he cheerfully pro-

nounced it the most important discovery ever made.

Unfortunately, the great discovery was soon followed by an ugly maelstrom of claims, counterclaims and slanders, now known in medical annals as "The Ether War." The altercation between Jackson and Morton grew exceptionally bitter. Dr. Crawford Long, who had first used sulphuric ether in a tumor excision in 1842, staked out a belated claim in 1849. Dr. Wells had committed suicide — but his widow continued to press her

husband's claim to priority. And all these contenders fought for their rights on the floor of Congress, where an award of $100,000 had been proposed, to be paid to Morton for his discovery. But the award was never made. The Civil War pushed the whole dispute into the background. It remained for Oliver Wendell Holmes, who had baptized the process as "anesthesia," to decide on the real winner with an enormously bad pun: "e (i) ther."

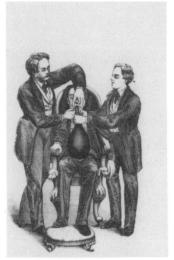

Patient inhales through mouth from rubber bag while his nose is pinched.

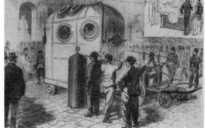

Anesthetic mixture pumped by crew into operating room on wheels.

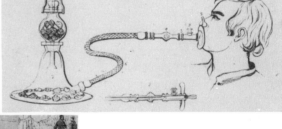

Early anesthetists dripped ether from a bottle into a handkerchief. To control effects of narcotics, various ether masks were devised. Air chamber was used later with mixture of nitrous oxide and oxygene pumped from outside into "operating room on wheels" (St. Louis Hospital, Paris).

256

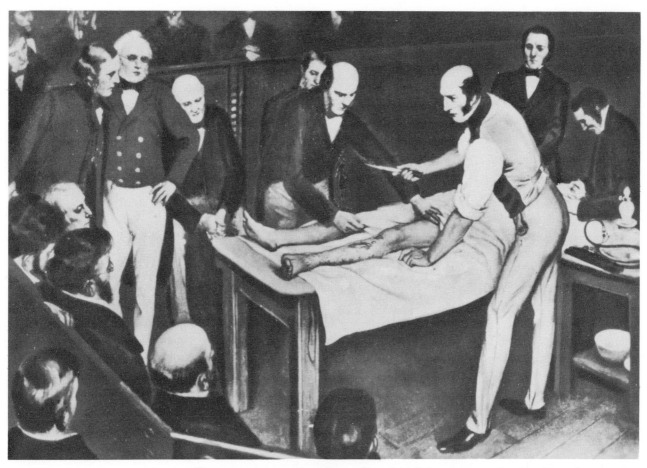

First amputation under ether performed by Robert Liston in London, December 21, 1846.

The news of ether-anesthesia spread quickly to Europe. A scant two months after Morton's triumph, Dr. Robert Liston, a bold English surgeon, was ready to test it before his class at University College, London. Once more the scene is melodramatic.

December 21, 1846: Liston, a strapping six-footer, enters his lecture room at the college. He removes his coat, then announces dryly to the class: "We are going to try a Yankee dodge today, gentlemen, for making men insensible." A few minutes later the patient, a 36-year-old butler named Frederick Churchill is brought in on a stretcher. As Peter Squire gives the patient ether from a makeshift inhaler, Liston prepares for an amputation of the thigh. As he is proud of his speed, he asks his assistants to time him. Then he starts to cut. Twenty-eight seconds later the severed leg hits the floor. When the patient revives, he asks in confusion: "When are you going to begin? Take me back, I can't have it done." They show him the severed stump and he falls back weeping. Liston stammers: "This Yankee dodge, gentlemen, beats mesmerism hollow."

There is an ironic twist to this operation: Frederick Churchill had come to Liston with a compound fracture. The surgeon had treated it with his bare hands, which, however dexterous, were unsterilized. Septicemia developed and amputation became necessary. As Victor Robinson put it, Churchill's leg was sacrificed to the ignorance of the age. But in the above illustration, young Joseph Lister is shown at the outer left, watching Liston operate. Two decades later Lister's discovery of antisepsis would help to avoid such tragedies.

SAVIORS OF MOTHERS

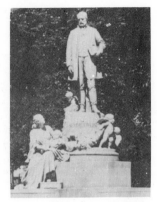

Semmelweis monument.

The same decade that was marked by the discovery of anesthesia saw the first effective attempts to prevent infection by contact. The man who made them probably knew little about bacteria; he simply preached asepsis from an empirical point of view. But by his crusading zeal, Ignatz Semmelweis, Hungarian obstetrician, saved the lives of innumerable women.

Unfortunately, the same zeal estranged him from his colleagues in Vienna and Budapest, who scoffed at his suggestions, and collectively opposed them. He had boldy asserted that the dirty hands of the doctors were carrying disease to parturient women. Such implications were an affront to professional pride. According to official theory, puerperal fever was caused by "hospital miasma." But though bad air was, no doubt, prevalent, Semmelweis was still able to prove his point.

In 1844, when he came to the maternity department of the Vienna General Hospital, the mortality figures were shocking. In Ward I, attended by medical students, the death-rate was over 10 per cent. But in Ward II, which was set aside for the training of midwives, the rate was only 3 per cent. Semmelweis concluded that students coming to the ward from the dissecting room transmitted cadaveric matter into the system of pregnant women.

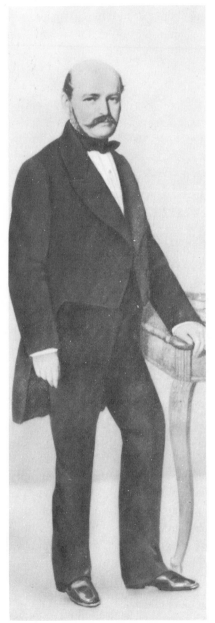

Semmelweis insisted that students wash hands before touching parturient patients.

The nurses in Ward II handled no autopsies, and this obviously accounted for the more favorable conditions there.

Semmelweis took exceedingly simple measures to stop the death-march in Ward I. In May, 1847, he asked his students to wash their hands in chlorinated lime water, and to scrub their fingernails with a handbrush before entering the ward. The death-rate in this ward then stood at 12.4 per cent. Within two months it fell to 1.27 per cent.

But his colleagues could not forgive Semmelweis the introduction of so simple a gadget as the hand brush. His zeal annoyed them even more. Semmelweis had called one doctor a murderer and a Nero; he had even blamed his own superior, Johann Klein, for the squalid conditions in the wards. His position became untenable. In 1850, without notice to his friends, he left the city.

Returning to Pest he became chief-obstetrician at the St. Rochus Hospital (1853). Here he reduced deaths from puerperal fever as he had in Vienna. Semmelweis died in 1865 in an insane asylum, probably from septicemia, the affliction that had given him the clue to his discovery in the first place.

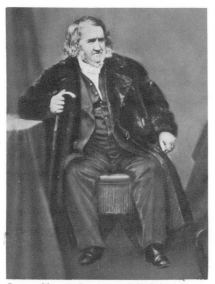

James Young Simpson, Edinburgh gynecologist, introduced chloroform.

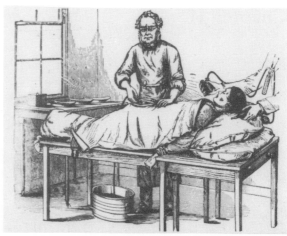

Anesthesia enabled Spencer Wells to explore uterine region, perform ovariotomies.
He insisted on absolute cleanliness of instruments and hands, operative discipline.

Gynecology advanced on other frontiers during this same period. With the aid of anesthesia, surgeons learned to alleviate more female troubles.

Now at last they could cut more deeply to reach abdominal and uterine regions. They could work at a slower pace, unhampered by the cries and struggles of their patients.

In January, 1847, a few months after Morton's demonstration, James Young Simpson (1811-1870) used ether to achieve painless childbirth. Then the indomitable Scotchman searched for other, more easily adaptable substances for obstetric practice. His living-room at Edinburgh was lined with vials containing soporifics. Simpson tried each one on himself. Finally, he hit upon chloroform, a liquid discovered independently by both Guthrie (a New York chemist) and Liebig. It had most of the advantages of ether, but lacked its disagreeable smell and cough-producing qualities.

Painless childbirth was vociferously opposed by religious circles. It was sacrilegious, they said, to oppose God's dictum: "In sorrow shalt thou bring forth children." But Simpson, an able polemicist, promptly replied that God himself was the first anesthetist: He had put Adam to sleep, then resected a rib to make Eve. The question was settled, however, in 1853, when Queen Victoria, attended by Dr. John Snow, gave painless birth to Prince Leopold. Since Victoria was said to rank close to God in England, religious opposition against "twilight slumber" was effectively dampened.

Simpson prospered as a gynecologist. His practice has been described graphically by Sir Robert Christison: "His two reception rooms were full of patients, there were more seated in the lobby, female faces stared from all the windows. Just the same he joined me, and let them kick their heels for two hours."

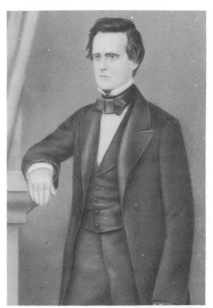

Marion Sims of South Carolina, repaired, in 1852, vesico-vaginal fistula (an abnormal communication between urinary and genital passages in women). This condition had defied surgical treatment for centuries. Sims' gynecological work received wide recognition in both Europe and America.

259

TRIUMPH OF MEDICAL SCIENCE

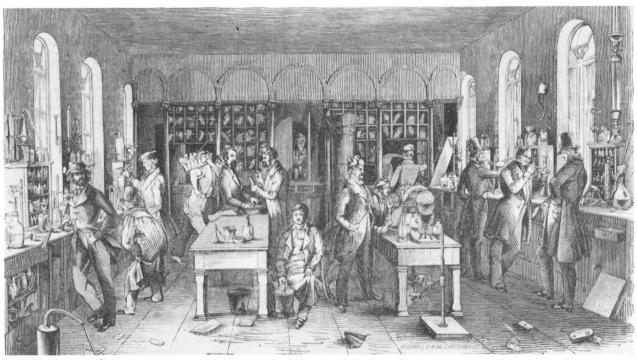

Liebig's chemical laboratory in Giessen (1845) provided students with facilities for experiment. It also stimulated the establishment of physiological laboratories which became, in turn, leading centers of scientific medicine.

German medicine burst out in the 1840s with a startling show of scientific vitality. On the surface, this complete about-face was unexpected, but actually it had been gathering force for some time. While the romantic philosophers were ruminating (often quite brilliantly) on the nature of medicine, their students were slipping off to Paris, where they were fed on solid empirical fare: dissections, experiments, statistics. When they returned home, they were ready to cut through the foggy layers of speculation.

Their efforts were aided by the existence of an unparalleled system of education. Each of the German petty states had excellent universities (in France, the sciences centered around Paris). As the old philosophers died off, young empiricists moved into their chairs. Thus, many of these schools were gradually converted into research centers. Interest in experimentation gathered such amazing impetus that Germany was able to seize and hold the lead in scientific medicine during the second half of the century.

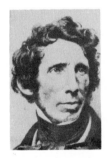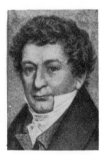

Wöhler (l.) produced urea chemically; Sertürner (r.) isolated, named, morphine.

REVEILLE IN   GERMANY

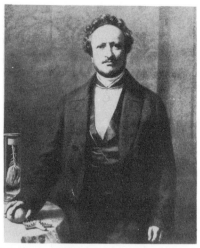

Within a few decades, the Germans had turned from their old do-nothing philosophical disciplines to the exact natural sciences. They had borrowed experimental methods from the chemist's laboratory, and applied them to problems of physiology, pathology and bacteriology. In these three fields, they had scored great triumphs. Moreover, they had snatched medical leadership from the French, and made laboratory medicine a German domain.

Johannes Peter Müller, the Rhenish physiologist, was a symbol of the transition from thinking to doing. He had started out as a confirmed Romanticist, but exposure to the teachings of the Swedish chemist, Berzelius, had turned him into an all-around naturalist. His investigations covered an amazing variety of phenomena. By indefatigable experiments with animals, he was able to vindicate Bell's idea of the function of the nervous system.

Johannes Müller and his pupils established physiology as a modern science.

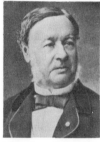
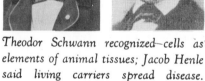

Theodor Schwann recognized cells as elements of animal tissues; Jacob Henle said living carriers spread disease.

At 26, he had formulated the theory of specific nerve energies, and had made a great many contributions to physiology. This latter science he regenerated almost single-handedly. He also gave it a magnificent textbook, his *Handbook of Human Physiology* (1833-1840).

While Müller made no epochal discoveries, he did exert a tremendous influence on his generation's thinking. Much of what happened in German medicine in the next half century — much by which the whole world has profited — was achieved by pupils of Müller. Müller taught Henle, for instance, and Henle taught Koch. Koch taught Welch and Ehrlich. A basic attitude bound all these men together. To solve physiological problems, they rigidly applied the standards of the laboratory sciences like chemistry and physics. They admitted as valid only what had been tested and proved irrefutable by experimentation.

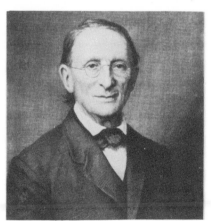

Carl Ludwig was most influential teacher of experimental physiology.

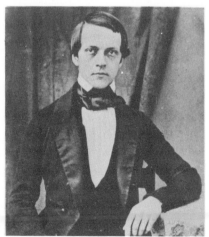

Hermann von Helmholtz explained hearing and vision in terms of physics.

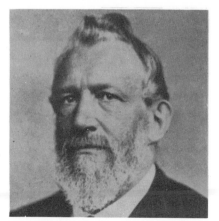

Emil Heinrich Du Bois Reymond became the founder of electro-physiology.

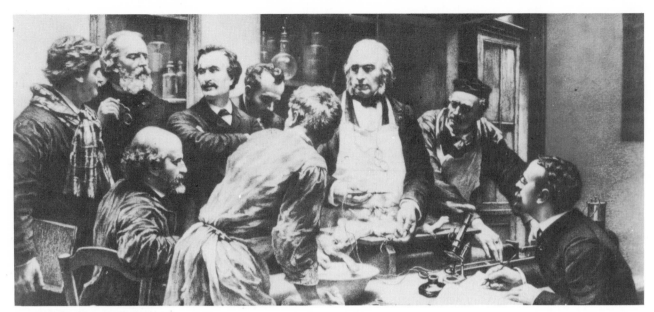

Claude Bernard during laboratory seminar in Sorbonne demonstrates function of vasomotor nerves.

MEDICAL SCIENCE: Continued

BERNARD AND VIRCHOW

In 1848 Claude Bernard began his lectures at the Collège de France with this remark: "Scientific medicine, which it ought to be my duty to teach, does not exist."

Compared with her brilliant clinics, laboratory facilities in France had indeed been poor. Consequently, Bernard had to begin work in a dingy cellar which he called "the tomb of the scientist." Later, his passion for experiment earned him a special chair of physiology at the Sorbonne, but it was not until 1864, after an interview with Louis Napoleon, that he was granted the use of appropriate laboratories.

Bernard's contributions to scientific medicine are as manifold as they are monumental. He shed new light on the workings of digestion by his research on the pancreatic juice. He proved that the liver is a sugar producing, sugar storing and distributing organ. These insights not only explained the nature of diabetes but helped to establish the concept of internal secretion. Bernard gave a new orientation to medicine by portraying the human body as a single functional entity, a balanced inter-play of body fluids.

Bernard put forth his epochal pronouncements only after rigid laboratory tests. He recharted medicine as an experimental science. "When entering a laboratory," he proclaimed, "leave theories in the cloakroom. Why think when you can experiment? . . . exhaust experiments and then think." When Bernard died in 1878, he was accorded a state funeral — the first man of science to receive such a tribute.

It is doubtful whether Bernard ever treated patients once he had begun his career as a physiologist. In contrast, Rudolf Virchow — another tireless proponent of laboratory medicine — always remained a physician and an aggressive champion of humanitarianism. "Physicians are the natural attorneys of the poor," he wrote in 1849, "and no small part of social problems comes under their jurisdiction."

All through his life, Virchow kept up a triple role of scientist, doctor and reformer. He founded the great scientific magazine: *Archiv für Pathologische Anatomie;* but scientific interest did not keep him from manning the Berlin barricades in the Revolution of 1848. This show of liberalism and a candid report on the disgraceful conditions in the typhus-stricken areas of Silesia led to his departure from Berlin's Charité

Hospital. After a stay at Würzburg, he returned in 1856 to Berlin in triumph to become the director of the first independent pathological institute.

Two years later Virchow published his revolutionary *Cellular Pathology*. Here he pronounced the cell the essential element of the living body and defined disease as the cell's reaction to altered conditions. The body, in Virchow's interpretation, is a humming "cell state" in which every cell is a citizen, and disease simply a "civil war between these citizens." William H. Welch called the cellular theory the greatest advance ever made in pathology.

The concept of the "cell state" re-mained valid for over half a century. While it still forms the basis of much work in histology, pathology and surgery Virchow's tenets have had to be somewhat modified by the exploration of intercellular structures.

Virchow accomplished a prodigious amount of work, in many fields. He conducted research in physical anthropology basing his deductions on census figures. In 1879 he went with Schliemann to Troy to explore her treasures. He gave many popular and scientific lectures — championed the cause of public hygiene, made laboratory studies of tumors, leukemia, thrombosis. At his Institute, Virchow trained hundreds of pathologists. Here he also collected and mounted personally some 23,000 specimens.

The small peppery professor was so busy every minute that his students had trouble to keep up with him. One candidate anxious to finish up his examination, caught Virchow dressed in tails, about to rush off to a session of the Berlin City Council. The candidate was invited to join him in his coach, where Virchow proceeded to quiz him. After a ride "Unter den Linden," they reached the famous Brandenburg Tor. Here Virchow served the student an abrupt notice: "Please get out, you failed."

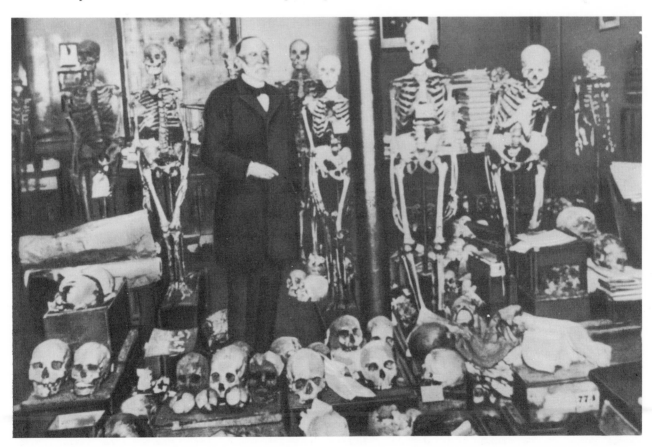

Virchow was a kindly, busy man, "who lunched on a bottle of beer and two sandwiches, amidst skeletons and skulls "   263

BACKWOODS DOCTORS

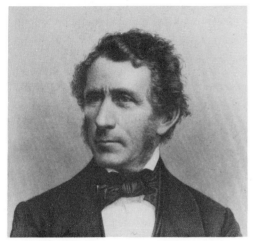

Daniel Drake campaigned for medical education.

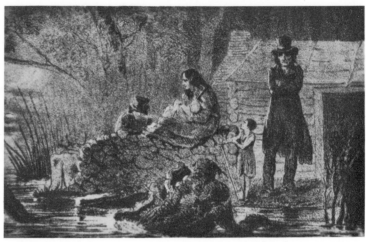

"He ain't sick, he only got the ager" (ague). Frontier quip on malaria.

The state of American medicine was still dismal in the 1850s. There were schools in the East, South and West, but their programs were hopelessly inadequate: lectures, three months a year, for two years, with little or no practical training. Students often sat through the same courses twice. They rarely saw patients. But these schools did have one advantage — tuition fees were modest. In 1851-52, one Thomas Wade was able to take his degree at Louisiana University for a total outlay of $146.50. At that time most tuition fees went to the professors who often owned medical schools.

In the West, the pioneer doctor had to forego any "book-learning." He relied instead on good sense, keen observation and a strong horse. His patients lived miles apart, through heavily forested areas. In Springfield, Illinois, visits averaged $1, with an extra 25c for each mile beyond a 4-mile radius. (If the horse was fed, the fee was cut in half.) Eyes, ears and nose were the doctor's principal tools, and his saddlebag served as the nearest drugstore. In it he carried Dover's Powder, Dragon's Blood (at 25c a dose), Peruvian Bark (at $1), and above all, Calomel. Bleeding, of course, was the main therapy. One pioneer doctor confessed that he could load the steamboat, Andrew Jackson, with all the Calomel he had prescribed, and float it on the blood he had drawn from his backwoods patients.

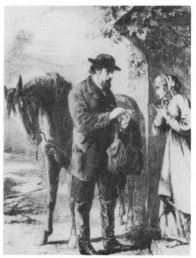

Dispensing medicine. Doctor's saddle bag was wilderness drugstore.

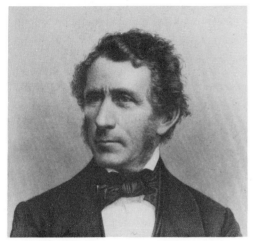

Pioneer doctor on his rounds. Consultation, $1. Double fee at night.

264

Science had no place on the frontier. Harsh experience gave the backwoods practitioner a store of worldly wisdom, and beyond that, he had no time for contemplation or experiment.

However, the best of the frontier doctors were painfully aware of their shortcomings, and tried to raise both their own standards and those of the profession. Unquestionably, the greatest of these physicians was Daniel Drake. He grew up in abject poverty on a Kentucky farm. But at 19, after apprenticeship with Dr. William Goforth of Cincinnati, he received the first diploma issued west of the Alleghenies. In two more decades he rose to leadership in the medical profession.

Drake was restless, energetic and intense: "hot and positive like the pole of an electric battery." He changed his residence seven times between Cincinnati, Louisville, Lexington (Ky.). In Cincinnati he founded two medical colleges, established the West's first medical journal, and championed a host of civic improvements. But medical education was his main concern. He was a superb lecturer, a master of the homely speech so characteristic of Lincoln. Unfortunately, his ardor led him into interminable squabbles — and occasional fistfights — with his colleagues. (He called it his "Thirty Years War.") At the end of his life Drake could truly confess: "Medical schools have consumed me." He was neither the first nor the last medical teacher to reach this conclusion.

During his travels up and down the Mississippi region — on foot, horseback and by boat, Drake compiled a monumental medical Baedeker: *Diseases of the Interior Valley of North America.* When Alfred Stillé reviewed its first volume (the second appeared posthumously) before the meeting of the A.M.A. in 1850, the author received so thunderous an ovation that he was touched to tears.

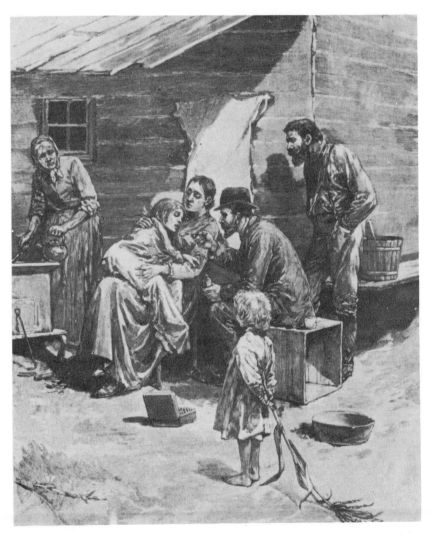

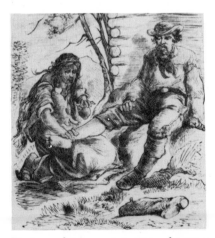

Doctor shortage prompts frontiersman to seek cure from Indian squaw.

Frontier children suffered from sickness and parental neglect. Little was done to alleviate whooping cough, measles, diphtheria. Infant mortality was high.

265

NEW TOOLS FOR DIAGNOSIS

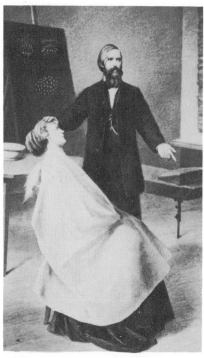

Albrecht von Graefe (1828-1870) was among the first to recognize importance of ophthalmoscope. He used it to diagnose eye afflictions, then developed appropriate surgical procedures.

While the American country doctor put his eyes and ears to work, new techniques of diagnosis were being developed in Europe. Physiologist Hermann von Helmholtz was now fashioning an instrument which permitted a glimpse of the hitherto hidden recesses of the eye. Other diagnostic aids soon followed. They enabled the doctor to concentrate his efforts with increasing effectiveness upon special organs. This led, in turn, to the rise of specialization as we know it today.

Helmholtz had started as a pupil of the great Johannes Müller. He was especially well grounded in physics, and happily combined this knowledge with his medical training. One result of this combination was his *Physiological Optics*, which has been called the greatest of all books on the physics of vision (1867). A similar work on acoustics had preceded it. But it was the "by-product" of such research which most markedly influenced the course of practical medicine.

Helmholtz has been called "the complete scientist." Though he began his career as a physiologist, he occupied in later years the chair of physics in Berlin. As a physicist, he was interested not only in persistent experimentation, but in the constant improvement of instruments which would help him to observe and measure his findings. To observe and measure the workings of the eye, for example, he invented the ophthalmometer and the ophthalmoscope.

Before 1851, ophthalmic operations had been confined almost entirely to the eye's optic surface. Now the ophthalmoscope allowed physicians to devise surgical operations which involved the perception of the eye's fundus. Great eye-doctors appeared on the scene, men like Albrecht von Graefe and the Dutchman F. C. Donders. In a short time, a whole new department of medical science grew up.

These ophthalmologists were much interested in establishing clinics, especially in view of the rapid growth of urban populations and the need for specialized therapy. Consequently, the number and importance of such institutions increased after the mid-century.

Specialists trained in Europe began to arrive in America, and this served to accelerate the trend. As George Rosen has shown in his study *Specialization in Medicine*, American ophthalmology advanced noticeably with the appearance of German doctors. They established eye surgery as a prominent specialty in the New World.

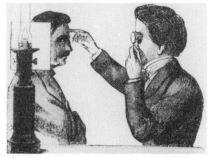

Ophthalmoscope (above) was invented by Helmholtz in 1851 to aid research.

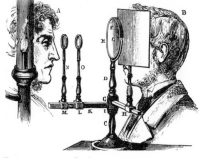

Ruet improved this instrument by use of concave mirror and condensing lens.

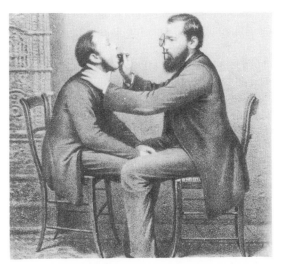

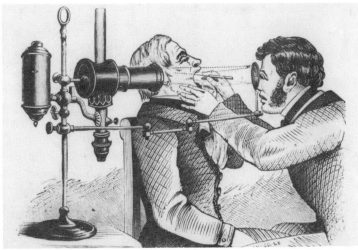

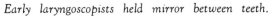

Early laryngoscopists held mirror between teeth.

Improved laryngoscope gave a clearer picture of obstructions

Laryngology in the modern sense began in this same decade.

A London singing teacher, Manuel Garcia, had invented the laryngoscope in 1854. Garcia was interested in the workings of the vocal cords from a pedagogical standpoint. But when he presented his discovery to the Royal Society in 1855, it attracted the attention of Ludwig Tűrck and Johann Czermak of Vienna. Both these men applied the laryngoscope independently to diagnostic problems. Their heated debate on the question of "priority" helped to arouse and sustain professional interest in the field.

Once the larynx and its lesions could be observed, surgical procedures were developed to alleviate such old nemeses as tumor of the larynx. This affliction had formerly meant death by suffocation. But now the surgeon could extirpate it with a fair chance of success. Unfortunately, he was still not always able to ascertain the exact nature of the lesion. This became all too evidént when later in the century, a *cause célèbre* stirred the profession.

Morell Mackenzie (1837-1892) was Britain's outstanding laryngologist when he was called to Berlin in 1887 to cope with the throat affliction of Crown Prince Frederick of Germany. After frantic attempts to decide on the proper treatment, the case was badly bungled. The growth, once removed, reappeared. Both Virchow and Mackenzie pronounced it benign, but 99 days after he became emperor, Frederick III died — of cancer of the throat.

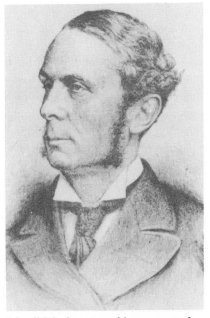

Morell Mackenzie used laryngoscope but failed to save Emperor Frederick III.

Marey's wrist sphygmograph (near right) was first instrument designed to register pulse graphically.

Politzer's tuning fork (far right) tested hearing via bone conduction.

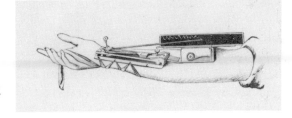

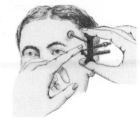

FLORENCE NIGHTINGALE

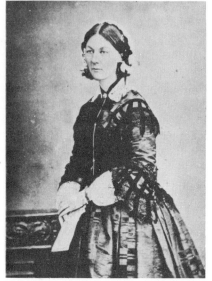

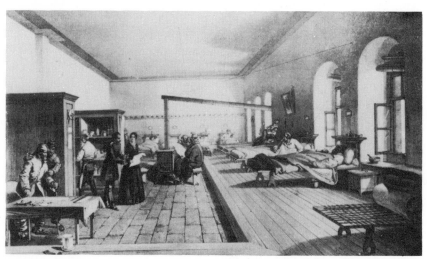

Soldiers tried "to catch a glimpse of her blessed shadow as she passed."

By the 1850's, the physician's knowledge of chest, heart and kidney diseases had been considerably extended, anesthesia and the stethoscope had been discovered, and new techniques were developing in the laboratory. Then came the Crimean War, and with it, a forceful reminder that medicine was not strictly a matter of science or techniques. Florence Nightingale — a woman with common sense, a talent for organization, and an abundance of simple human kindness — forced medical attention to focus once more on the care of the patient.

It has been said, with some justification, that Miss Nightingale accomplished more during the Crimean War than the entire British medical department. Her work at Skutari Hospital was almost miraculous. With 37 assistants (plus a system of nightly rounds), she was able to cut the death rates from 42% to 2% — a feat unmatched, at that time, in the annals of practical medicine. Miss Nightingale and her audacious charges used soap, water, clean linen and humane treatment in wards where cholera and dysentery ran rampant, where the wounded had hitherto died of malnutrition and the squalor rivalled that of the London slums. But in the midst of her work, one medical superior smugly warned her "not to spoil the brutes" (her patients).

Florence Nightingale (1820-1910) at the time of her departure for the Crimea.

The British people were proud of the lady with the lamp. When she returned home in 1856, they prepared a tremendous welcome for her in London. But Miss Nightingale dodged it and confined herself to a quiet call on Queen Victoria. "Such a head," said Victoria to Albert when she left, "I wish we had her at the War Office."

Unfortunately, Miss Nightingale was to remain an invalid and a recluse, for the next 60 years. From her lonely chamber, she continued her fight to place nursing on a professional basis. With £44,000 from her grateful countrymen, she established at St. Thomas Hospital the first professional school for nurses.

Hospital ward at Skutari refurnished by Florence Nightingale. She worked 20 hours a day, requisitioning clothing, bedding, food wherever it could be found.

268

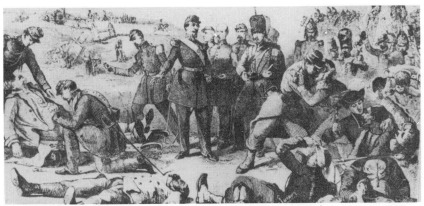

Butchery at Solferino where 30,000 died, gave Dunant idea of "relief societies."

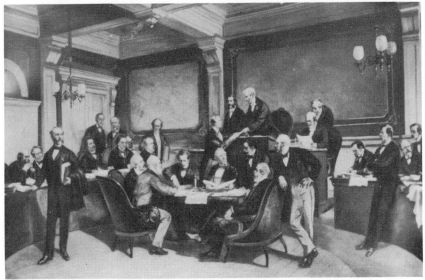

Geneva Convention, August 1864, marks beginning of International Red Cross.

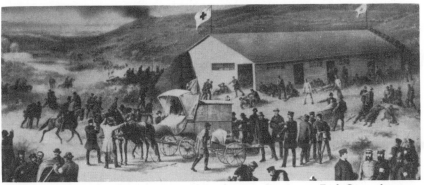

Field hospital during Danish War, 1864, first conflict to see Red Cross function.

In June, 1859, three years after Florence Nightingale's return from the Crimea, an investment banker from Geneva — J. Henri Dunant — went to Italy with the intention of gaining an audience with Napoleon III. The French Emperor was then battling the Austrians at Solferino, and Dunant was caught up in the war's most bloody battle. This sensitive man was horrified by the neglect of the soldiers: there were only two doctors for 6,000 wounded men. The Austrian prisoners among them were terribly mistreated. To alleviate all this misery, Dunant organized a makeshift nursing service. His admonition, *"sono fratelli"* (We Are All Brothers), moved the local populace to bring water, bandages and food to the sufferers.

Three years later, in his famous *Recollections of Solferino*, Dunant proposed the establishment of permanent relief societies which could take immediate action in case of war; he also proposed a neutral zone for hospitals, doctors and nurses at the scene of battle. These ideas were incorporated in the Geneva Convention, which was signed by 12 governments on August 22, 1864. On that day, the International Red Cross was born.

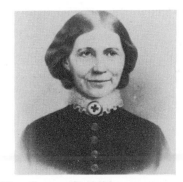

Clara Barton, Civil War nurse, aroused American interest in the Red Cross.

CIVIL WAR MEDICINE

MORE SOLDIERS DIED OF DISEASE THAN FROM BULLETS

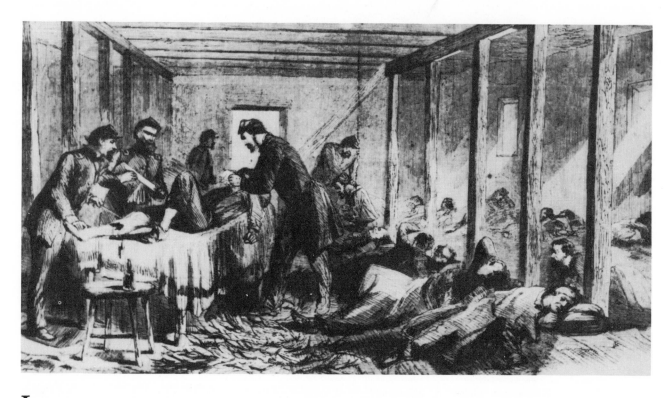

It was largely without the blessings of medical progress that the Civil War was fought. Pasteur was conducting experiments in bacteriology as the guns roared along the Potomac; Lister was working on the relief of post-operative putrefaction. But the benefits from such discoveries belonged to the future.

Among the more available blessings, the ambulance corps proved, at first, to be little more than a touring service for Washington idlers. After the first battle of Bull Run (1861) the wounded lay for three days before help came.

Anesthesia was administered about 80,000 times in the North, mainly with chloroform, yet not on a broad enough basis. General Grant had assigned Dr. Morton of ether fame to give courses in anesthesia. Even he could not overcome an old prejudice: many surgeons believed that "surgical shock" was essential for the success of an operation. They would rather amputate during the heat of battle, when the patient's heart was at great tension. Surgical shock was dangerously lessened by anesthesia, they felt, and so most wounded went without it.

There was another blessing only dimly understood: blood transfusion. It was applied exactly twice during the war. One recipient probably died from it, the other survived.

No less tragic was the ignorance in matters of wound infection. As Dr. W. W. Keen, later a pioneer of aseptic surgery confessed: "We operated in our pus-stained coats . . . we used undisinfected instruments from undisinfected plush cases . . . Surgeons . . . nearly always imperiled life and often actually caused death."

All together dysentery, typhoid fever and tetanus took a much heavier toll than actual combat. Statistics, far from complete, hold that total Union losses amounted to 300,000 men — one third due to wounds, two thirds due to sickness. For the South the picture was equally dismal.

If northern medical care was poor, conditions proved much worse in the South. The shortage of trained surgeons grew so desperate there that callow graduates were shoved out into the field. The Civil War experience of Dr. Simon Baruch (father of Bernard Baruch) is probably typical: "Before ever treating a sick person, and still under the age of 22, I was put in charge of a batallion of 500 infantry."

If surgeons were scarce, medical instruments were mostly non-existant. Kitchen knives had to do duty as scalpels. Dr. Joseph Jones, after the war a prominent surgeon in New Orleans, was reputed to be the only doctor on the confederate side who could boast of a clinical thermometer.

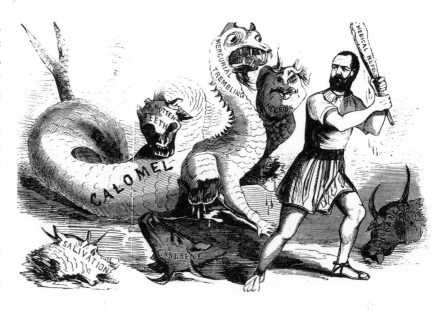

Over-drugging with calomel was curtailed by Dr. William A. Hammond, who became U. S. Surgeon General at 34. He reformed Union medical services (above).

Smuggling medicines into the South (below); to alleviate drug shortage, Southern ladies went North, returning with opium, morphine sewn into their hoopskirts

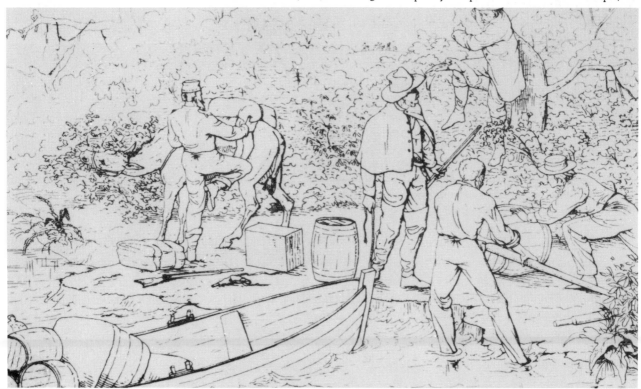

PSYCHIATRY TAKES ROOT

CHARCOT—HYSTERIA AND HYPNOTISM

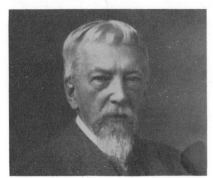

S. Weir Mitchell (1829-1914) studied neurological cases during Civil War.

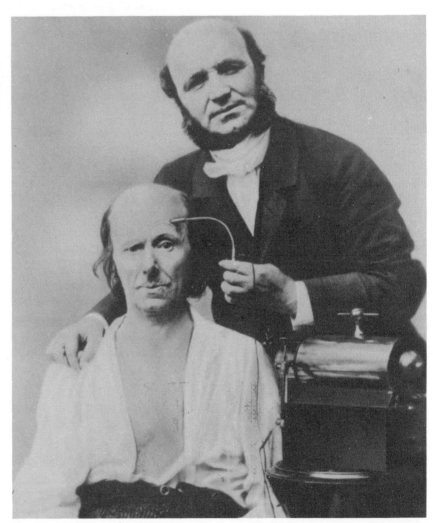

Civil War medicine has been called, with some justification, "the last flowering of the medical Middle Ages." But the conflict at least served to point up mistakes and assess experiences. Both were brilliantly recorded in the North's *Medical and Surgical History of the War of the Rebellion*. In spite of dismal failures the war had opened up new fields of therapy and research — especially in neurology.

At Turner's Lane Hospital in Philadelphia, Silas Weir Mitchell was able to set aside a ward (with Surgeon-General Hammond's blessings) for shock and hysteria cases. The studies conducted here resulted in Mitchell's classic book, *The Injuries of Nerves and Their Consequences*, which laid the basis for modern neurosurgery. Mitchell also developed a rest cure for nervous diseases, known as the "Weir Mitchell Treatment."

During the same period, the picturesque Duchenne of Boulogne (1806-1875) applied electricity to the diagnosis and treatment of nervous conditions. With his own "faradic" machinery — and entirely without an official assignment — he wandered through the wards of Paris Hospitals. Photographic studies helped him to record results (see above). His findings enabled him to define the neural basis of many afflictions — among them muscular atrophy, tabes dorsalis, infantile paralysis.

Jean-Martin Charcot was easily the foremost neurologist of his day. After his arrival at the Salpêtrière in 1862, he rapidly turned it into the leading center for neuroclinical research. Its 3000 patients offered him ample material which he used for clinical studies and impressive demonstrations. Charcot was a good diagnostician, and a sensitive psychiatrist but his interpretations of psychic disease proved by no means irrefutable, especially his teachings on the subject of hysteria. He applied hypnotism to treat this affliction. To treat the psyche was a daring move in the age of laboratory medicine. Mesmerism had then fallen into disrepute. Surgeons used it, sporadically, to effect anesthesia, but most scientists pooh-poohed it. They also pooh-poohed the whole idea of psychic phenomena. Many doctors still excised the womb (hystera) to cure hysteria. But Charcot removed the symptoms of hysteria by hypnosis. His cures were seldom permanent, though, and his interpretation of

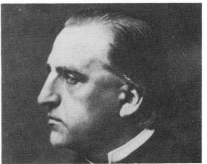

Charcot (1825-1893) made La Salpêtrière in Paris center of psychiatric research.

the phenomenon was faulty. Yet, Charcot's influence proved revolutionary, especially on one of his students — Sigmund Freud.

Freud was deeply impressed with Charcot's mode of treatment. Like the master, he experimented, at first, with electrotherapy, but soon discarded it as useless. Then Freud used hypnosis on his patients to bring repressed memories to the surface. Such memories, he held, were the cause of psychic trauma. Later on, he developed psychoanalysis as an approach to psychoneurosis more effective than hypnosis. Charcot's teachings served Freud as the point of departure for a whole new system of psychiatric treatment.

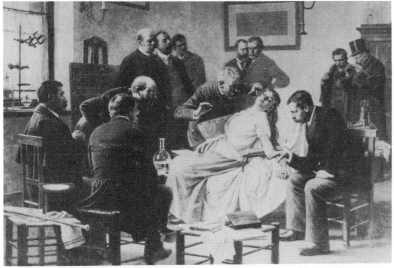

Hypnotism became the subject of intense study by medical men after Charcot had demonstrated its efficacy in relieving the symptoms of hysteria.

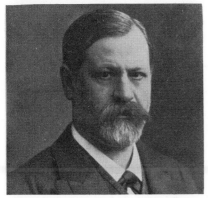

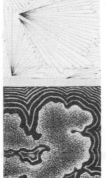

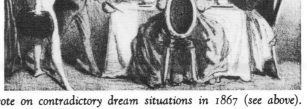

Sigmund Freud studied under Charcot (1885), was impressed with hypnosis.

Marquis d'Hervey wrote on contradictory dream situations in 1867 (see above). Later, Freud interpreted such dreams as symptoms of repressed sexual desires.

LISTER CURBS SEPSIS

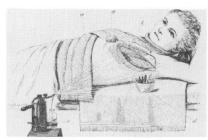

Carbolic spray.

With pain dulled by anesthesia, the surgeon could cut deeper into the human body. But at the same time, postoperative complications set in with increasing frequency. Wounds rarely healed without pus-formation, and about 50 per cent of the operations resulted in overt blood-poisoning. In addition, erysipelas and hospital gangrene now threatened to wipe out the

more chances of death than the English soldier on the field of Waterloo."

Yet the solution to the whole problem had been available since 1847 when Semmelweis had urged the obstetricians to disinfect and clean their hands. Surgeons still refused to do so. Semmelweis and his teachings had been completely sidetracked. Even young Joseph Lister, hard at work on the problem

pared him well for his future attack against infection in surgical wounds.

Lister himself was a painstaking and reasonably successful surgeon, but he was not content with his results. His Quaker conscience was aroused by the death toll from blood-poisoning. Septicemia was particularly flagrant then in cases of compound fracture, where the skin was ruptured with the bone

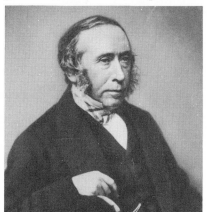

James Syme, Edinburgh surgeon; Lister was his aid, son-in-law, successor.

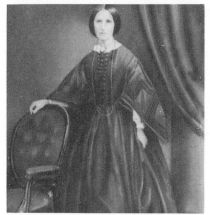

Agnes Syme Lister was throughout life her husband's untiring helpmate.

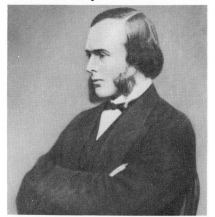

Joseph Lister during his stay at Glasgow, where he developed antiseptic surgery.

recent advances in the surgical art.

These terrors of the operating table were well understood. One mother, while consenting to her daughter's operation, asked the surgeon (Sir Frederick Treves) in perfect innocence: "but who will take care of her funeral?" James Young Simpson said: "A man laid on the operating table in one of our surgical hospitals is exposed to

of inflammation, scarcely had grasped their significance.

Lister had studied at University College Hospital in London, but he spent the first seven years of his career (1853-1860) working for James Syme at Edinburgh. (He also married Syme's daughter, Agnes.) Under Syme, Lister began to examine blood coagulation and wound-inflammation. Such studies pre-

ends exposed to the air. Blood-poisoning seemed unavoidable in such cases — so surgeons speedily amputated the limb. But in simple fractures, where the wound was unexposed, healing was usually effected without complication. Lister reasoned, as the "miasma-believers" had reasoned before him, that the air caused putrefaction.

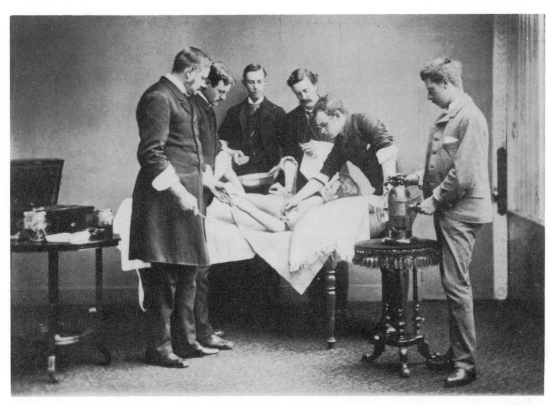

Antiseptic Method: surgeons operate while carbolic spray (on velvet trimmed table) wards off airborne microbes.

Lister had continued his studies with much zeal after he had become professor of surgery in Glasgow in 1860. In 1865 his theory received vindication from an unexpected quarter. Pasteur had just discovered that microscopic organisms caused fermentation in wine. Lister immediately seized on the similarity between fermentation and pus-formation to "confirm" his theory: not air, but airborne bacteria caused wound infections. To ward off the invaders, Lister devised the carbolic spray. To kill bacteria in open wounds he developed a lint bandage soaked in carbolic acid. He applied it first in August 1865 — and so started the age of antisepsis.

Though sterilization of the air was later discounted, Lister did call attention to the presence of germs in the operative field. He therefore advised that the surgeon touching wounds wash his hands carefully in a 1:20 carbolic acid solution. He insisted, moreover, that wound-dressings be kept clean. Such procedures set the precedent for today's high standards in aseptic surgery.

But once introduced, the "spray and gauze" method caused an immediate and violent reaction. Lister was surrounded by a band of faithful students, yet as one of them put it: "The non-Listerians looked at (us) as crazy believers in vain things like germs." Theodore Billroth (a late "convert") wrote to his friend Volkmann in 1874:

"If you were not so energetic a supporter of this antiseptic method I should say the whole thing was a swindle." Older surgeons were especially recalcitrant. They felt silly operating under a continuous spray of carbolic acid. Thus, when Lister returned to London in 1877 to head the University College Hospital, he met with discouraging opposition.

Later discoveries in bacteriology placed emphasis on asepsis rather than antisepsis, and Lister's carbolic donkey engine was consigned to the surgical museum. But his principles had made the development of asepsis possible. It was he who expounded the doctrine which at long last made all surgical procedures "safe."

275

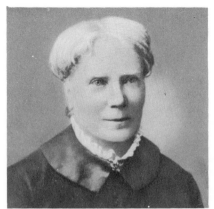

Elizabeth Blackwell, first academically-trained U. S. woman doctor; founded New York Infirmary for Women, 1857.

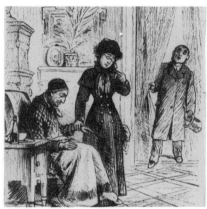

Cartoon of 1860s shows a resentful male physician watching his female competitor make pulse check-up.

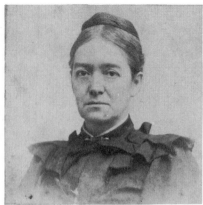

Mary Putnam Jacobi, Paris-trained pediatrician, writer, lecturer; she organized post-graduate school in New York.

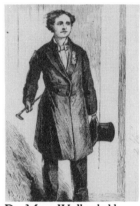

Dr. Mary Walker held commission as assistant surgeon during Civil War.

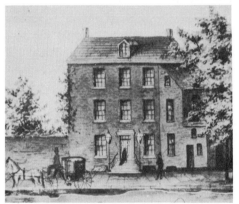

First Woman's Medical College opened in Philadelphia, 1850, guided by Dr. Anne Preston; men had called lady-doctors "too delicate."

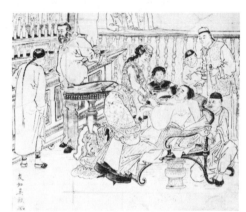

Dr. Reifsnyder, graduate of Woman's Medical College of Pennsylvania, performed daring operations in China; see cutting of tumor above.

"THERAPY IN BLOOMERS"

In the face of much mockery and discouragement, women doctors made considerable headway in the decades following the Civil War. Their advance was strikingly illustrated at President Arthur's New Year's Reception in 1881. The center of interest here were not the diamond-studded dresses of the diplomat's wives, but the strange attire of one Dr. Mary Walker. The doctor — as was her habit — wore trousers. Congress supposedly had consented to her appearance in male attire, but the records yield no evidence. Dr. Walker, who had been commissioned a lieutenant and an assistant surgeon during the Civil War, was the first woman to serve officially on the staff of any army in wartime. When taken prisoner, she was exchanged for a soldier and awarded a medal. Afterward, she paid occasional surprise visits to Washington circles from her habitat in Rome, N. Y.

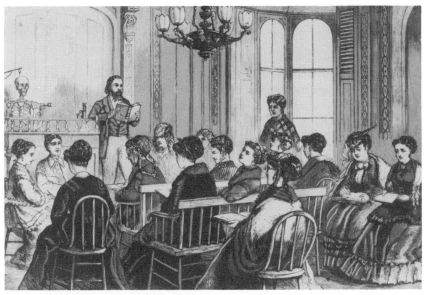

Lecture at Woman's Medical College at the New York Infirmary, 1870.

Dr. Walker had been preceded in her profession by Elizabeth Blackwell, who won her diploma from Geneva Medical College on January 23, 1849. Rejected by a host of schools, she had entered Geneva backed by the unanimous vote of the student body. Later, she worked at La Maternité in Paris. After losing an eye from an accidental infection, she returned home undaunted, and started her own dispensary in a rented room near Tompkins Square in New York. In 1857 this humble establishment became the New York Infirmary for Women and Children, to this day a bright spot in New York's medical picture.

Earlier in the century, the Philadelphia County Medical Society had solemnly pronounced women unfit for the profession, "due to their delicate organization and predominance of the nervous system." But the ladies refused to be delicate. In 1850, they founded the first real training center for women, the Woman's Medical College of Pennsylvania, an institution which still flourishes.

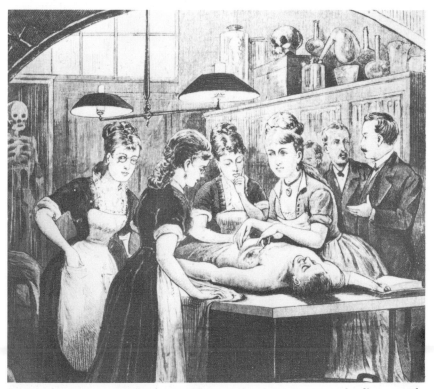

Women students during dissection. Their study of anatomy was loudly opposed.

Fine women doctors continued to appear as the century wore on. A French writer observed that woman doctors, "Therapy in Bloomers," were a definite feature of the American scene. Among them, Mary Putnam, deserves especial mention. She took her degree in Paris, joined the New York County Medical Society, married its president, Dr. Abraham Jacobi, and later became the first woman member of the New York Academy of Medicine. By the 20th century, women had made headway in almost every field of medical endeavor.

277

IN PRAISE OF
THE COUNTRY DOCTOR

COMPANION FROM THE CRADLE
TO THE GRAVE

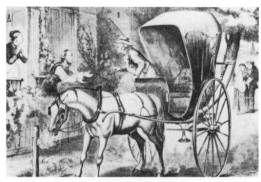

"*Doctor, come quickly!*" *An emergency call, 1871.*

It is doubtful whether the old-time country practitioner could hold his own in matters of science against a modern first-year medical student. But if the horse and buggy doctor lacked technical knowledge, he made up for it with intuitive discernment. He knew his patients intimately — their background, their character; he treated people rather than afflictions. And because of his sympathy toward human suffering — which Osler has called the mainspring of all good medicine — he brought solace and comradeship to troubled homes. In the community, he held an exalted position; the people looked on him almost as an arbiter of Life and Death.

Unquestionably, the modern doctor, with his instruments and knowledge, can do incomparably more for his patients, but for all-around medical wisdom, the old-time practitioner has set a great example. His selfless service to man remains an inspiration to this day.

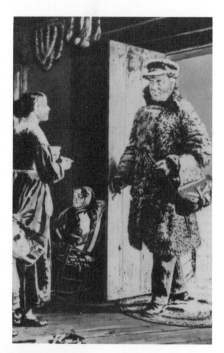

Worried New England mother welcomes doctor. Painting by Thomas W. Wood (right); "Let's see what the trouble is." Pen and ink drawing by A. B. Frost (below, left); Outdoor office hours. Country doctor on horseback dispenses counsel and medicine to rural patients (below right).

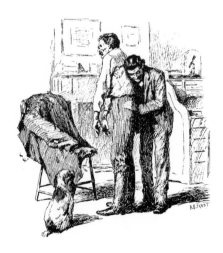

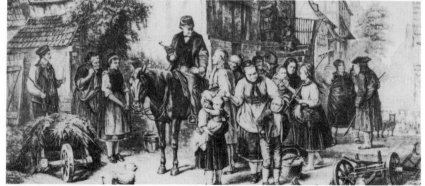

278

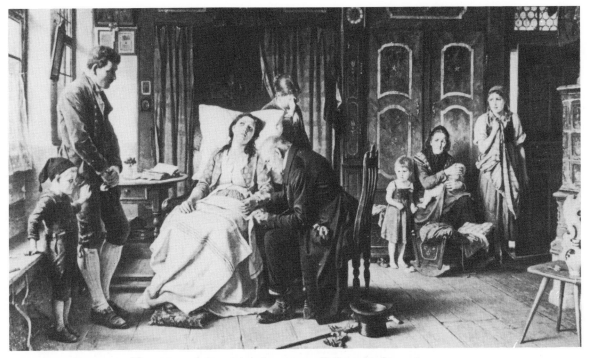

The country doctor in his classic pose: Dedicated to his patients —
but helpless in the face of afflictions such as heart attack (see
painting, above, by Benjamin Vautier) and diphtheria (painting,
below, by Sir Luke Fildes).

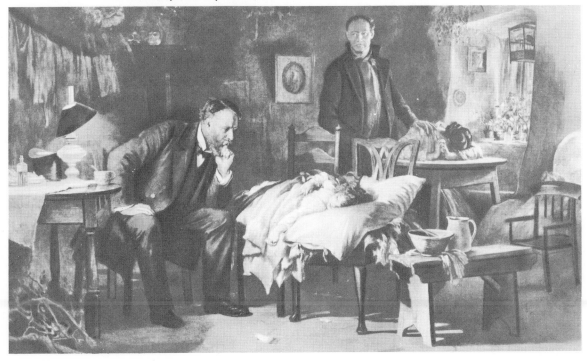

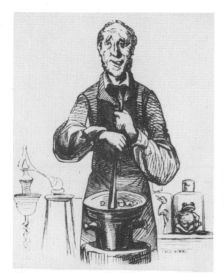

FOR ALL THESE ILLS . . .

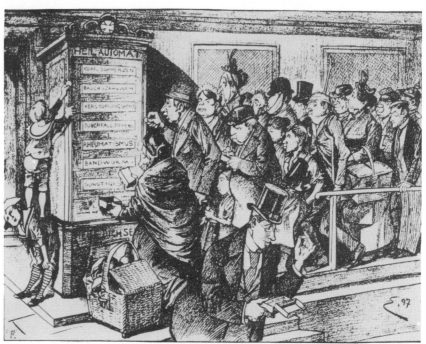

Heal automat: German cartoon shows mechanical dispensing machine with "cures for headache, indigestion, rheumatism" at the drop of a nickel.

In all ages, the sick have clamored for quick cures, and medical sectists, faddists, or downright quacks have answered the call. The advancing Age of Science proved no different in this respect, unless perchance, it proved worse. Talk of the "wonders of science" was in the air. Popular magazines bulged with new "discoveries," and their advertising pages carried heartening news: from now on, if the promises were to be believed, healing was to be by pills . . . and the doctor appeared all but obsolete.

Quackery became big business after the Civil War, when the amateur peddlers of the '40s were outdistanced by manufacturers of patent medicines. On the printed pages, sure cure drugs were now praised to the skies. Some were harmless — others were not. Shipped all over the country, the people swallowed them, literally and figuratively, because they wanted the solace which the medical profession could not honestly give them.

The questionable right to deceive the public went unchallenged until the early 20th century. At that time, an aroused and reorganized American Medical Association helped to expose the shady manipulations that had made many a medicine maker a millionaire. The Pure Food and Drug Acts soon followed, backed by the manufacturers of ethical products. Meanwhile, the American people had suffered a great deal. Yet as Arthur Schlesinger has remarked, the whole episode was almost a tribute to the robustness of the homo americanus. A less sturdy nation might have been exterminated!

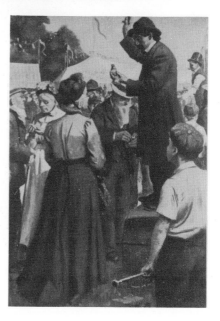

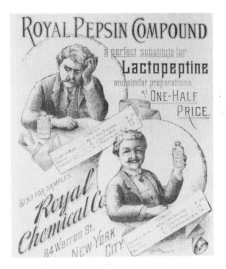

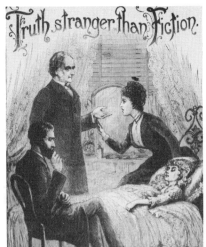

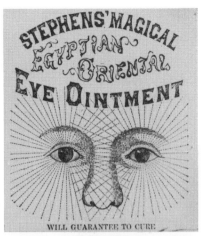

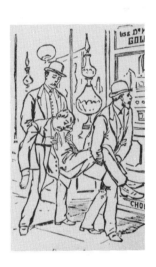

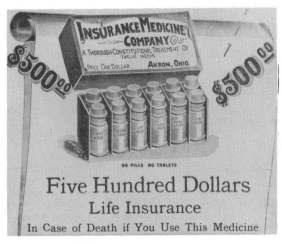

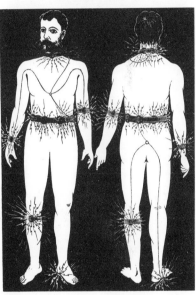

Five Hundred Dollars
Life Insurance
In Case of Death if You Use This Medicine

For all these Ills

Costiveness and Biliousness,
Sour Stomach, Flatulence,
Foul Breath, and Colics,
Failure of Appetite,
Constipation,
Eruptions,

Clogged Liver, Bilious Fevers,
Deterioration of Kidneys,
Enlargement of Liver,
Indigestion, Dropsy,
Jaundice, Piles,
Rheumatism,

**TAKE
AYER'S
PILLS**

Dysentery,
Anæmia, Nausea,
Diarrhœa, Worms,
Pimples, Sties, Boils,
Inflammation of Bowels,
Nervousness, Ennui, Insomnia,

Dyspepsia,
Melancholia,
Nervous Debility,
Torpidity of the Liver,
Heart Disease, Headaches,
Stomach, Back and Side Pains.

Rescue FOR Weak Men

Prof. Jules Laborde's Wonderful French Preparation of
"CALTHOS" that Restores Lost Manhood.

FIVE DAYS' TRIAL TREATMENT
Absolutely **Free** by Sealed Mail.

NO C.O.D. OR DEPOSIT SCHEME.

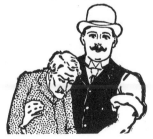

The marvelous French remedy, "CALTHOS,"
recently introduced in this country by the Von
Mohl Co., of Cincinnati, Ohio, one of the largest,
richest and most responsible business firms in the
United States, has attracted the attention of the
entire medical profession because of the wonder-

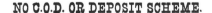

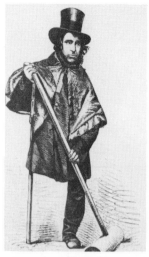

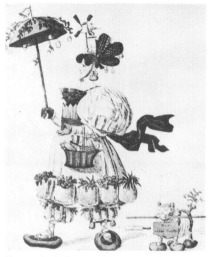

SANITATION
FOR CITIES - -
AT LAST

Before rise of municipal hygiene only feeble attempts had been . made to remove filth from streets.

Fear of cholera since 1830's led Europeans to try ridiculous protective measures such as "anti-cholera garb."

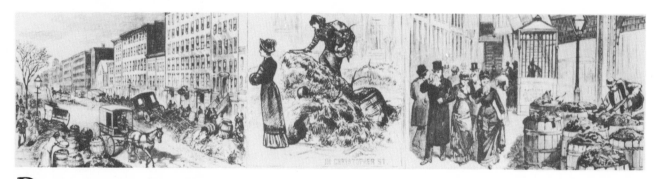

During the midcentury medicine expanded its work in a new direction. The doctor, always a servant of man, now became a servant of cities, nations and humanity as a whole. The age of Public Health had dawned.

Since the late 18th century there had been a growing concentration of people in the manufacturing centers Slum districts had grown alarmingly. The resultant squalor was unmatched in history. The humanitarians were shocked by it, the sanitarians saw it as a breeding ground for mass affliction. Both groups banded together and

backed by doctors embarked on a crusade for better community health.

The sanitary movement quickly gained momentum throughout industrial Europe. It was in England, however, where conditions were worst that its most outspoken leaders appeared Edwin Chadwick (1800-1890) awakened the British people and the government to check the health hazards of the cities. He demanded proper drainage, removal of refuse and an adequate water supply. Chadwick enforced the impact of his message by the employment of vital statistics. They showed irrefutably

how slum clearance and the control of social environment could stamp out wholesale tragedy and economic loss. Chadwick joined forces with Dr. T. Southwood Smith to formulate the fundamental credo of modern preventive medicine: that the health of the individual is indivisibly tied up with the health of the populace at large. In 1848 the British Government under pressure of the Health of Towns Pioneers finally took action. It set up a General Board of Health with both Chadwick and Dr. T. Southwood Smith as commissioners.

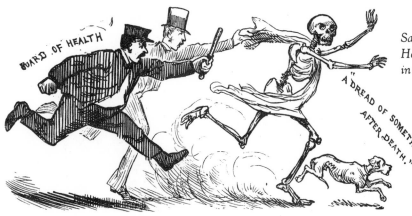

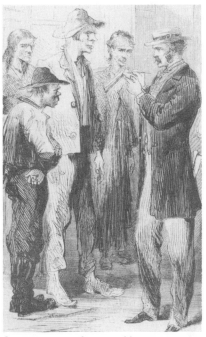

Sanitary reforms effected by New York Health Bill of 1866, received accolade in Harper's Weekly cartoon (left).

In America, the sanitary committees met with the usual public indifference. In addition, these groups had to overcome the obstacle of political finagling. Big city bosses used jobs in the street-cleaning department as political plums. Influential saloon-keepers were made health wardens. If health boards were established, they were staffed by aldermen or inefficient stooges. When New York City was threatened by cholera, for example, Mayor Fernando Wood refused to call out the board. "I consider the Board more dangerous to the city," he said, "than the Cholera."

At the same time, New York City harboured 100,000 slum dwellers and about 20,000 "damp-cellar inhabitants." The stench and filth in the downtown district made breathing almost impossible.

Statistics on slums sold sanitary reforms to citizens. From its start in 1847, A.M.A. had backed slum clearing.

The connection between disease and filth was evident, but the city fathers ignored it until Stephen Smith and a committee of irate citizens finally pried open their eyes.

In February, 1866, the Metropolitan Health Bill was passed. It provided for a nine-man Board of Health — three of them physicians. This group was given full responsibility to bring about sanitary reform. Their energetic clean-up measures (see illustrations on this page) set the pattern for the establishment of permanent health administrations in many other cities and states.

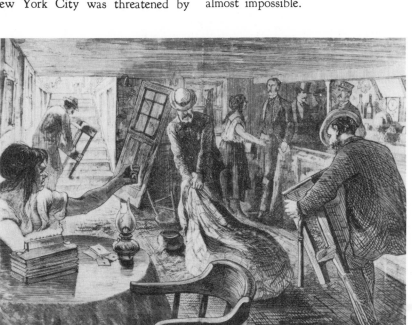

"Cave Dweller" is evicted by officials of New York City Health Department.

YELLOW FEVER RIPS THE SOUTH
ITS RAVAGES SPEED SANITARY REFORM

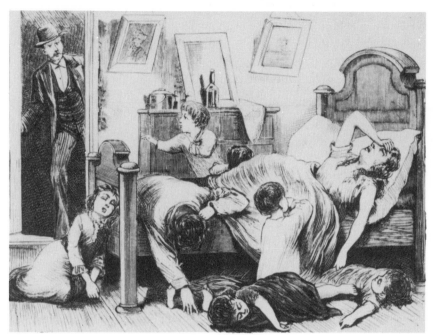

"The children rolled around on the floor and screamed" (Leslie's Weekly).

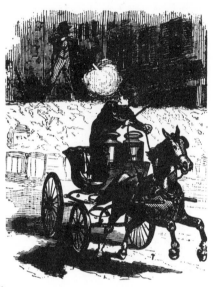

Shooting evaders of quarantine (Memphis).

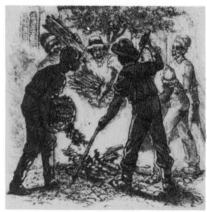

"Fires are burned at night for the purification of the atmosphere . . ."

Soon after its inception in 1866, the New York City Board of Health faced its first crucial test. A wave of cholera threatened the city. But thanks to the clean-up measures recently instituted, cholera failed to assume epidemic proportions. This success did much to propagate the idea of sanitation. The gospel caught on in the North, but the Southern states, exhausted by four years of war, and unable to raise their hygienic standards, remained easy prey to epidemics.

Yellow Fever had never been quite absent from the Southern coastal regions. In 1878, it struck across the Gulf States with unusual fury.

In retrospect, this quickfire spread seems easy to explain. The sanitary conditions in Memphis and other Southern cities had reached an all-time low. Pavements had decayed to the point where "the soil was reeking with offal and excreta of ten-thousand families." There were no garbage or refuse collection systems to speak of, but there were plenty of corrupt politicians. As Keating wrote at the time: "The glamours of the gutter politicians are more effective than the warnings and appeals of skilled sanitarians." In Memphis, New Orleans and Vicksburg, the cities which were hardest hit, boards of health existed in name only. No wonder that the scenes that ensued when yellow fever broke out were essentially like those of the famous London Plague of 1665, only now the caskets came by the trainload instead of the cartload. About 90 to 100 victims died each day in each of the three major cities. Local and state governments were unprepared to take any effective steps to alleviate the suffering.

Volunteers disinfected stricken homes, and destroyed the blankets, sheets, pillows and clothing of the dead. But all to no avail. Later, a Senate committee called for the tightening of quarantine measures, since the "affliction was indubitably transmitted by passengers from tropical countries." Unwittingly, a reporter for *Frank Leslie's Illustrated Newspaper* came much closer to the truth. He described a Memphis home in which the mother had just died and the children were brought in to say goodbye: "She had the black vomit, and they were told they had better not kiss her, but they did, and as they came up one after the other, and gave her the last kiss on earth, their lips were stained with that horrible stream of death. And what is almost miraculous, none of them have caught the fever yet." About twenty years later, the "miracle" was explained dramatically.

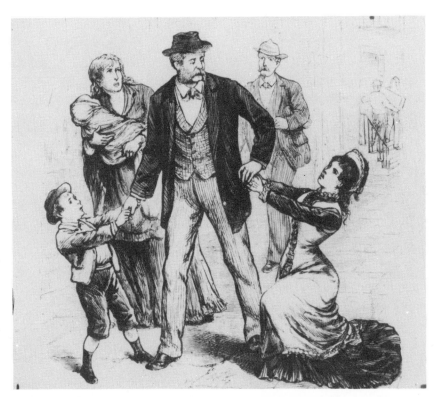

A doctor with too many patients: "I have seen women and children on their knees begging him to come to their homes — some of them trying to drag him in."

EPILOGUE: REED AND GORGAS

During the Spanish-American War, American soldiers were dying at the rate of 200 a day, but not from enemy action. Like the people of Memphis, they were victims of yellow fever. In 1900, the U. S. Government sent a commission to Cuba to solve the riddle of this disease and to wipe it out if possible. The commission decided to follow the much contested theory of Dr. Carlos Finlay, a Cuban physician, who held that an insect carrier was involved. This theory led Dr. Jesse Lazear to produce the disease in test cases via insect bites. Tragically, he died while proving his point (Sept. 25, 1900). But Walter Reed, inspired by Lazear's notebook, closed the loop-

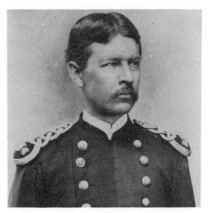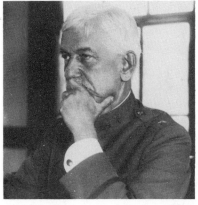

Major Walter Reed (left) backed by research of Dr. Lazear pronounced mosquito carrier of yellow fever. General Gorgas (right) freed Cuba, Panama of scourge.

holes in the commission's argument. Controlled experiments proved that yellow fever was not transmitted by black vomit, stricken persons, or contaminated clothing, but by a mosquito, Aedes Aegypti. Once it was known that the mosquito served as the vector of yellow fever, Chief Sanitary Officer Gorgas was able to clear Cuba of the dread disease in three short months.

285

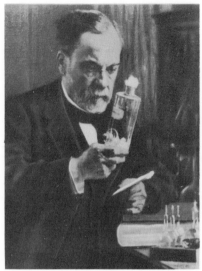

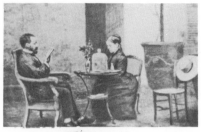

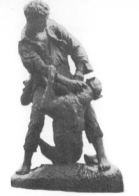

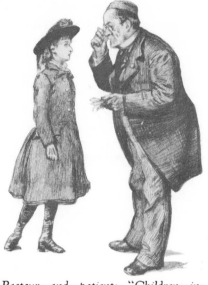

Louis Pasteur (1822-1895). "Chance only favors the mind that is prepared."

Pasteur and patient: "Children inspired him with a loving solicitude."

PASTEUR - PEER OF PREVENTIVE MEDICINE

While their intentions were praiseworthy, the Sanitarians could do only half the job of wiping out mass afflictions. The other half — actual prevention of epidemic diseases — was left undone because next to nothing was known about their causes. So people continued to die in droves when epidemics struck.

However, in the '60s and '70s, Louis Pasteur, a French chemist, was at work on a bold plan of action. His experiments in wine and beer fermentation had already given Lister enough insight to lessen putrefaction in surgical wounds. Now Pasteur himself traced out the germ theory of infection and thereby gave a new direction to the fight against disease. His crusade for preventive medicine eventually supplanted the more defensive approach of sanitation.

Pasteur was well-equipped to lead such a crusade. First, he was a laboratory scientist, with no stomach for armchair theories. Words like miasma, humours, and spontaneous generation did not exist in his vocabulary. Second, he was a practical and a social scientist. While Faraday fled from the siren call of industry, Pasteur answered it. He put his talents to work for the big national industries, be it beer, wine, silk, or cattle. This helped to impress his skeptical countrymen with the importance of science. Third and last, Pasteur was an ardent and excellent propagandist. He fought, he talked, he demonstrated. And so, with the aid of all these qualities, he was able to prove and publicize his momentous theories: that specific microbes were at the root of specific diseases, and that such diseases could be combatted by

their own causative microbes in weakened form.

Pasteur's transfer from practical chemistry to medical science is an oft-told and dramatic episode. In the 1850s, the French wine and vinegar industries had been troubled by "sick" vats. Pasteur had been engaged to "cure" their products, and he had done so, first, by pointing out that some microbes produced healthy wine or vinegar, and that others spoiled the product; second, he had recommended practical measures for killing off the "bad" microbes, which descended upon the vats from the air. All microbes had parents, he said; they did not burst upon the scene spontaneously. This theory aroused the wrath of that "titanic" chemist Baron von Liebig. The baron said fermentation was strictly an inorganic, chemical reaction; worse yet, he refused to look at microbes under a microscope. In the battle which followed, Pasteur convinced his fellow scientists that he was right and the baron wrong.

The wine and vinegar industries saved, Pasteur was led to his second basic tenet: that disease, like fermentation, is a putrefactive process caused by microbes. Lister had acted on this ingenious equation in 1865 without proof, and long before that, Robert Boyle had stated that whoever controlled fermentation could also control disease. But Pasteur had the good fortune to put the theory to a practical test. Although he was an absolute novice in the field he undertook to save the million-dollar French silk industry (1865-1868). Technical experts had failed before him, but the indefatigable chemist found the guilty parasite, and showed his clients how to avoid further catastrophes.

Pasteur revolutionized both industry and medicine by using laboratory methods to fight disease. Through these methods he saved his country millions — enough, it has been estimated, to cover the indemnity paid by France to Germany after the Franco-Prussian War in 1871.

The work Pasteur had done in the silk region served him as an excellent introduction into other problems of animal and human pathology.

By the early 1880s, Pasteur had developed a vaccine from weakened bacilli to use against anthrax, a carbuncle disease of cattle. He announced his discovery in a brilliant public demonstration at Mélun in May, 1881. Its impact was hardly lessened when Koch, the great German scientist,

quietly and methodically proved that the vaccine was not very reliable. More important, Pasteur had worked out the principle of fighting microbes with microbes, and he carried this valuable insight into his research on rabies.

In 1884-85, Pasteur's laboratories re-echoed with the howls of mad dogs. He had learned to keep the hydrophobic virus in supply by injecting it into the brains of laboratory animals. Then, from the dried-out spinal tissues of such animals, he was able to produce a vaccine which made other laboratory animals gradually immune to rabic infection. This discovery was the magic key to disease prevention and it made the 1880s "the most wonderful period in medicine."

On July 6, 1885, Pasteur was asked to save the life of 9-year-old Joseph Meister, who had been gashed in 14 places by a mad dog. Pasteur prevented the boy's death with 14 injections. From then on, his laboratory took on all the characteristics of a dispensary. A picturesque and polyglot crowd of "bitten" people assembled there and begged Pasteur to save them. Infected children were sent from America. From Russia 19 men arrived terribly maimed by a mad wolf on the rampage.

Now that the new principle of immunity had been established, the fight against disease could move forward on the broad front of preventive medicine, and it was here that the Pasteurians carried the master's torch to greater triumphs.

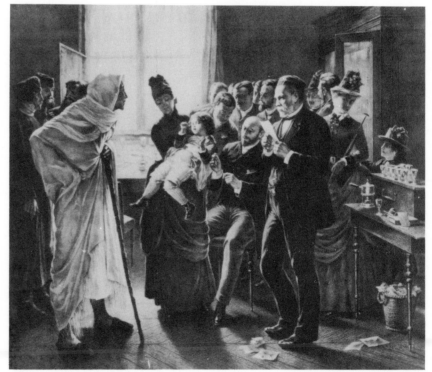

Pasteur supervising antirabic injection of patients bitten by mad animals. Successful treatments at Pasteur Institute, Paris, helped to establish science of immunity.

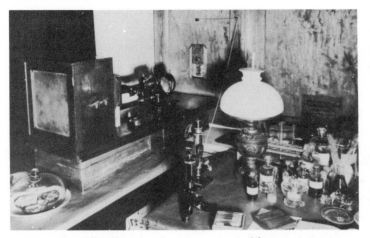

Koch's office at Wollstein, with camera to record bacteria.

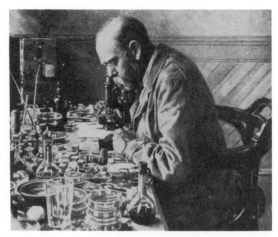

Koch looking for Rinderpest (cattle plague) microbe.

KOCH TRACKS DOWN TUBERCULOSIS

Great times are said to produce great men, or vice-versa. Whatever the case, the decades between 1870 and 1890, were certainly boom-times for great microbe hunters. In those years, Pasteur and Robert Koch changed the entire course of medical thinking. Yet two more strikingly different men would be hard to find. Pasteur, the ex-chemist, was intuitive and brilliant; Koch, the ex-doctor, was methodical, if devastating, in his experiments. If

Pasteur had made bacteriology a science — Koch made it an exact one. One pulled and capered, the other pushed, and so the chariot of medical progress began to roll with gathering speed toward a triumphant *fin de siècle.*

Koch became a self-made bacteriologist after a year's work as district physician in Wollstein, Silesia. His laboratory experience was limited and his equipment simple, except perhaps for the microscope which Frau Koch had given him on his 30th birthday in 1873. In a corner of his office he set out to examine the blood of animals which had died in a local epidemic of anthrax. First, he tracked down its causative bacillus; then he succeeded in breeding it in a "pure culture." From this culture, he could infect other animals at will. This closed the circle of evidence and proved that anthrax was caused by a specific microbe.

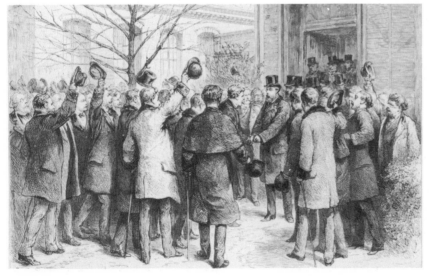

Dr. Koch cheered for discovery of tuberculin (1890). Hopes that it would cure tuberculosis were unfulfilled. It proved useful in diagnosing this disease.

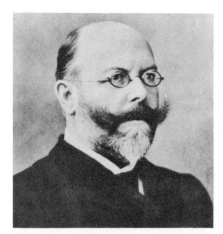

F. A. J. Loeffler, Koch's assistant at Berlin Institute for Infectious Diseases.

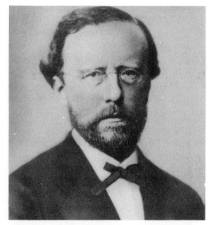

Theodor Klebs discovered, with Loeffler, bacillus causing diphtheria (1884).

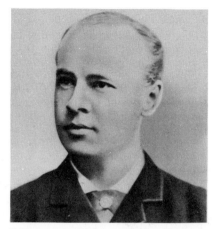

William H. Welch studied with Koch, introduced his teachings in America.

Koch demonstrated his findings on April 29, 1876 before a group of scientists of the University of Breslau. Proof for his epochal verdict that specific diseases were caused by specific germs was so compelling that pathologist Julius Cohnheim, rushed to his laboratory admonishing his students, "Drop everything and go at once to Koch. I consider this the greatest discovery yet made in bacteriology."

In the following years Dr. Koch made rapid progress. Called to the Reichsgesundheitsamt in Berlin in 1880 he was able to pursue his research under more favorable conditions and with the aid of competent assistants. This group embarked on a fast and furious hunt and succeeded in tracking down microbes that caused gonorrhoea, diphtheria, typhoid fever, gangrene and many other diseases.

Of all his triumphs it was Koch's discovery of the tubercle bacillus that had perhaps the greatest impact on human welfare. Koch showed the true cause of the White Plague — and pointed the way to its extermination. With the aid of microscopes, municipal

physicians could now single out afflicted slum-dwellers and remove them from crowded quarters.

Through experiments in Egypt and India, Koch found the comma bacillus the true cause of cholera. He erred in 1890 when he announced his tuberculine as a "cure" for tuberculosis. (It proved a valuable diagnostic aid.) Just the same his contribution to medical science was magnificent, permanent, and beyond reproach.

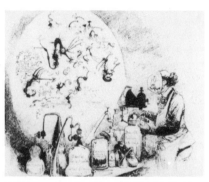

"Discovering Bacillus of Health." Cartoon on "bug hunting mania" (Robida).

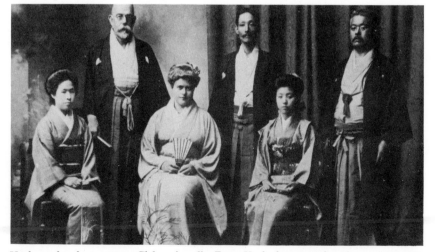

Koch on his last trip to Tokyo (1908); Frau Koch, his second wife, 29 years his junior, at his left; Kitasato, his Japanese pupil, antitoxin pioneer, is at far right.

THE ASEPTIC METHOD

CLEAN HANDS - - GERM-FREE INSTRUMENTS

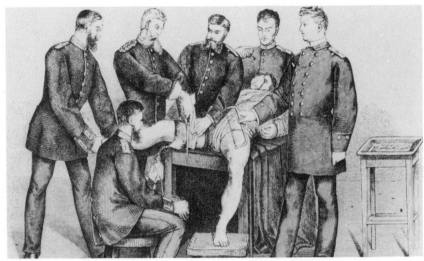

Esmarch performs amputation during Franco-Prussian War (1870-1871).

A great change in operative technique took place between 1880 and 1900. The revelations of Pasteur and Koch on the nature of bacteria led to a renewed attack against wound infection.

Earlier, Lister had cried out against descending airborne germs; he had devised a carbolic spray to protect wounds during operations but when the airborne germs proved rather harmless he abandoned his spraygun (1887).

Less irritating ways to prevent infection were soon developed in Germany. At von Bergmann's clinic in Berlin, surgeons became men-in-white; their hands were thoroughly disinfected before each operation; instruments, towels, gowns — all the paraphernalia of the operating table — were "pasteurized" by the simple expedient of boiling them in that very symbol of the aseptic age: the sterilizer.

In 1874 Dr. John Erichsen of University Hospital, London, had solemnly declared the intestinal region "forever shut from the intrusion of the wise and humane surgeon." But as the dangers of infection decreased, the abdominal cavity became what W. W. Keen has called "the surgeon's playground." Von Bergmann, Billroth and von Mikulicz fairly romped there.

In Central Europe, aseptic surgery received its strongest impetus from Theodor Billroth, a rare blend of artist and surgeon. During his most productive years in Vienna (1867-1893) he brought visceral surgery into its own. He was the first to excise cancer of the stomach and he devised many other important operations in the abdominal region.

Billroth cherished as the greatest compliment the remark of a gentleman who approached him after a clinic. "You have given your students the complete truth as one rarely hears it." The gentleman was Dr. Samuel Gross, dean of American surgery.

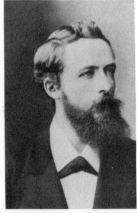 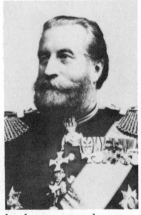 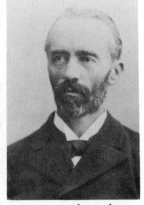

Von Mikulicz (left) specialized in intestinal surgery; wore cotton gloves during operation; Ernst von Bergmann (center) headed Berlin School, introduced sterilizer; Theodore Kocher (right), Swiss surgeon and pathologist was first to excise thyroid.

290

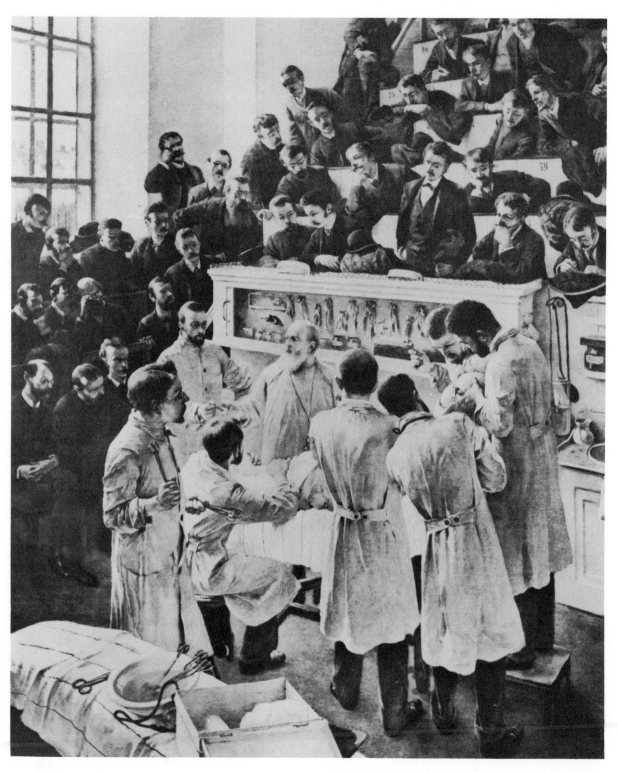

Billroth in Vienna amphitheatre. German surgeons introduced asepsis, made abdomen "surgeon's playground."   291

SURGERY: Continued
AMERICA

Dr. Samuel D. Gross, Philadelphia surgeon during operation at Jefferson College (note frock coat). Painting by Thomas Eakins, 1875. This famed surgeon preached and practiced high professional ideals — his integrity and benevolence made him a symbol of medicine in the native American grain.

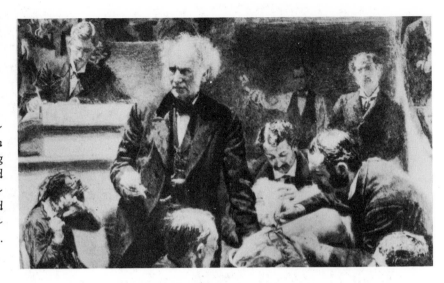

On the whole, the surgeons of America were a progressive group. Their native ingenuity and pluck made them daring but unruffled operators in the famous "McDowell tradition." Even the old-world leaders in scientific medicine had to admit this. Dr. Samuel D. Gross, of Philadelphia, was lionized in Paris; Valentine Mott of New York received a call to Constantinople to extirpate a wen on the Sultan's head — while trembling court physicians applauded; and Dr. Marion Sims, the gynecological surgeon, was said to be so famous that he could settle in any capital of Europe and immediately be swamped with patients.

But these men were slow to adopt antisepsis. When Lister came to America for the 1876 Centennial, he was merely received politely. There was no marked progress in the prevention of infection. Frock coats still prevailed in the operating room. It was not until the 1880's that Listerian principles were established, at Mount Sinai Hospital, New York, through the pioneer work of Dr. Arpad Gerster.

Other doctors made a partial, if superstitious, adknowledgment of Lister's doctrine: they consulted the weather to fix the day of operation — a northeast wind was supposed to bear erysipela germs. No responsible surgeon would dare to touch a knife. But an ill wind with all its evils occasionally does blow some good — even for surgery.

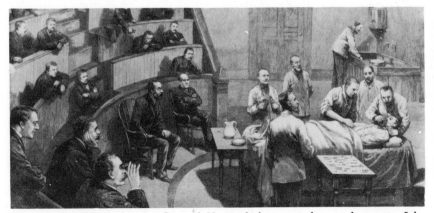

Operation in Massachusetts General Hospital shows trend toward asepsis. John C. Warren, grandson of anæsthesia sponsor and a Lister student, was surgeon here.

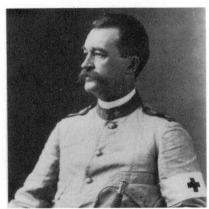

Nicholas Senn, Chicago Intestinal surgeon, operated on pancreatic cyst.

On August 21, 1883 a cyclone struck Rochester, Minnesota. One-third of the frontier town was destroyed. There were no hospital facilities for the injured, so Dr. William W. Mayo, the local practitioner, was asked to set up an emergency medical service. He acquitted himself so well that the nuns from the nearby Convent of St. Francis offered to build him a permanent establishment. In this way, St. Mary's Hospital, the first unit of the Mayo Clinic was founded. The 40-bed hospital (cost: $75,000) opened in Rochester on October 1, 1889.

When the fateful cyclone struck in 1883, Dr. Mayo's sons, William and Charles, were "dissecting a beef's eye" at a butcher shop in nearby Clayton, Minnesota. The two boys had acquired an interest in surgery while accompanying their father on his rounds. A Mayo family legend holds that Charlie gave anesthesia when only nine, standing on a cracker-box. During the 1890's the Mayo brothers became an amazing surgical team, as well as ingenious hospital administrators. By the turn of the century, they were handling an impressive number of operations — 3151 in 1904 alone. The Mayos adapted the new aseptic procedures and made many original contributions to surgical technique. In addition they provided for a close cooperation between operating room and laboratory. It is this vital union that has made the Mayo Clinic one of the greatest clinical and research institutions in the world.

Aseptic surgery was fully developed by early 1900's. Dr. Charles McBurney, famed for appendix incision, during operation Roosevelt Hospital, New York.

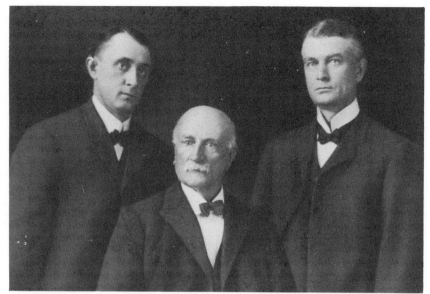

The Doctors Mayo of Rochester, Minnesota: Charles, William Sr., and William.

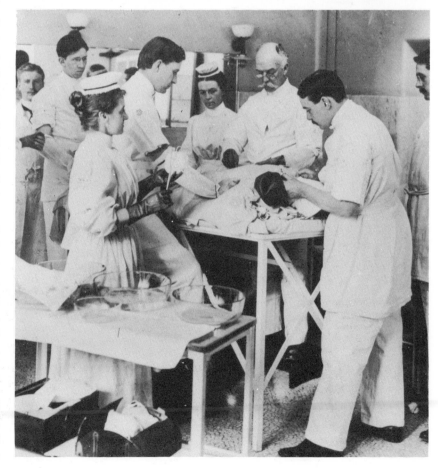

NURSES ARE NEEDED

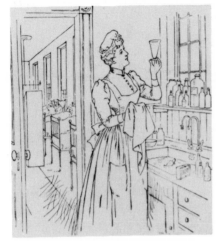

Advent of aseptic method increased need for nurses trained in ward, laboratory.

Lister's antiseptic methods were opposed with vehemence by many of the hospitals; they wanted to avoid the fuss and bother of carbolic sprays. Then too, there was the problem of personnel. Most hospitals were understaffed. Trained nurses were essential to carry through antiseptic — and later aseptic procedures. At first the doctors did not take much interest in the training of hospital aids. They even voiced the uncomfortable feeling that enlightened nurses would meddle in the doctor's domain.

Dr. Samuel Gross tried to demolish this prejudice in 1869 with a manifesto to the American Medical Association. He emphatically declared: "The medical profession needs nurses," and he called on physicians to cheerfully contribute to their training. "Nursing in its more exalted sense," he continued, "is as much of an art and a science as medicine."

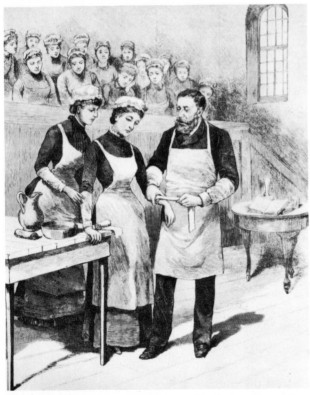

Physician gives practical course in bandaging for student-nurses at Old Blockley Hospital, Philadelphia, 1885.

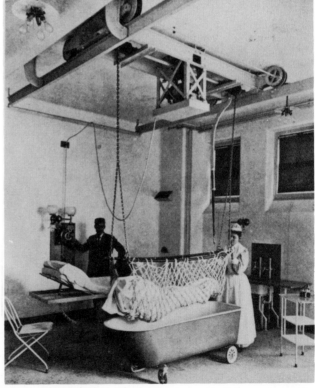

Nurses at New York Hospital use crane to lower sunstroke victim into cold water bath (circa 1880).

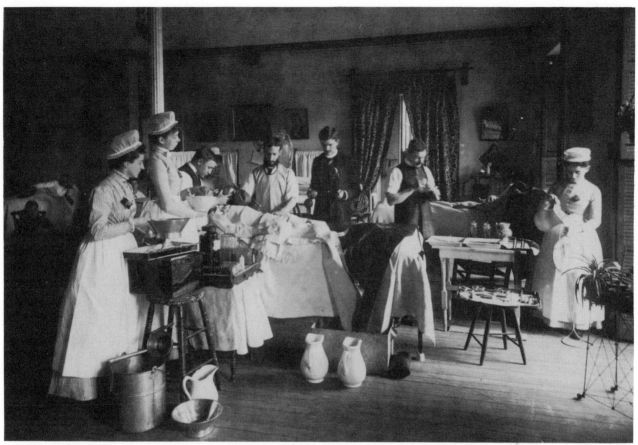

Operation in ward of Bellevue Hospital (circa 1880). Nurses' caps and striped blouses were introduced here in 1876.

But in 1869 there was as yet nothing exalted about nursing. The average hospital was a rather filthy place; its patients were poor and its nurses little more than wardmaids. At Bellevue, "10-day women" — drunk and disorderly "gamps" — were allowed to work off their sentences as nurses' aids.

Such conditions gave impetus to the struggle for improvement, especially at Bellevue. Here student nurses chipped in $1 of their $12 monthly allowance to improve teaching facilities. After 1873, when regular training had started at Bellevue, a number of other nursing schools opened their

doors. The profession developed in efficiency and self-assurance. Women of high calibre joined it, and often led the way toward hospital reform. Like-minded doctors and administrators helped to transform many hospitals from places of horror into centers of socio-medical progress.

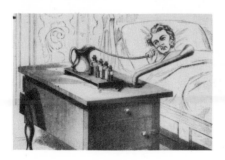

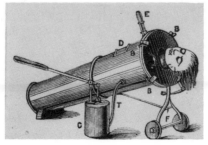

Mechanized Nursing: Unattended patient obtains medicine from nursing table. Patented 1869 (far left).

Forerunner of the iron lung (near left): Spirophore was used to restore asphyxiated persons and newborn infants.

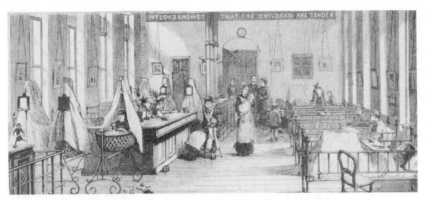

East London Hospital for Children was early center of pediatric research.

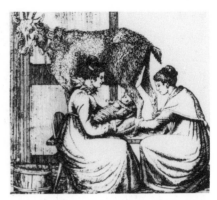

"Fresh Milk" before Age of Pasteur.

CHILD CARE - - - A NEW SCIENCE

In almost every age, reformers had striven to alleviate the suffering of children. But in spite of their efforts, child mortality had remained fearfully high. Doctors did not know enough about the causes of infant diseases, consequently, mothers had to stand by helplessly and watch their children die from attacks by invisible foes.

The discoveries in the field of bacteriology changed this condition. Preventive measures were developed against diphtheria and other children's diseases; ways were found to diagnose tuberculosis, and in time to test susceptibility to scarlet fever.

Though Pasteur's work was accountable for most of these advances, he ranks as the child's greatest benefactor for still another reason. The process of "pasteurization" made possible a controlled supply of germ-free milk. Before its introduction, milk-borne epidemics were common. Each summer thousands of city children died from *cholera infantum*, or suffered from

lesser afflictions. All this was gradually eliminated as pasteurization became widely adopted — and legally enforced.

Once cows' milk had been made safe, chemical researchers were able to modify its components and adapt them

to the needs of the individual infant. This was especially helpful in cases where mother's milk was not available, or perhaps inadvisable. Until the adoption of these and other blessings, pediatricians had to struggle long and hard to gain academic recognition.

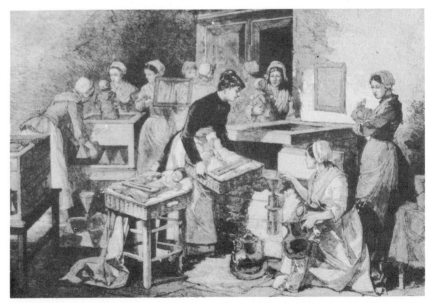

Incubators warmed by kerosene flame were first used at La Maternité in Paris, 1884.

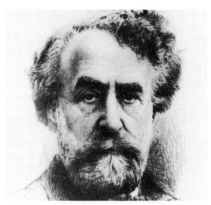

Dr. Abraham Jacobi, Dean of pediatrics.

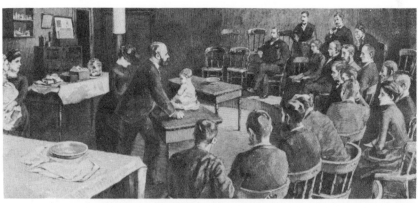

Children's Clinic at the New York Polyclinic School of Medicine, 1890.

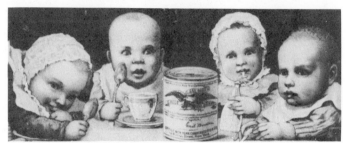

Condensed milk helped to simplify infant feeding. Borden, 1886.

In American medical schools, pediatrics was taught (if taught at all) as part of gynecology. Then, during the 1860's, a vertible one-man revolution took place. In 1853, Dr. Abraham Jacobi had arrived from Germany to settle in New York. Here he pursued the problems of pediatrics with humanitarian zeal and medical acumen. In 1870 he was appointed to the chair of clinical pediatrics at Columbia University. (It was 30 years before he became a full professor.

When pasteurization was vindicated, he made "boil the milk until you see the bubbles" his most effective slogan in fighting an old prejudice: that only raw milk had any benefit. Jacobi used intubation in cases of diptheria — to keep the larynx open — a technique developed by his colleague, Joseph P. O'Dwyer. When diphtheria antitoxin became available, Jacobi advocated its use. Still vigorous in advanced age, he delivered a masterful address as the newly-elected president of the American Medical Association when he was 82.

RISE OF THE FORMULA

To fulfill the infant's nutritional needs, Dr. Jacobi recommended that milk should be diluted. But that was as far as he would go; he wanted no part of the new-fangled process of "percentage feeding." The baby's stomach, he said, was no reagent bottle.

Yet infant mortality was effectively reduced by the exact adjustment of milk-content to the child's metabolism. Thomas M. Rotch of Harvard was the first to develop this percentage feeding theory — the direct precursor of the modern formula. He based it on the amount of fat, protein and carbohydrate which an infant needs. By removing some cream from the milk and adding sugar, the percentage was properly adjusted. But the procedure was often discouragingly complicated, for example: in 1904 a book on the subject offered two pages of algebraic equations to aid the perplexed practitioner.

Things are simpler now. The percentage theory has been replaced by the caloric theory, which is based on the infant's need for 50 calories per pound of bodyweight per day. In the ideal formula — which still has its percentage aspects — the emphasis is on the supply of calories: 50% from carbohydrates, 35% from fats, and 15% from proteins.

In this same period, condensed milk was to become an additional boon to mothers. Introduced in 1856 by Gail Borden, manufacturing methods were gradually standardized. Condensed milk soon proved a sterile, highly digestible food for children.

297

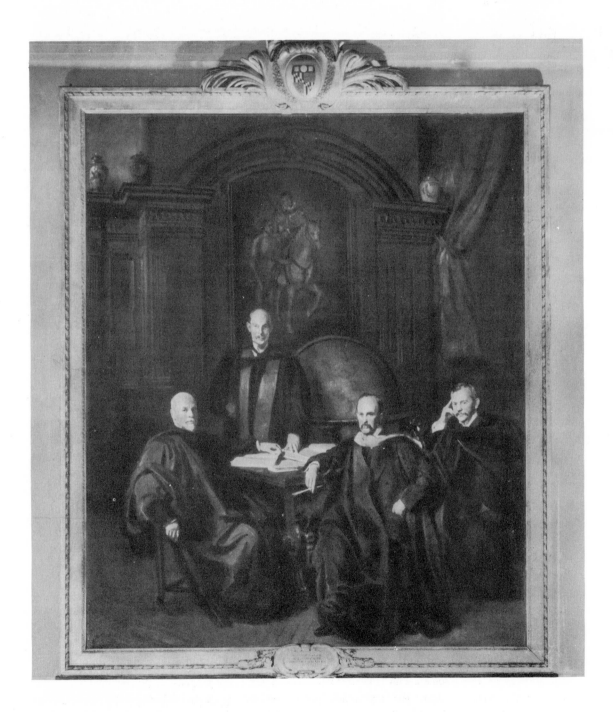

The Four Doctors: W. H. Welch, pathology, W. S. Halsted, surgery; W. Osler, med-
icine; H. A. Kelly, gynecology. (Painting by Sargent, Welch Medical Library.)

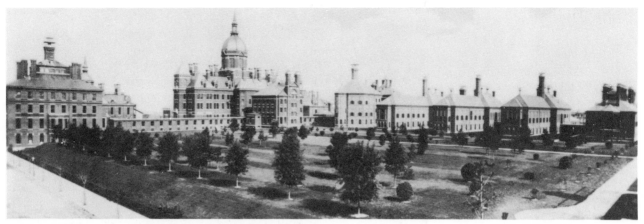

The Johns Hopkins Hospital at the time of its opening, 1889.

GREAT DOCTORS - - GREAT TEACHERS

"We have broken completely with the idea that reading books and listening to lectures is an adequate training for doctors."
— William H. Welch

Throughout the 19th century a regrettable laxity prevailed in the training of American doctors. Many medical schools indulged in what Osler politely called the "unrestricted manufacture of diplomas." In Baltimore alone, there were five medical schools before the Hopkins opened its doors, and one of them granted the right to practice after a two-year course.

Johns Hopkins, a Quaker philanthropist, had something better in mind. His will provided for the founding of a medical school with university standing linked closely with a hospital to be erected at the same time. Both institutions were to unite in the education of doctors and in the training of medical scientists equipped to do original research. The program was a novel one, and the men who were called upon to carry it through made it an inspiring success.

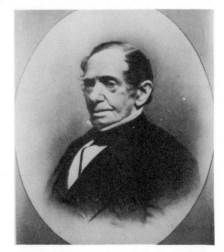

Johns Hopkins (1795-1873) endowed medical school integrated with hospital.

The trustees under the leadership of President Gilman selected a "senior staff" consisting of young but brilliant men: William H. Welch was 34, William Osler 39, William S. Halsted 37, Howard A. Kelly only 31. The head of each hospital department was to direct the corresponding section of the school. There were great medical teachers in other universities such as Philadelphia, Northwestern, Harvard, New York, but their work was hampered by the lack of a unified plan and by the paucity of laboratory equipment. The Hopkins set out to give doctors a background, on a par with European standards and it provided the instrumentalities to achieve this purpose. It tried to attract young men of high caliber, well versed already in the preclinical subjects. In fact, admissions standards were so high that the staff first doubted whether enough acceptable aspirants could be found. As Osler said to Welch: "We were lucky to get in as professors, for I am sure that neither you nor I would ever get in as students."

Work at the Johns Hopkins Medical School had already begun before the Hospital opened its doors in 1889. The Pathology Institute as the other departments, Medicine, Surgery and Gynecology, first served for postgraduate studies. In 1893 the graduates moved in and in 1895 the first full courses for undergraduates began:

JOHNS HOPKINS: Cont.
WELCH and HALSTED

Dr. William Welch arrived in Baltimore in 1885 to take up his duties as Chief Pathologist at Johns Hopkins. A year later, his favorite dream came true: he set up a postgraduate course in the newly equipped Pathology Laboratory.

The young professor had long discerned the widening gulf between American medical practice and the new scientific approach in Europe. As a student at the New York College of Physicians and Surgeons, he had listened to some excellent lectures, worked in a somewhat rickety laboratory, and visited a clinic each Saturday afternoon. After graduation, he had served a two-week internship. All of which seemed very inadequate to Welch.

The young pathologist took two trips to the Continent, worked there

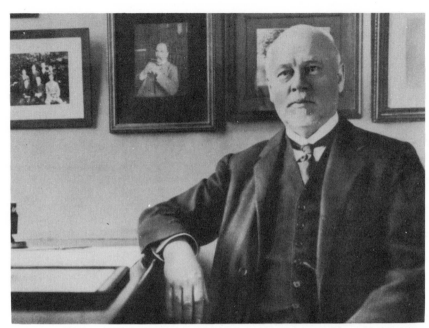

William "Popsy" Welch, pathologist. He was as stubby as he was erudite. It was said of him that nobody could prove legally that he had a neck.

in Cohnheim's laboratories at Breslau, and later with Koch, Klebs and Weigert. He watched Ludwig teach physiology at Leipzig, with the accent on experimental research. Between trips, he tried to introduce European teaching methods at Bellevue Hospital Medical College in New York. In 1878 three far-off rooms were placed at his disposal, plus "fully $25" for new equipment. When the class needed frogs, his sister caught them in the upstate marshes of New York. As the Flexners commented, "It was a banner day when the boxes of damp grass arrived croaking with their live cargo." When the Hopkins appointment came in 1884, and with it Welch's big chance, he took his second trip to Europe.

After studies in Vienna, Budapest, Prague and Leipzig, Welch arrived at the high point of his grand tour. In July 1885 he enrolled at the Institute of Koch in Berlin. His one month

laboratory course with the great bacteriologist had a lasting effect on Welch. He returned home with the burning conviction that American medical education has to be brought up to the standards of German laboratory medicine.

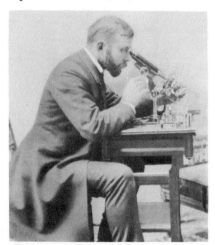

Student microscopist, ca. 1885. Welch after his studies in Germany taught young doctors scientific medicine.

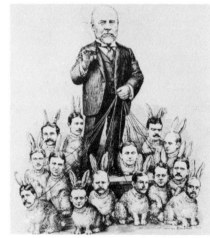

"Welch's Rabbits:" generation of scientists trained at the Hopkins. Cartoon by Max Broedel, medical illustrator.

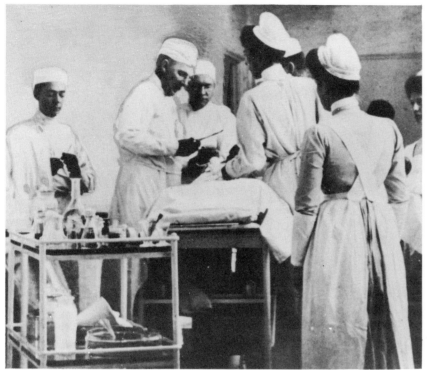
Halsted operating: the aloof "Professor" raised surgery at the Hopkins to a fine art. He often spent four painstaking hours on a "simple" operation.

At Johns Hopkins, Welch put his knowledge of scientific medicine to work. Students learned by doing; they were given a chance at experimental research, usually in close connection with hospital cases. This alliance with practical medicine was made even closer by personal ties among the faculty. Students and house surgeons attended Welch's autopsies. Frequently Drs. Osler and Halsted added their comments to the demonstrations. Thus, Welch conducted the first *truly* pathological seminar in America. This seminar became the backbone of teaching at the Hopkins, and it also stimulated reform at other institutions. In Welch's own words, "it transformed the laboratory side of our teaching from the weakest to the strongest feature of the medical curriculum."

Welch also made his influence felt in the selection of the Johns Hopkins faculty. Much to his credit, he advocated the appointment of Dr. William Halsted as head of Surgery. Halsted, a dynamic New York surgeon, had been in grave danger of falling victim to a cocaine addiction which he had contracted during self-experimentation in local anesthesia. Two years of research work with Welch at the Hopkins redeemed him. In 1890 the trustees made him Surgeon-in-Chief.

Halsted fitted well into the Johns Hopkins mold. He was thoroughly convinced that surgery must be practiced and taught along scientific lines. Wards and operating rooms, he said, were "laboratories in the highest sense," and the operation itself only a small part of surgical procedure.

Halsted studied healing processes under the microscope; he searched insistently for safer operating techniques, and was meticulously slow in his own surgery. Other surgeons thought him a bit eccentric: "four hours to do a breast! four solid hours for an operation that ought to take an hour and a half at the most." But Halsted continued to take his time. He tied each blood vessel to keep the operation almost bloodless; he tried to match each wrinkle of the skin when suturing; and he kept his amphitheatre strictly aseptic.

It was this same passion for aseptic methods that brought about the introduction of rubber gloves into surgery. Halsted's head nurse, Miss Caroline Hampton, was using an antiseptic which irritated her hands. Halsted ordered some long rubber gloves for Miss Hampton. Then, on an aid's insistence, he adopted them himself during operations. Later on, Miss Hampton became Mrs. Halsted. So the advent of rubber gloves was, as John Finney — a Halsted associate put it — "a case where Venus rendered great aid to Aesculapius."

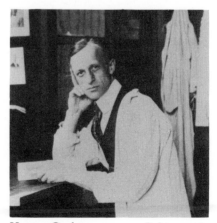
Harvey Cushing came to Baltimore in 1896 as Halstead's assistant and became much interested in bacteriology.

301

OSLER: GIANT OF THE WARDS

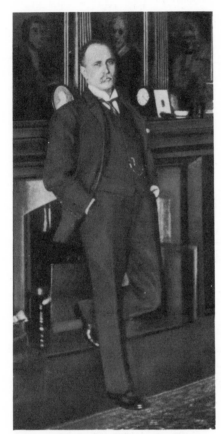

Osler at Oxford where he taught from 1905 until his death in 1919.

How did Osler look? Sargent wrestled with this question when he painted The Four Doctors (see pg. 298). Welch, Kelly and Halsted came to life on canvas at the first sitting. But Osler, "with an olive green forehead," seemed to change like a chameleon; Sargent had to make many sketches till he finally caught his subject. Some saw Osler as the physician incarnate; others as a "wonderful pirate."

302

Dr. William Osler came to Johns Hopkins in 1889 as Professor of Medicine and Physician-in-Chief. He was probably the most illustrious of the "four saints" and the institution's collective pulse quickened noticeably upon his arrival. During his 17 years in Baltimore, his warm personality did much to make faculty and students a "happy band of fellow-workers."

Osler was a many-sided man. To enumerate and appraise his contributions and traits puts one almost in a mood of despair. Even Cushing — who, in his 3 volume biography — neglected no postal card or dinner date with Osler, could not exhaust the subject.

Pathologist, clinician, educator, bibliophile, sanitarian, philosopher, writer of the most quotable English — Osler defies any simple description. As his own epitaph, he proposed: "He taught medical students in the wards;" and indeed, this was his most important contribution to the Hopkins plan.

To counteract the "nickel in the slot" attitude of textbook medicine, Osler brought his fourth-year students into direct contact with patients. They accompanied him on his famous rounds, and this undoubtedly marked the highpoint in their training. Osler's grand entrance into the wards, three times a week, became a popular ritual.

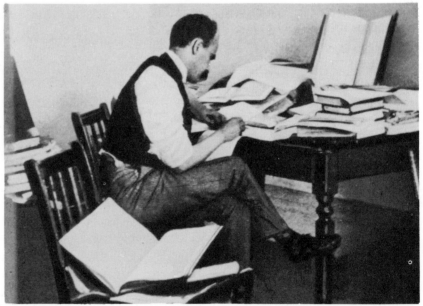

"Parturit Osler — nascitur Liber:" Osler in his study (1891) writing Principles and Practice of Medicine. In this book he succeeded to make "a scientific treatise literature." Reading it gave Fred L. Gates the inspiration to suggest to Mr. John D. Rockefeller the founding of the Rockefeller Institute for Medical Research.

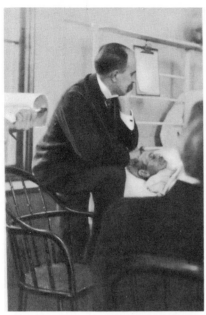

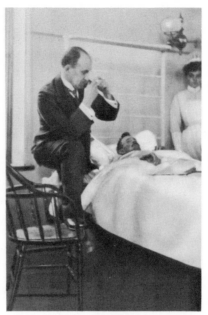

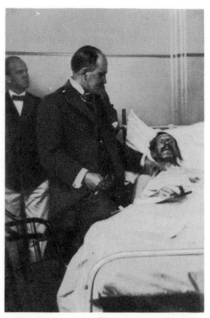

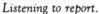

| *Listening to report.* | *Looking at specimen.* | *Examining a patient.* |

A WARD ROUND WITH THE "CHIEF"

Trailed by his assistants, nurses, and students, Osler would sit down at a bedside, always with a cheerful remark to the patient, and listen to the clinical report. Then he would launch into a thorough, lucid discussion of the case, not without quips and occasionally downright banter.

On Saturday nights, Osler held medical soirées at his home. Here he discussed both clinical and human problems with a remarkable grasp of the broader aspects of the medical profession. In his talks as in his writings bon mots were frequent and memorable: about medicine — "an art, not a trade; a calling, not a business, a calling in which your heart will be equally used as your head"; about patients who ignore good advice —

"Dame Nature gives long credit, but always sends in her bill;" and about doctors — "Medicine is seen at its best in men whose faculties have had the most harmonious culture."

This latter motto was especially true of Osler. It also has particular meaning for the modern doctor.

Today, when medicine is in danger of blind reliance on laboratory products or diagnostic machinery, Osler's work and words can serve as a powerful antidote against over-specialization. A true humanist Osler saw medicine whole and he saw it as part of the spectre of life. In his love for medicine, Osler never forgot the patient. With Dr. Parry of Bath, he believed it was "much more important to know what sort of patient has a disease than what sort of disease a patient has."

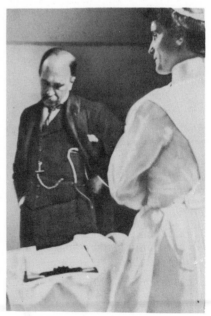

Osler said medicine "should begin with the patient, continue with the patient, and end with the patient."

303

RAYS OF HOPE

RADIATION - - - A NEW ERA
IN THERAPY AND DIAGNOSIS

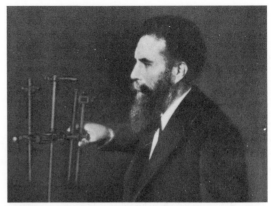

William Roentgen found "new kind of rays," enabling the doctor to see the inner man.

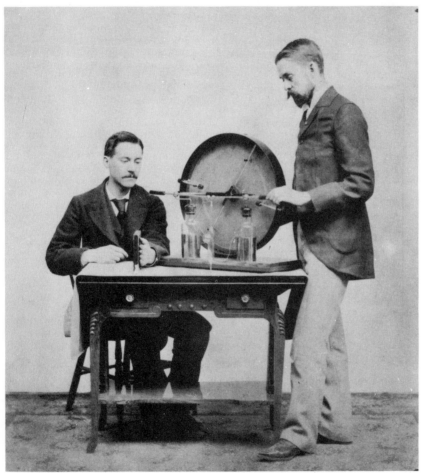

Dr. Ed. C. Jerman, X-ray pioneer operates static machine 1896. X-ray photos had to be exposed for as long as an hour; tubes were cranky, erratic, undependable, "just like women," as early roentgenologists said in jest.

Among the discoveries that now followed each other like a chain reaction — none was more portentious for medicine than the utilization of x-rays. All that had been accomplished in the field of diagnosis before its arrival was literally so much stumbling in the dark. Doctors felt their way about the body's surface, checking overt symptoms against an accumulated stock of clinical lore. But now a mysterious penetrating beacon opened the "inner man" to medical inspection. The application of x-rays would soon exert a more profound influence on medical practice than almost any other factor in the history of the healing art.

Wilhelm Roentgen, a physics professor at Würzburg University, had presented a paper "*On A New Kind of Rays*" to the Würzburg Physico-Medical Society in 1895. He hardly could anticipate that his research on "conduction of electricity through low vacuum tubes" would have world-wide repercussions. In fact, he resented the immediate sound and fury with which the public greeted what he took to be a discovery of academic interest.

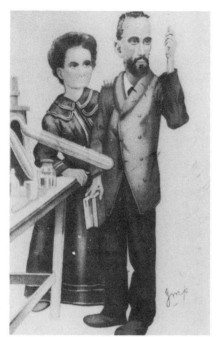

Pierre and Marie Curié (from cartoon in Spy). Radium's "rays of hope" were closely related to Roentgen rays.

note of it, and to show how it could extend man's vision. Once it became known that x-rays could be produced easily, a great many amateurs rigged up their own makeshift installations. One of them even produced the shadow-gram of a mouse with a tube made from the chimney of a kerosene lamp.

Before long the doctors began to test the machine for its diagnostic value. In their enthusiasm, they received terrible burns, or lost their lives, because the enigmatic rays produced cancer. Paradoxically, under certain conditions, the rays also counteracted its growth. Roentgen therapy and diagnosis grew apace in the 20th century, and a new specialty — Roentgenology — was born. Almost every department of medicine — surgery, gynecology, dermatology, chest and abdominal therapy, etc. —

advanced with the aid of this wonderful discovery.

Niels Ryberg Finsen, a Danish physician, was studying the use of radiation in medicine three years before Roentgen discovered the x-rays. The healing qualities of sunlight had impressed Finsen, but he knew that heliotherapy was impractical in a northern country. So instead of the sun he used arc lamps. With a special lens, he filtered out their heat and light rays, and concentrated the remaining "ultraviolet" radiation upon lupus and other skin afflictions. His treatments proved successful, and in 1896 the Finsen Medical Light Institute was founded — as a center for ultraviolet therapy and experiment. Finsen died in 1904, one year after he had received the Nobel Prize for his discovery.

The news that a solid-penetrating ray had been discovered swept through Europe and America. Comedians and cartoonists had a field day. One London firm offered "x-ray proof underwear" to prevent exposure of the private regions. Acting on hearsay, Assembly-man Reed of New Jersey introduced a bill to prohibit the use of x-rays in opera glasses. About the only luke-warm segment of the public — the medical profession — had been fooled too often to get hastily excited about anything.

All this uproar was about something which had always existed — a form of radiation which could pass through bodily obstacles. Roentgen called it x-rays because its nature was so mysterious. He was the first to take

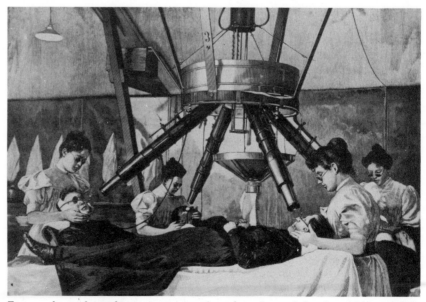

Finsen ultraviolet radiation treatment for tuberculosis of the skin. Heat and light rays from arc lamp were filtered out through quartz lenses mounted in tubes, the ultraviolet rays thus isolated proved therapeutically valuable.

TOWARDS CHEMOTHERAPY

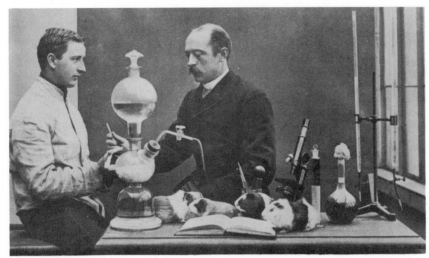

Behring injecting guinea pigs with tetanus germs to produce lockjaw antitoxin.

In the "germ-hunt" of the 1880's, the bacteria that cause tetanus, cholera, pneumonia and diphtheria had "popped up like corn in a pan" (Cushing). But their discovery could not be fully explored without some knowledge of the mechanics of immunity. What really happened when a specific germ entered the bloodstream? The immunologists worked hard to provide an answer.

They found that an intruding bacillus releases a poison into the bloodstream which produces an excess of counter-poison in the affected body. This "anti-toxin" is carried by the blood. It creates an immunity by counteracting the toxic effect of bacterial invasions. Once this was known, Emil von Behring was able to produce his famous anti-diphtheria serum. He injected horses with increasingly strong doses of diphtheria germs. As the horses developed immunity, he bled them, collected the blood in a bowl, and allowed it to coagulate. The liquid part of it, the serum, held the antitoxin. In 1891 this antitoxin was first used on a diphtheria-stricken child — with successful results.

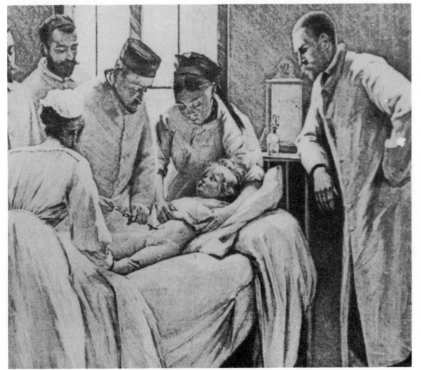

Emile Roux (right) proved that antitoxin could be effective even after onset of diphtheria: here he supervises injection in Paris Children's Hospital.

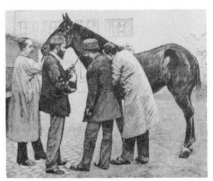

Four-legged serum plant: "immunized" horses supplied diphtheria antitoxin.

Behring and Kitasato also were able to produce in rabbits a tetanus antitoxin which could neutralize the toxin causing lockjaw — even when injected after the onset of the disease. Here was true immunity. Still, the knowledge of serotherapy was far from complete — especially in view of the fact that it proved impossible to produce in animals sera of a unified quality. This lack of standardization hampered further research. It was Paul Ehrlich who found a way out of this impasse.

Behring and Ehrlich were decidedly of the same generation. They were born one day apart in March, 1854, and both were disciples of Koch. But in the question of antitoxins they differed widely. Behring held that effective sera could only be produced organically, by way of animals. He called any inner disinfection by way of chemical substances "chymerical." These substances, he predicted, would kill the patient before they could counteract the disease producing toxins. But Ehrlich proved that chemotherapy was sound in principle and practice.

In his early years, the ingenious chemist-doctor-histologist had explored the reaction of body tissues to chemical substances. Some of them affected the cells — others did not. Inspired by his uncle, Carl Weigert, he had stained living cells with dyes — and these dyes made cell reactions and affinities visually discernable. The study of affinities enabled Ehrlich to produce substances which would counteract specific bacterial poisons, without harming the patient's organism. This trend of research led eventually to his discovery of salvarsan, the first controlled synthetic drug against syphilis. How Ehrlich performed this Promethean feat is one of the inspiring and well-known chapters of medical history. It marks the beginning of the new age of chemotherapy — an age that was to bestow new and untold blessings on the sick.

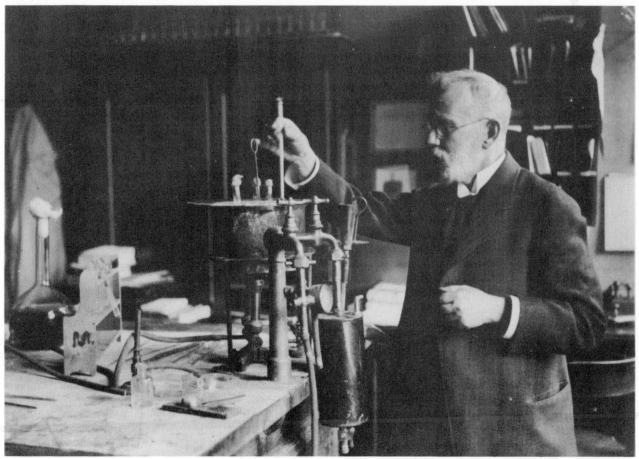

Paul Ehrlich (1854-1915), set test pattern for chemotherapy with salvarsan, synthetic drug against syphilis 307

ACKNOWLEDGMENTS

The assembling of the picture and text material for this book has led me through innumerable libraries and museums the world over. In all my travels I have found the most ready cooperation from medical librarians . . . In particular I must acknowledge my indebtedness to The New York Academy of Medicine. Special thanks are due to the Misses Annan and Delahanty of the Rare Book Room and to all the members of the library staff.

Many institutions and publishers have supplied me with illustrations and permitted the use of quotations:

The generosity of the following organizations is gratefully acknowledged.

Ashmolean Museum:
p. 96 top r.

Bellevue School of Nursing:
p. 293 top

Bibliothèque Nationale:
p. 183 top, p. 74 bottom r.

Blakiston Co.:
Osler quot. p. 232

Bodleian Library:
p. 85 top l.

Boston Medical Library:
p. 254

British Journal of Ophthalmology:
p. 132 top

British Medical Journal:
p. 19 top r.

British Museum:
p. 27 top

Ciba Aktiengesellschaf Basle:
p. 115 c.

Dutton & Company:
quot. p. 225

Edinburgh Medical Journal:
p. 201

General Electric X-ray Corp.:
p. 304 bottom

Guy's Hospital London:
p. 193

The Johns Hopkins Hospital:
p. 298, p. 303

The Johns Hopkins Univ. Press:
p. 179 upper r.

Hutchinson & Co.:
p. 65 top

Alfred A. Knopf:
Shryock, Mod. Med. quot. p. 247

Kunstsammlung Basel:
p. 137 center l.

London Electrotype Agency:
p. 34 top

MacMillan & Co. Ltd.:
p. 218 center

Metropolitan Museum:
p. 62 top, p. 40 bottom, p. 292 top

Missouri Botanical Garden:
p. 159 top

Dr. C. O. McCormick:
p. 258 upper r.

Morgan Library:
p. 75 bottom

National Portrait Gallery:
p. 157, top, p. 209 bottom

New York Historical Society:
p. 6 center

New York Hospital:
p. 294 bottom r.

Osler Library, Montreal
p. 300-301

Pennsylvania Hospital:
p. 226 top, p. 222 bottom

Rijksmuseum Amsterdam:
p. 154 center, p. 184 top

Rijksmuseum der Natuurweteunschappen:
p. 153 lower

Royal College of Physicians:
p. 145 top

Royal College of Surgeons of England:
p. 210, p. 111 bottom, p. 187 top l.

Royal Humane Society:
p. 219 top

Royal Medical Society Edinburgh:
p. 208 center

School of Medicine and Dentistry, University of Rochester:
p. 303

Scottish National Portrait Gallery:
p. 188 bottom l.

Stadtarchiv, Lindau:
p. 131-132

Stadt-und Hochschul Bibliothek, Bern:
p. 67 bottom r.

U. S. Army Medical Library:
p. 273 bottom

University of Chicago Press:
Edwin Smith Papyrus quot. p. 6

University College Hospital, London:
p. 257

William Welch Medical Library:
p. 185 bottom, p. 296

Wellcome Historical Medical Museum:
p. 212 top r. (2)

Winthrop-Stearns Inc.
p. 216 l. (courtesy of Dr. Frank
Stockman).

Woman's Medical College of Pa.:
p. 276 center

Zentralbibliothek Zurich:
p. 72

To the following individuals I wish
to proffer sincere thanks for assistance,
suggestions and photographs.

F. B. Adams Jr.
Adri Ames
Edward Arnold

Helen Baine
Dr. Roland H. Bainton
James F. Ballard
Dr. Walter R. Bett
Dr. Ernest Bettmann
W. J. Bishop
Dr. George Blumer

Dr. Edward Churchill
Margaret Clark
H. A. Clegg

Janet Doe
Dr. T. G. H. Drake
Barbara M. Duncum

Blanche Edwards
Dr. S. Epstein

Dr. Albert Fields
C. J. Foley
Dr. W. W. Francis
Magdalen Freyder

Dr. Iago Galdston
David Goodman
Beverly Gray
Florence M. Greim

Al Marston Hamlin
Richard Hatch
Cora F. Holbrook
George Hornby
James Horne

Edward E. James

Joseph B. Kelly
Dr. Walter Kempner
Allen Klein
M. R. Kneifl
Janet Koudelka

Dr. Sanford V. Larkey
W. R. Le Fanu

Dr. C. O. McCormick
Dr. W. B. McDaniel II
M. Ruth MacDonald
Virginia F. Maldoon
Charles B. Moore

Sol Novinsky

Betty Paulis
Dr. Curt Proskauer

B. Lee Reed
Dr. Philip Reichert
Dr. M. Rooseboom
Dr. Dorothy Schullian
Dr. Charles Singer
Mark Spilka
Dr. A. O. Stolze
Deborah Stolzman

Dr. Owsei Temkin

Dr. Ashwood Underwood

Dr. Henry Viets

Mildred E. Walter
Dr. Jerome Wilson

To list the books and articles I have read and consulted would fill a book in itself. Every page would bulge with references. Since this is principally a graphic survey of medicine's past we had to dispense with footnotes. A short bibliography is given on the following pages — a help, we hope, for readers who may want to make a further study of topics we could treat but briefly. There is no need to repeat the detailed bibliographies that can be found in the standard ·textbooks of medical history.

No endeavor in this field can be undertaken without having on one's elbows the classic accounts of Garrison, Castiglione, Sigerist and Sudhoff. Of the older histories of the profession I have always been partial to that of Withington (Medical History from the Earliest Times. London 1894.) The newest arrival in the field, Dr. Ralph Major's: A History of Medicine (2 vols. Springfield, Ill. 1955) is a thoroughly reliable and handy guide, selective in its approach, written with warmth and lucidity.

A few decades ago medical history was almost synonymous with medical bibliography. More recently medicine's past has been presented in the context of the great social and cultural movements. By applying this broader viewpoint historians like Henry Sigerist, Richard Shryock and George Rosen have made medical history more alive and meaningful. Throughout my work on this book I have derived much inspiration from their writings.

*

BIBLIOGRAPHY

Abbreviations:

A. M. H. — Annals of Medical History.

B. H. M. — Bulletin of the Institute of the History of Medicine, Baltimore.

p. 1

W. Osler: *The Evolution of Medicine.* New Haven, 1921. p. 15.

pp. 2-3

E. M. Guest: *Ancient Egyptian Physicians.* Brit. Med. Journal, 1926/I:706.

W. Dawson: *The Beginnings: Egypt and Assyria.* (Clio Medica), New York, 1930.

pp. 4-5

G. E. Smith & W. Dawson: *Egyptian Mummies.* London, 1924.

H. Ranke: *Medicine and Surgery in Ancient Egypt.* B. H. M. vol. 1:237, 1933.

pp. 6-7

C. L. Leake: *The Old Egyptian Medical Papyri.* Lawrence, Kansas, 1952.

pp. 8-9

M. Jastrow: *Babylonian-Assyrian Medicine.* A. M. H. vol. 1:231, 1927.

pp. 10-13

C. J. Brim: *Med. in the Bible.* N. Y., 1936.

pp. 16-19

H. L. Arnold: *The Caduceus & U. S. Army Med. Dept.* B. H. M. vol. 13:627, 1943.

E. & L. Edelstein: *Asclepius.* Balt., 1945.

A. Walton: *The Cult of Asclepios.* Boston, 1894.

pp. 20-21

W. H. S. Jones: *Philosophy & Medicine in Ancient Greece.* Baltimore, 1946.

pp. 22-25

W. A. Heidel: *Hippocratic Med.* N. Y., 1941.

W. H. S. Jones: *The Doctor's Oath.* Lond., 1924.

W. F. Petersen: *Hippocratic Wisdom.* Springfield, Ill., 1946.

pp. 26-27

J. R. Oliver: *Greek Med. & Greek Civilization.* B. H. M. vol. 3:623, 1935.

pp. 32-33

T. C. Allbutt: *Greek Med. in Rome.* London, 1921.

pp. 24-25

H. Gossen: *The Physician in Ancient Rome.* Ciba Symposia, vol. 1:2, 1939.

pp. 40-41

S. McKay: *The Hist. of Ancient Gynecology.* New York, 1901.

pp. 42-45

G. Sarton: *Galen of Pergamon.* Kansas City, Kansas, 1954.

J. Walsh: *Galen Clashes with the Medical Sects of Rome.* Med. Life, vol. 35:408, 1928.

pp. 46-47

S. D'Irsay: *Patristic Medicine.* A. M. H. vol. 9:364, 1927.

pp. 48-49

W. K. Hobart: *The Medical Language of St. Luke.* Dublin, 1882.

pp. 50-51

G. F. Fort: *Hist. of Med. Economy during the Middle Ages.* New York, 1883.

D. Riesman: *The Story of Medicine in the Middle Ages.* New York, 1935.

pp. 52-53

G. L. Walton: *The Saints Cosmas and Damian.* Proc. Charaka Club, Vol. 4: 15, 1916.

pp. 56-57

E. G. Browne: *Arabian Medicine.* Cambridge, 1921.

D. Campbell: *Arabian Medicine.* London, 1926.

A. O. Whipple: *The Med. School at Gondisapor.* Proc. Charaka Club, vol. 9:95, 1938.

pp. 58-59

O. C. Gruner: *The Canon of Avicenna.* London, 1930.

pp. 60-61

Spanish Infl. on the Progr. of Med. & Science. Wellcome Found., London, 1935.

pp. 62-63

E. Kremers & G. Urdang: *History of Pharmacy.* Philadelphia, 1940.

pp. 64-65

D. I. Macht: *Moses Maimonides.* B. H. M. vol. 3:585, 1935.

pp. 66-69

P. O. Kristeller: *The School of Salerno.* B. H. M. vol. 17:138, 1945.

pp. 70-71

F. R. Packard: *Regimen Sanitatis Salernitanum.* N. Y., 1920.

pp. 72-75

D. Riesman: *The Story of Medicine in the Middle Ages.* N. Y. 1935.

pp. 76-77

G. Franchini: *Origin of the Univ. of Bologna.* A. M. H. n. s. vol. 4:187, 1932.

M. N. Alston: *The Attitude of the Church towards Dissection.* B. M. H. 16:221, 1944.

pp. 78-79

T. C. Allbutt: *The Hist. Relations of Medicine & Surgery.* London, 1905.

pp. 80-81

W. A. Brennan: *Guy de Chauliac on Wounds.* Chicago, 1923.

pp. 84-85

J. Arderne: *Treatises of Fistula in Ano.* ed. D'Arcy Power. London, 1910.

pp. 90-91

C. A. Mercer: *Leper Houses.* London, 1915.

pp. 92-93

A. M. Campbell: *The Black Death and the Men of Learning*. N. Y., 1931.

R. Crawfurd: *Plague and Pestilence in Literature and Art*. Oxford, 1914.

pp. 94-95

A. Castiglioni: *The Renaissance of Med. in Italy*. Baltimore, 1934.

pp. 96-97

A. E. C. MacCurdy: *Leonardo da Vinci's Notebooks*. London, 1910.

pp. 98-101

R. S. Munger: *Guaiacum*. Journal of the Hist. of Med., vol. 4:196, 1949.

W. A. Pusey: *The History & Epidemiology of Syphilis*. Springfield, 1933.

pp. 104-105

J. C. Allbutt: *Hist. Relations of Med. & Surgery*. London, 1905.

E. M. Bick: *Source Book of Orthopedics*. Baltimore, 1948.

pp. 106-107

J. L. Miller: *Renaissance Midwifery*. Lect. on the Hist. of Med., Mayo Found., 1932.

pp. 108-109

G. de Francisco: *The Power of the Charlatan*. New Haven, 1939.

pp. 110-111

W. Osler: *Linacre*. Cambridge, 1908.

pp. 112-115

H. E. Sigerist (ed): *Four Treatises of Paracelsus*. Baltimore, 1941.

I. Galdston: *Psychiatry of Paracelsus*. B. H. M. vol. 24:205, 1950.

pp. 116-117

C. L. Dana: *Story of a Great Consultation*. A. M. H. ser. 1, vol. 3:122, 1921.

pp. 118-119

D. Slaughter: *Med. in the Life of Rabelais*. A. M. H. s. 3, vol. 1:396, 438, 1939.

pp. 120-123

Saunders & O'Malley: *The Illustrations from the Works of Vesalius*. Cleveland, 1950.

R. H. Bainton: *Hunted Heretic*. Boston, 1953.

pp. 124-127

S. Paget: *Ambroise Pare*. London, 1897.

G. Keynes (ed): *Apologie and Treatise of A. Pare*. Chicago, 1952.

pp. 128-129

J. L. Miller: *Joyfull Newes*. Lectures on Hist. of Med. Mayo Found., 1932.

pp. 134-135

J. Webster & M. T. Gundi: *The Life & Times of Tagliacozzi*. N. Y., 1951.

pp. 136-137

G. Zilboorg: *The Med. Man & the Witch during the Renaissance*. Baltimore, 1935.

pp. 140-141

R. H. Shryock: *The Development of Modern Medicine*. N. Y., 1947.

R. H. Major: *Santorio Santorio*. A. M. H. n. s. 3, vol. 10:369, 1938.

pp. 144-147

A. Malloch: *William Harvey*. N. Y. 1929.

pp. 148-149

H. S. Redgrove: *Van Helmont*. London, 1922.

pp. 152-153

E. Hollander: *Die Medizin in der Klassischen Malerei*. Stuttgart, 1903.

pp. 154-155

H. R. Catchpole: *Reignier de Graaf*. B. H. M. vol. 8:1261, 1940.

pp. 156-157

D. Riesman: *Sydenham, Clinician*. A. M. H. vol. 7:171, 1925.

pp. 158-159

A. W. Haggis: *Errors in the Early History of Cinchona*. B. H. M. vol. 10:47, 1941.

pp. 160-161

J. Nohl: *The Black Death*. London, 1926.

pp. 162-163

R. Crawfurd: *The King's Evil*. Oxford, 1911.

C. J. S. Thompson: *The Quacks of Old London*. London, 1928.

pp. 164-165

C. Dobell: *Leeuwenhoek*. N. Y., 1931.

R. H. Major: *Athanasius Kircher*. A. M. H. s. 3, vol. 1:105, 1939.

pp. 166-169

G. Keynes: *The History of Blood Transfusion*. Brit. Journ. Surg. vol. 31:41, 1943.

H. Brown: *Jean Denis and Transfusion of Blood*. Isis vol. 39:15, 1948.

pp. 170-173

F. Packard: *Guy Patin*. New York, 1925.

J. W. Courtney: *Moliere and the Faculty*. A. M. H. s. 1, vol. 5:309, 1939.

H. W. Haggard: *Med. in the Days of the Grand Monarch*. (Medicine & Mankind, 1936.)

pp. 174-175

G. Parker: *The Early History of Surgery in Great Britain*. London, 1920.

pp. 176-177

H. Cushing: *Dr. Garth*. Johns Hopkins Hosp. Bull. vol. 17:1, 1906.

pp. 178-179

R. Viets: *A Brief History of Medicine in Massachusetts*. Boston, 1930.

W. B. Blanton: *Medicine in Virginia in the 17th Century*. Richmond, 1930.

pp. 186-187

S. W. Simon: *The Influence of the Monros*. A. M. H. vol. 9:244, 1927.

pp. 194-197

E. Caulfield: *The Infant Welfare Movement*. New York, 1931.

pp. 198-199

L. Baumgartner: *John Howard & the Public Health Move.* B. H. M. vol. 5:489, 1937.

A. E. Clark-Kennedy: *Stephen Hales.* Cambridge, 1929.

pp. 200-201

B. Ramazzini: *Diseases of Workers.* transl by W. C. Wright. Chicago, 1940.

pp. 202-203

L. Auenbrugger: *On Percussion.* ed. H. E. Sigerist. B. H. M. 4:373, 1936.

pp. 206-207

F. Beckman: *Brit. Surgery in the 18th Cent.* A. M. H. n. s. vol. 9:549, 1937.

pp. 208-209

W. F. Mengert: *The Origin of the Male Midwife.* A. M. H. n. s. vol. 4:453, 1932.

pp. 210-213

S. R. Cloyne: *John Hunter.* Baltimore, 1950.

pp. 214-215

I. Galdston: *Progress in Med.* N. Y., 1940.

pp. 216-217

L. J. Moorman: *William Withering.* B. H. M. vol. 12:355, 1942.

pp. 218-219

R. H. Fox: *Dr. J. Fothergill.* London, 1919.
J. J. Abrahams: *Lettsom.* London, 1933.

pp. 222-227

M. Kraus: *Am. & Europ. Med. in the 18th Cent.* B. H. M. vol. 8:679, 1940.

N. G. Goodman: *Benjamin Rush.* Phila., 1934.

W. F. Norwood: *Medical Education before the Civil War.* Philadelphia, 1944.

C. E. Heaton: *Med. in N. Y. during Colonial Period.* B. H. M. vol. 17:9, 1945.

pp. 228-229

R. de Saussure: *French Psychiatry in the 18th Cent.* Ciba Symp. 11:1221, 1950.

pp. 230-231

W. R. Le Fanu: *A Bio-Bibliography of Edward Jenner.* Philadelphia, 1952.

pp. 234-235

Napoleon and His Physicians. Ciba Symposia, vol. 3:964, 1941.

pp. 238-239

L. Brown: *The Story of Clinical Pulmonary Tuberculosis.* Baltimore, 1941.

pp. 242-243

J. M. Ball: *The Sack 'Em Up Men.* Edinburgh, 1928.

pp. 244-245

W. Osler: *William Beaumont.* Oxford, 1929.

J. T. Flexner: *Doctors on Horseback.* N. Y., 1938.

pp. 248-249

R. H. Major: *Classic Descriptions of Disease.* Springfield, Ill., 1948.

pp. 252-253

V. Robinson: *Triumph over Pain.* N. Y., 1946.

pp. 254-257

Th. E. Keys: *The History of Surgical Anesthesia.* N. Y., 1945.

pp. 258-259

F. Slaughter: *Immortal Magyar.* N. Y., 1950.

H. L. Gordon: *James Simpson.* Lond., 1897.

pp. 262-263

M. Foster: *Claude Bernard.* Lond., 1899.

E. H. Ackerknecht: *Rudolf Virchow.* Madison, Wisc., 1953.

pp. 264-265

M. E. Pickard & R. C. Buley: *The Midwestern Pioneer.* N. Y., 1946.

pp. 266-267

J. H. Bryan: *Hist. of Laryngology.* A. M. H. n. s. vol. 5:151, 1933.

pp. 268-269

C. Woodham-Smith: *Nightingale.* N. Y., 1951.

pp. 270-271

G. W. Gray: *Doctors in Blue.* N. Y., 1952.

pp. 272-273

G. Zilboorg & G. Henry: *A History of Medical Psychology.* N. Y., 1941.

pp. 274-275

W. W. Cheyne: *Lister.* Lond., 1925.

pp. 276-277

K. C. Hurd-Mead: *A History of Women in America.* Haddam, 1938.

pp. 282-283

H. Kramer: *Early Boards of Health.* B. H. M. vol. 24:503, 1950.

pp. 286-287

R. J. Dubos: *Pasteur.* N. Y., 1950.

pp. 288-289

L. Brown: *Robert Koch.* A. M. H. n. s. vol. 7:99, 292, 385, 1935.

pp. 290-291

E. R. Wise: *Theodor Billroth.* A. M. H. s. 1, vol. 10:278, 1928.

pp. 292-293

H. Clapsattle: *The Doctors Mayo.* Rochester, Minn., 1941.

pp. 294-295

V. Robinson: *White Caps.* Phila., 1946.

pp. 298-303

A. M. Chesney: The Johns Hopkins Hosp. & School of Med. vol. 1, Balt., 1943.

S. & J. T. Flexner: *William Henry Welch.* New York, 1941.

W. G. MacCallum: *William S. Halsted.* Baltimore, 1930.

H. Cushing: *The Life of William Osler.* New York, 1924.

pp. 306-307

I. Galdston: *Behind the Sulfa Drugs.* New York, 1943.

INDEX

315

317